The Management of Lithiasis

DEDICATION

To our families and mentors, and especially to Mr Robert J. McCormack, FRCS, and Mr W. Selby Tulloch, FRCS, master craftsmen and teachers extraordinary.

Developments in Nephrology

Volume 38

A list of the titles in this series can be found at the end of the book.

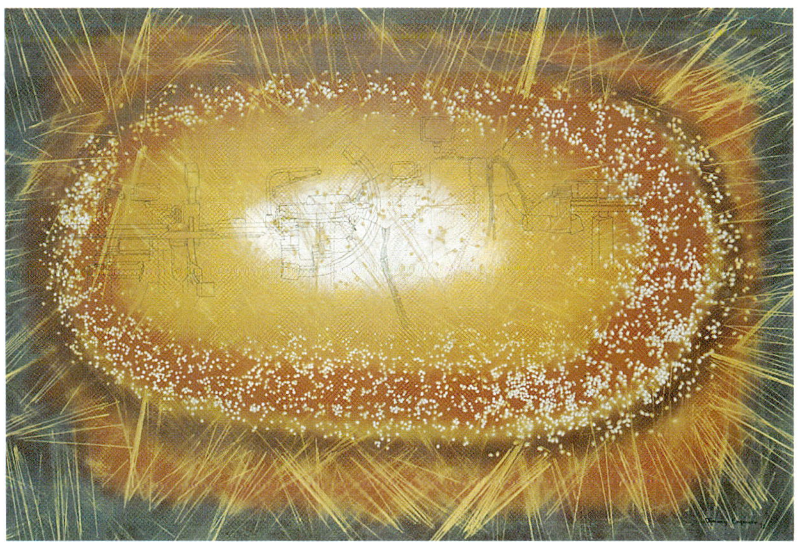

Frontispiece: Artist's impression of lithotripsy [Jimmy Engineer] (This painting was commissioned for the book and the original hangs in the corridors of the Lithotripsy suite at the Aga Khan University Medical Center).

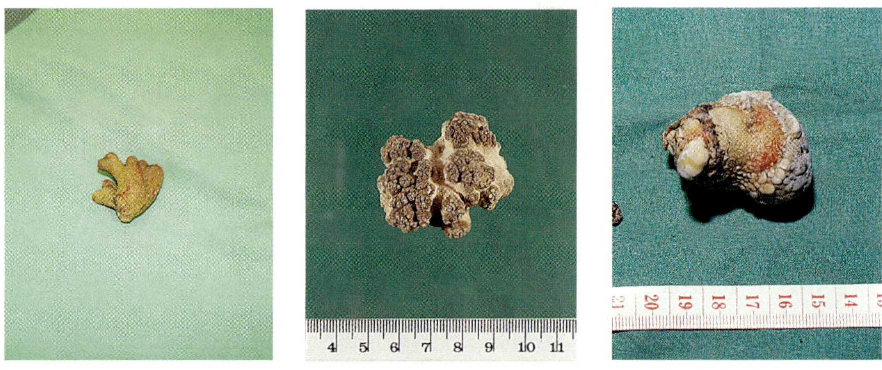

Figures 1.9–1.11 Varying morphological characteristics of renal calculi.

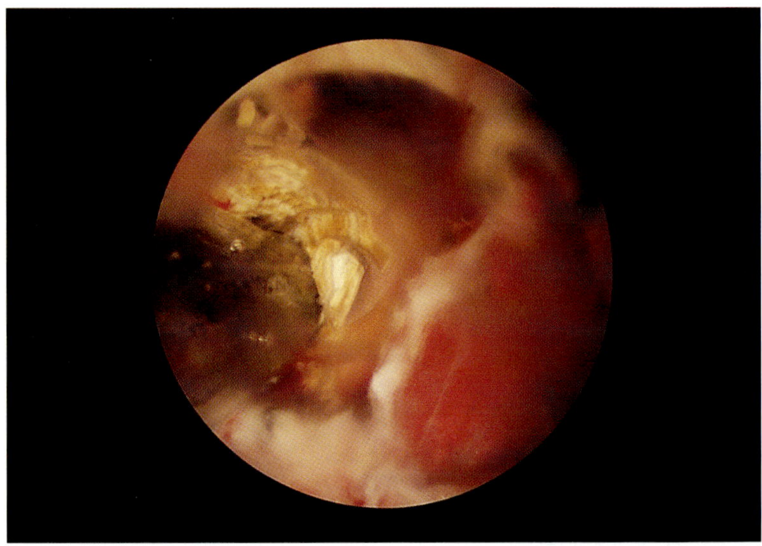

Figure 17.1 Stone as viewed through the nephroscope

The Management of Lithiasis
The Rational Deployment of Technology

EDITED BY

Jamsheer Talati
Roger A.L. Sutton
Farhat Moazam
Mushtaq Ahmed

The Aga Khan University Medical Center,
Karachi, Pakistan

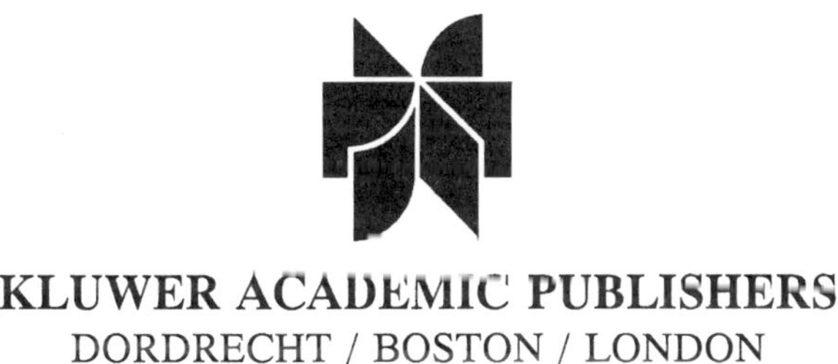

KLUWER ACADEMIC PUBLISHERS
DORDRECHT / BOSTON / LONDON

Library of Congress Cataloging-in-Publication Data is available.

ISBN 0-7923-4198-8

Published by Kluwer Academic Publishers,
P.O. Box 17, 3300 AA Dordrecht, The Netherlands.

Kluwer Academic Publishers incorporates
the publishing programmes of
D. Reidel, Martinus Nijhoff, Dr W. Junk and MTP Press.

Sold and distributed in the U.S.A. and Canada
by Kluwer Academic Publishers,
101 Philip Drive, Norwell, MA 02061, U.S.A.

In all other countries, sold and distributed
by Kluwer Academic Publishers Group,
P.O. Box 322, 3300 AH Dordrecht, The Netherlands.

Printed on acid-free paper

Typeset by EXPO Holdings, Malaysia

Printed and bound in Great Britain by Hartnolls Ltd., Bodmin, Cornwall.

Contents

Section I: EPIDEMIOLOGY AND AETIOLOGY OF URINARY TRACT CALCULI

Section II: CHOICES IN THE MANAGEMENT OF URINARY TRACT CALCULI

Section III: ENHANCEMENT OF EFFICACY AND SAFETY OF TREATMENT

Section IV: HIGH TECHNOLOGY AT AFFORDABLE COST

Section V: PREVENTION OF URINARY TRACT CALCULI

Section VI: PAEDIATRIC UROLITHIASIS

Section VII: BILIARY TRACT STONES

List of contributors

Farhat Abbas, MBBS, FCPS, FRCS
Assistant Professor, Department of Surgery, The Aga Khan University Medical Center, Karachi, Pakistan

Salman Adil, MBBS
Lithotripsy resident, Department of Surgery, The Aga Khan University Medical Center, Karachi, Pakistan

Mushtaq Ahmed, MBBS, FRCS
Hassanali Sajan Professor of Surgery, Chief of General Surgery, Department of Surgery, The Aga Khan University Medical Center, Karachi, Pakistan

Muneer Amanullah, MBBS
Resident, Department of Surgery, The Aga Khan University Medical Center, Karachi, Pakistan

Salma H. Badruddin, PhD
Dietitian, Associate Professor, Departments of Medicine and Community Health Sciences, The Aga Khan University Medical Center, Karachi, Pakistan

Nageeb Basir, MBBS, MRCP
Assistant Professor, Department of Medicine, The Aga Khan University Medical Center, Karachi, Pakistan

John A. Belis, MD
Professor of Urology, The Milton S Hershey Medical Center, Hershey University, Hershey, Pennsylvania, USA

S. Raziuddin Biyabani, MBBS, FCPS
Instructor, Department of Surgery (Urology), The Aga Khan University Medical Center, Karachi, Pakistan

Noshir F. Dabhoiwala, MD, FRCS
Attending Urologist, Boerhave Kliniek and Teacher in Urology, Academisch Centrum, University of Amsterdam, Amsterdam, The Netherlands

Mansur Dhanani
Materials Manager, The Aga Khan University Medical Center, Karachi, Pakistan

Hermie Drago, MBBS
General Practitioner, Mirpurkhas, Sindh, Pakistan

Salah R El-Faqih, MD, FRCS (Eng), FRCS (Ed)
Chairman, Department of Surgery and Professor and Consultant Urologist, King Saud University Faculty of Medicine, Riyadh, Saudi Arabia

Lucas Greiner, Dr Med.
Professor, Director Medical Klinik A, Klinikum Wuppertal GmbH, Universität Witten-Herdecke, D-42283 Wuppertal, Germany

Gregory Halenda, MD
Urologist, The Milton S Hershey Medical Center, Hershey University, Hershey, Pennsylvania, USA

Karim Hamawy, MD
Fellow, Department of Radiology, Boston University Medical Center, Boston, USA

Timothy S. Harrison, MD
Emeritus Professor of Surgery and Physiology, The Milton S Hershey Medical Center, Hershey University, Hershey, Pennsylvania, USA

Ziaul Amin Hotiana, MBBS, FRCS
Assistant Professor, Department of Surgery (Urology), The Aga Khan University Medical Center, Karachi, Pakistan

Imtiaz Hussain, MD, FRCS
Consultant Urologist, Bedford District General Hospital, Bedford, UK; formerly Professor and Chief of Urological Surgery, Department of Surgery, College of Medicine, Riyadh, Saudi Arabia

Sarwat Hussain, MD, FRCR
Head, General Radiology, Boston University Medical Center, Boston, USA

Z.X. Jiang
Lecturer, Laser Physics Department, University of Leeds, Leeds, UK

Meher Kakalia
Student, London School of Economics, London, UK

Farakh Khan, MBBS, FRCS, DU
Professor and Chairman, Department of Urology, The King Edward Medical College, Lahore, Pakistan

Nadeem Mustafa Khan
Director, Professional Services, The Aga Khan University Medical Center, Karachi, Pakistan

Naeemuz Zafar Khan, MBBS, FRCS
Professor and Chief of Pediatric Surgery, Children's Hospital, Pakistan Institute of Medical Sciences, Islamabad, Pakistan

Mohammed Khursheed, MBBS, MRCPath
Professor and Chairman, Department of Pathology, The Aga Khan University Medical Center, Karachi, Pakistan

Ernest Lall, MBBS
Chief of Surgery, The Christian Hospital, Taxila, Pakistan

James E. Lingeman, MD
Director of Research, Methodist Hospital, Unit for Kidney Stone Disease,
Indianapolis, Indiana, USA

Amanullah Memon, MBBS, FRCS
Assistant Professor, Department of Surgery (Urology), The Aga Khan University
Medical Center, Karachi, Pakistan

Farhat Moazam, MBBS, FACS
Quaid-i-Azam Professor of Surgery, Chairperson, Department of Surgery, Chief of
Pediatric Surgery, Associate Dean for Postgraduate Education, The Aga Khan
University Medical Center, Karachi, Pakistan

Zafar Nazir, MBBS, FCPS, FRCS
Assistant Professor, The Aga Khan University Medical Center, Karachi, Pakistan

Joop W. Noordzij, MD
Urological Surgeon, Military Hospital, Utrecht, The Netherlands

Yvonne M. O'Meara, MD
Director Clinical Nephrology, Boston University Medical Center, Boston, USA

Turab Pishori, MBBS, FCPS
Senior Instructor, Department of Surgery, The Aga Khan University Medical
Center, Karachi, Pakistan

Sarfaraz K. Qureshi, PhD
Executive Director, Pakistan Institute of Development Economics, Quaid-i-Azam
University, Islamabad

Th.M. de Reijke, MD
Consultant Urologist, Academic Center, Amsterdam, The Netherlands

Tariq K. Shah, MD, FRCS
Consultant Urologist, Bradford District Hospital, Bradford, UK; formerly Assistant
Professor of Surgery (Urology), Department of Surgery, The Aga Khan University
Medical Center, Karachi, Pakistan; Lecturer and Research Fellow, Institute of
Urology, London, UK; and Consultant Urologist, Lister Hospital, Stevenage, UK

Roger A.L. Sutton, DM, FRCP, FRCPC
Professor and Chairman, Department of Medicine, The Aga Khan University
Medical Center, Karachi, Pakistan; formerly Professor and Chairman, Department
of Medicine, University of British Columbia, Vancouver, British Columbia,
Canada

Ardesheer Talati, BA
PhD Student, Cornell University, New York, USA

Jamsheer Talati, MBBS, FRCS
Habiba Sabjaali Jiva Professor of Surgery, Chief of Urological Surgery, Department of Surgery, The Aga Khan University Medical Center, Karachi, Pakistan

R. Vleeming, MD
Urologist, Academic Centre, Amsterdam, The Netherlands

Grace Warren, MD, FRCAS, Dame
Leprologist, Minoram Leprosy Hospital, Minoram, Thailand; Chief Leprosy Consultant, Leprosy Mission, London; Leprosy consultant to Mission Hospital, Minoram, Thailand; Leprosy consultant to Marie Adelaide Hospital and Manghopir Leprosy KMC Hospital, Karachi; formerly Leprosy Surgeon, Chang Mai Hospital, Hong Kong

Graham Watson, MD, FRCS
Consultant Urologist, Eastbourne District Hospital, Eastbourne, UK; formerly Senior Lecturer and Honorary Consultant and Research Fellow, Institute of Urology, London, UK

Foreword

The last twenty years has seen the biggest revolution in the treatment of renal tract stone that has ever been experienced in the history of urolithiasis. The treatment of upper tract renal stone has progressed from the days of a very traumatic and morbid procedure to the relatively innocuous, walk in/walk out therapy of extracorporeal lithotripsy.

This progression of events has resulted in a complete reappraisal of management of all types of urinary calculi. From an initial reluctance to treat many stones because of the trauma involved, we have now passed to a situation where smaller and asymptomatic stones may be pre-emptively treated before the treatment of serious clinical problems. It is true to say that in Westernized societies the problem of urolithiasis has almost completely been solved by the advent of advanced technology.

In this volume, attention is drawn to the fact that there are still persistent difficulties in treating urolithiasis in the less developed and less affluent societies. The differences in epidemiology of urolithiasis in various areas of the world are highlighted, noting a rapid decrease in the incidence of bladder calculi in impoverished areas where affluence increases. Coupled with this progression of affluence however is the well documented increase in the incidence of upper tract renal stones of oxalate nature. This scenario has been almost universal across all countries in the last few decades.

Whilst in the ideal situation it is possible to clear practically all urolithiasis atraumatically by either endoscopy or extracorporeal lithotripsy, it is obviously not rational to recommend such treatment to patients where facilities are not available. Installation of expensive extracorporeal lithotriptors is obviously impossible because of their prohibitive price and for poorly affluent countries, alternative means of therapy still need to be addressed. This consequently means that it is still necessary for many patients to be treated by open renal surgical techniques. As experience develops however, it should gradually be possible for more and more endoscopic procedures to be carried out even if extracorporeal lithotriptors cannot be afforded.

The book also highlights the problems of treating patients in diffuse areas where it is difficult for patients to come to the treatment centre, in contrast to those in large urban conurbations where patients can easily access centres for lithotripsy or endoscopic surgery. In more rural areas there would appear to be some benefit in taking treatment facilities direct to the patient, utilizing mobile lithotriptors and mobile teams of physicians.

This volume also explores the metabolic actiology and the medical control of calculus disease in difficult climatic and economic conditions. The cost of all medical therapies is now coming under immense scrutiny, especially in the more affluent areas. Therapies are being examined both for evidence of their efficacy and their cost effectiveness. There is little doubt in the area of stone disease described in this volume that endoscopic stone removal and extracorporeal lithotripsy have more than justified their place in the surgical armamentarium on the grounds of outstanding efficiency and cost effectiveness when compared with previous methods of open surgery. Such effective new technology, saving as it does much expense, must surely be the way forward for any society, particularly where resources are radically cost contained and difficult to access for the poorer members of the community.

Hopefully in the next twenty years economies will have improved so that a full range of interventional therapy for urolithiasis will become available to all populations in all parts of the world. Under the guidance of such enlightened physicians as Dr Talati and his colleagues, I am sure this will come about.

This volume is surely to be commended to all who must deal with the multitude of problems within urolithiasis and will be an invaluable guide to the best possible management.

Professor J.E.A. Wickham
MS, MD, BSc, FRCS, FRCP, FRCR
The London Clinic and Guy's Hospital, London;
Former Dean, Institute of Urology, London

Preface

Urinary bladder calculi in children and infective biliary stones in adults have been afflicting populations in developing countries long before the transition to Western diseases. Now with the addition of renal stones and cholesterol gallstones the disease burden has doubled in developing countries. The Western world has developed minimal access surgery to deal with diseases. The technology to accomplish this is expensive and in order to make it available to deserving patients, developed nations have had to resort to overall cost savings in health care. Hence concepts such as managed care, practice guidelines and evidence based medicine have come into prominence.

With the world now reduced to a global village it does not take long for the technology to permeate to developing countries. The private sector in developing countries avidly takes up such advances in technology; the public sector, unable to bear the costs, remains deprived. In the absence of a price regulatory mechanism, it is obvious that only the rich can afford to purchase sophisticated care. For the management of calculus disease two social classes are likely to emerge: those that can afford minimally invasive procedures and those that can only afford conventional surgery.

This book is a reflection of the times and prevalent concerns in developed as well as developing countries about the management of stone disease. The prevention of urinary calculi is discussed. Money spent on health education and disease prevention is likely to have a more even impact on populations irrespective of social class. Knowledge of the scientific basis of extracorporeal shock wave lithotripsy (ESWL) should enable health care providers to select equipment to suit their specific needs and circumstances. Considerable emphasis has been given to rational use of minimally invasive procedures. Suggestions are offered for lowering costs by elimination of unnecessary investigations and treatment. Results from minimally invasive procedures are compared with those from conventional surgery to permit decisions based on cost–benefit analyses. Indications are prioritized for the use of minimally invasive procedures to enable referral systems to develop in poor countries such that the most deserving patients are not denied access. Use of instrumentation and equipment across specialities could be the basis of developing a cost-effective service for minimally invasive surgery. The implications on surgical training of the modern 'high tech' approach is another area demanding attention and is alluded to in this book.

This book on calculus disease therefore offers its readers a chance to pause and think as we enter the twenty-first century with rapidly advancing technology, soaring costs of health care the world over and attempts to disseminate technology to developing countries where huge populations live under widely disparate conditions and the disease burden is compounded by changing life styles.

J. Talati
R.A.L. Sutton
F. Moazam
M. Ahmed

Acknowledgements

The editors are very grateful to the authors, who have dedicated time and effort in spite of their busy schedules; to Dr Raziuddin Biyabani, for help with checking references; to Ms Martha Travas, Ms Seema T. Khan, Mr Murad Bana and especially Jack Fernandes who shouldered the major secretarial and organizational load; to Messrs Aslam Bashir, Aamir Tariq and Shamsuddin Qureshi in the audiovisual centre of the Aga Khan University for their help in producing illustrations, tables and photographs; to Ms Nynke Coutinho, Phil Johnstone and Boudewijn Commandeur at Kluwer Academic Publishers, for their patient and understanding help; and to the Aga Khan University and the University Hospital, whose critical and thoughtful environment fed, fired, and stoked this book.

We are grateful to the following publishers for permission to reprint material from journals and texts: Plenum Press, New York; Blackwell Science Limited, Oxford; Ferozesons (Pvt) Ltd, Lahore; and Williams and Wilkins, Baltimore.

We are especially grateful to Dr Timothy S. Harrison, whose enthusiasm for publishing material on critical analysis of treatment regimes with special reference to work in constrained circumstances, directed our efforts to this publication; to Drs James Wickham, Scott McDougall, Stephen Dretler, Sarwat Hussain, Imtiaz Hussain and John Belis, who each in their own way has supported this work and made this publication possible.

The editors

Section I
Epidemiology and Aetiology of Urinary Tract Calculi

1. Urolithiasis: Composition, symptomatology and pathology

AMANULLAH MEMON and JAMSHEER TALATI

Urinary tract stones come in all shapes and sizes. They may lie in the pelvis, calyces, ureter, bladder or urethra. Those in the ureter are usually spindle shaped. Some may resemble an ice-cream cone, with a dimple at the top suggesting the site of previous attachment to a renal papilla. In the bladder, they may be rounded and multiple when they form in a post-prostatic pouch, in older men. In children the stone may assume a jack stone appearance or become ovoid, depending on whether it is composed of oxalates or urates.

Calculi may fill the renal pelvis, and assume resemblance to a stag's antlers (hence the term staghorn calculi). Those which incompletely fill the calyces in addition to the pelvis are called partial staghorns. Stones in the bladder may grow to more than 5 g in weight, though these will be seen in children over 4 years old. As stone mass and distribution in the pelvicalyceal system are important determinants

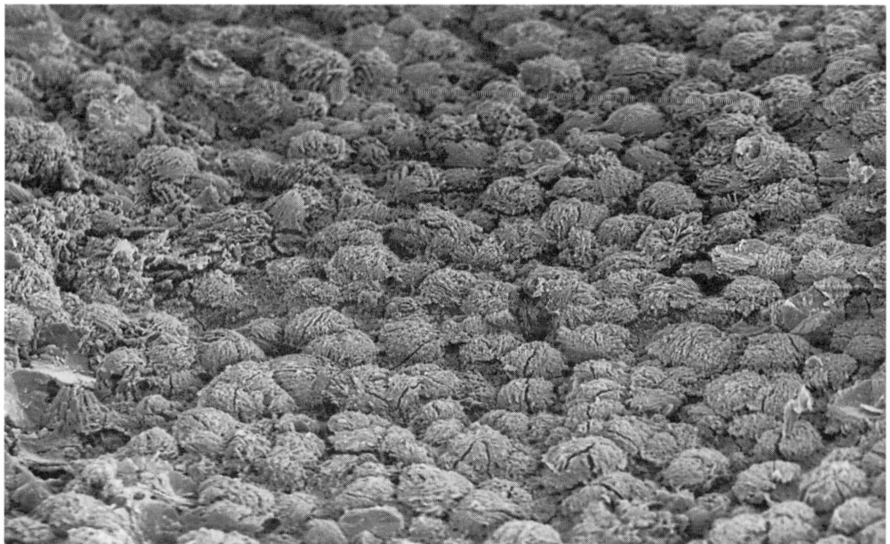

Figure 1.1
Figures 1.1–1.8 represent electron microscopy photographs of stones (courtesy Dr Vicar Zaman)

J. Talati et al. (eds) The Management of Lithiasis, 3–10
© 1997 Kluwer Academic Publishers. Printed in Great Britain.

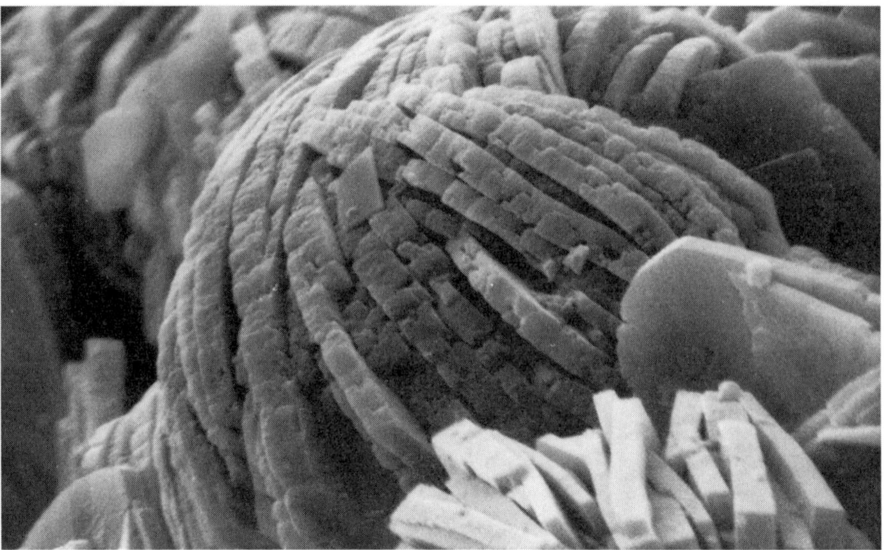

Figure 1.2

of treatment outcomes, many [1, 2] have tried to establish measurement guidelines which include consideration of morphology, site, size, parenchymal function and unique anatomical defects.

Urinary calculi are the consequence of temporary, periodic or permanent disorders in the composition of urine which lead to nucleation and birth of a calculus. Factors affecting growth may be dissimilar to the initial event of the nucleation [3, 4] aptly shown by the dissimilarity between the chemical composition of core and covering [5].

Stones are composed of a variety of crystals, the relative frequency of which varies from country to country. Table 1.1 shows the composition of stones in children in Pakistan as compared to the West [6]. Figure 1.1–1.8 demonstrate the appearance of the variety of crystals found in stones. Figures 1.9–1.11 (see p. iv) show the varying morphological characteristics of stones.

Table 1.1   Percentage contribution of different varieties of stones in children in Pakistan and the West

	Pakistan	N. America	W. Europe
Ca oxalate/phosphate	50.0	57.6	37.1
Struvite/carbonate	8.7	25.3	54.0
Uric acid	8.7	7.6	1.3
Ammonium urate	26.1	1.8	0.9
Xanthine	2.1	–	–
Mixed/unidentified	4.4	1.5	3.8
Cystine	–	6.2	2.9

The North American and the European data are from the *Pediatric Clinics of North America* 1987;34:683–709 (stones from Pakistan were analysed by infrared spectroscopy in Japan). Table reproduced by permission from the *Pakistan Journal of Surgery* [6].

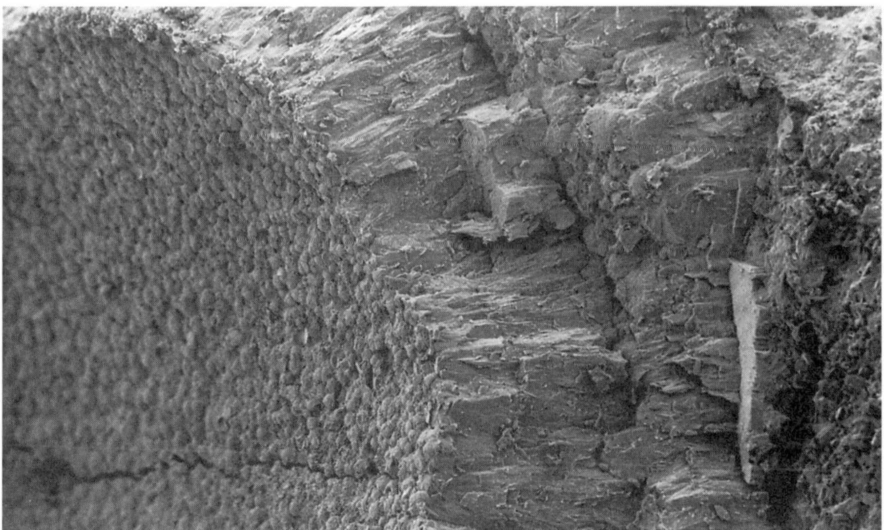

Figure 1.3

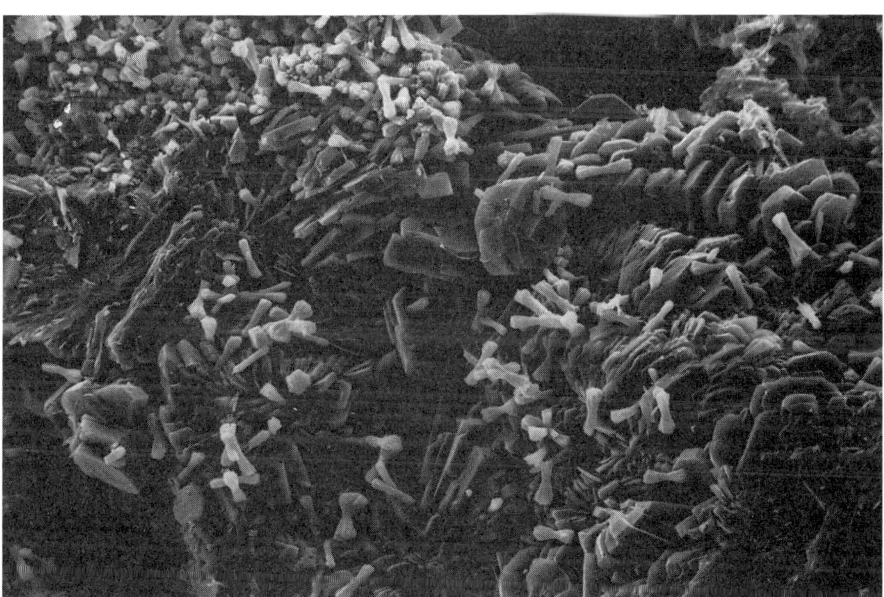

Figure 1.4

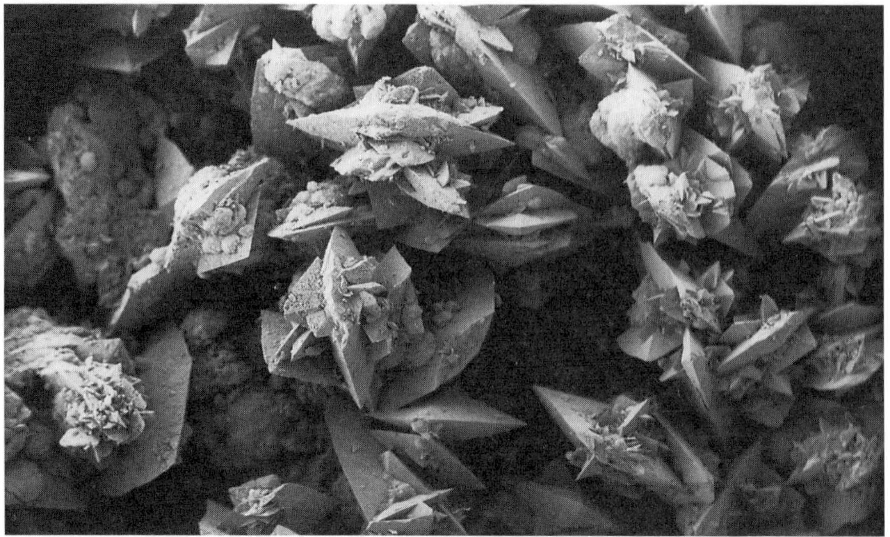

Figure 1.5

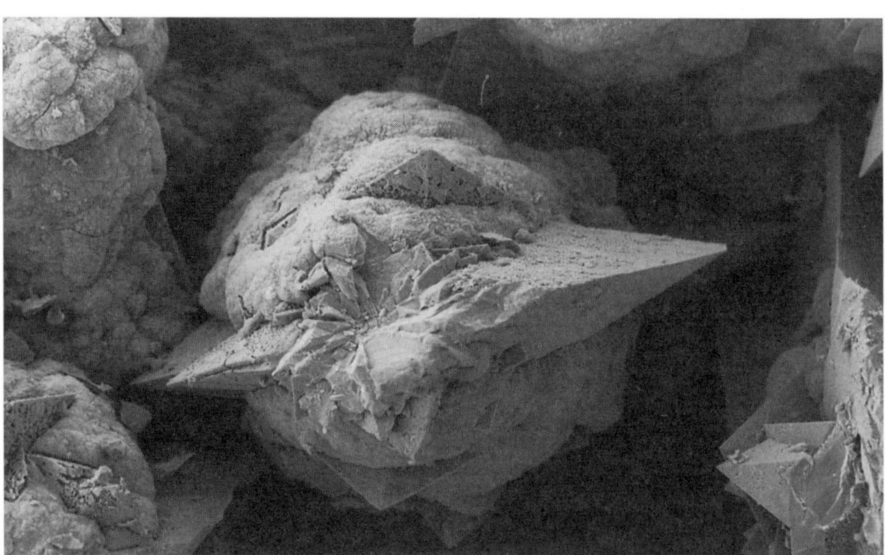

Figure 1.6

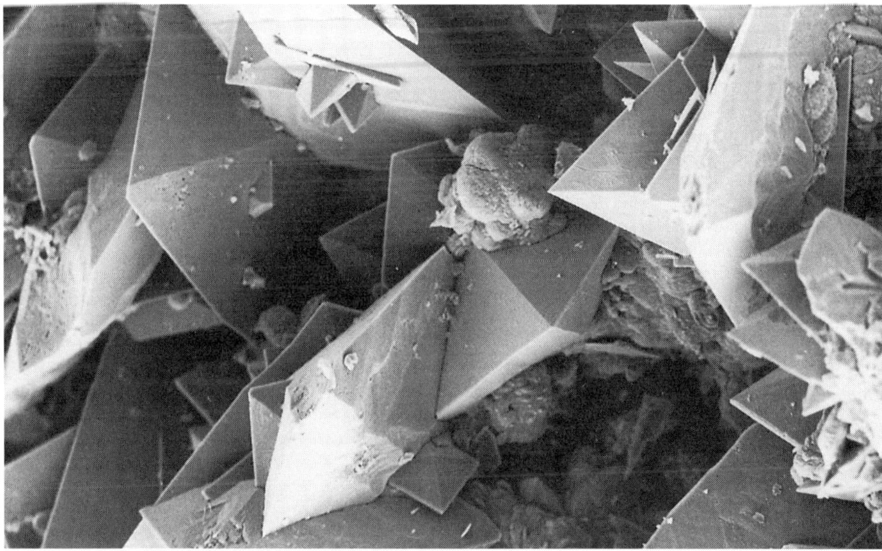

Figure 1.7

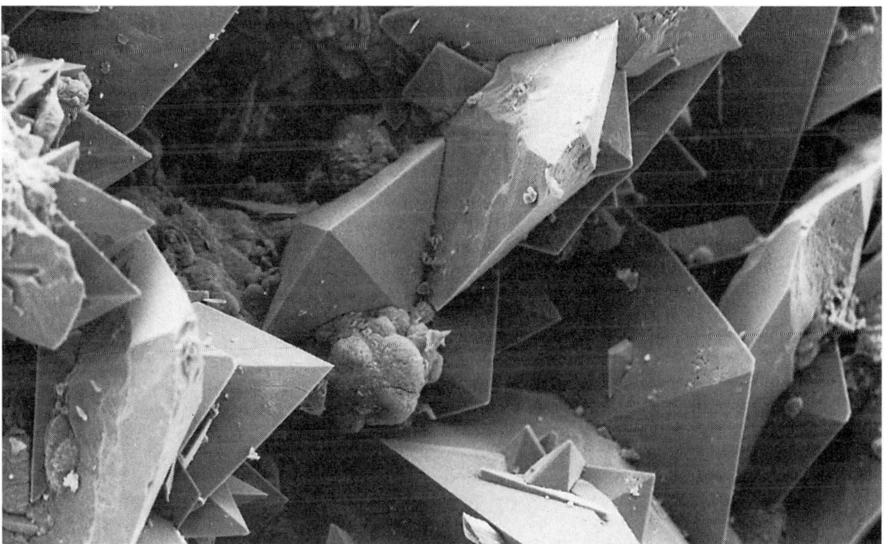

Figure 1.8

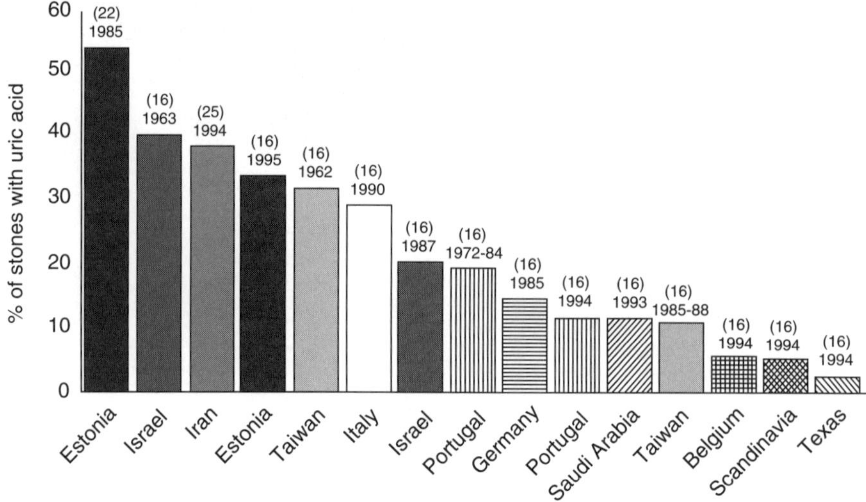

Figure 1.12 Percentage of stones which are composed of uric acid in different countries at various times in their development (numbers in parentheses refer to references)

The composition of bladder stones is less variable. Khan [7] reports from Hazara (in north-west Pakistan) that the nucleus contains a mix of calcium oxalate (CaOx) and ammonium urate in 50%, CaOx struvite and ammonium urate in 21.6%, and CaOx only, CaOx and struvite, CaOx struvite and brushite or CaOx apatite and ammonium urate in 7% each. The outer layer contains CaOx and ammonium urate in 50%, CaOx struvite and ammonium urate in 14%, pure CaOx in 14%, and other constituents as above in 7% each [7].

Renal stones at our hospital, the Aga Khan University Medical Centre (AKUMC), are predominantly CaOx stones. Eighty-eight per cent of stones contain > 30% oxalate, 64% contain > 30% calcium, 42% contain some urate, and 75% have more than 80% of their bulk composed of calcium oxalate.

In Hyderabad, a town 100 miles to the north of Karachi, they are predominantly phosphatic [8]. Fifty per cent of (30) bilateral stones were composed of phosphate in a rapidly industrializing town of Faisalabad in Punjab, where 44% of the patients came from rural areas [9]. Quantitative chemical analysis on our AKUMC 1990 stone population in urban Karachi showed that only 9% contained > 50% phosphate. This difference in the phosphate content of stones from the urban and rural areas has also been noted by Yoshida [10] in Japan. Infrared analysis of stones at the Sindh Institute of Urology and Transplantation, which draws a large number of patients from rural Sindh, has however shown that recently the most common crystal type is whewellite, seen both in the nucleus (in 63%) and in the outer layers (in 66%) [11].

The frequency of uric acid stones varies inversely with the per capita income. Thus uric acid stones are seen in only 3.9% of stone formers in Germany today [12], 2% in the USA, and 4% in Scandinavian countries, but constitute 23%, 27%,

30% and 37%, respectively, of the stones seen in Sudan, Pakistan, Thailand and Iran [13]. In Israel, 40% were composed of uric acid 25 years ago; today only 19% are uric acid stones. In 1963, 50% of the urate stones were pure urate; the figure is now only 0.7% [13]. Exceptions to this relationship exist – uric acid stones were seen in 11.5% [13] to 20% [14] in Saudi Arabia; in 26% in Italy [15] and 14% in Germany in the 1980s [14]. All are affluent countries.

Ammonium urate is a common component of paediatric bladder stones; surprisingly it is present in 44% of calcium oxalate stones in Macedonia [17]; it has now reappeared in the West in patients who use excessive laxatives, and in those with ileal resections and ileostomies, as a result of dehydration, low urinary citrate and high ammonia.

Symptomatology and pathology

If arrested in the urethra, stones cause difficulty in micturition and retention of urine. Arrested in the ureter they produce typical renal/ureteric colic or a dull kidney pain in the loin, flank or the anterior fixed renal pain area, at the tip of the ninth costal cartilage. Anuria may result from blockade to both ureters or the ureter of a sole functioning kidney. Bladder stones may cause variable frequency and intermittent obstruction. In the child, they cause pain which the child tries to relieve by a characteristic tugging at the penis. In the adult, the stones may cause a sudden temporary interruption of the urinary stream. Whewellite stones appear to pass spontaneously more frequently; they also require surgery more often [18].

Stones obstruct and cause infection. Pyelonephritis and cortical atrophy may result. Xanthogranulomatous pyelonephritis is a serious end result requiring nephrectomy, as is end-stage renal failure. Twelve per cent of admissions to a nephrourological unit in Pakistan are for renal failure from calculus disease [19]. Ten per cent of end-stage renal disease in Pakistan is due to stones, compared to 3% in the West [20]. In a series of 30 patients with bilateral stones, 6% had anuria, and an additional 7% had an elevated creatinine level [9]; 2–7% of patients had chronic neglected renal stones present in renal failure.

Because of the disastrous consequences – loss of kidney, loss of life and the number of days off work – and the frequency of the problem, every effort must be made to prevent stone disease and treat it promptly.

References

1. Griffith PD, Valiquette L, Pica Burden. A staging system for upper tract urinary stones. J Urol 1987;138:253–7.
2. Rocco F, Larches P, Mandressi A *et al*. A new classification of reno-ureteral calculi. Arch Ital Urol Nefrol Androl 1989;61:355–9
3. Finlayson B. Renal lithiasis in review. Urol Clin N Am 1974;1:181–212.
4. Vermeulen CW, Lyn ES. Mechanisms of genesis and growth of calculi. Am J Med 1968;45:684–92.

5. Naqvi SA, Rizvi SA, Shahjehan S. Bladder stone disease in children; clinical studies. J Pak Med Assoc 1984;34:94–101.
6. Khan MN, Islam S, Afzal S *et al.* Urolithiasis in children, a comparison of Western and Pakistani data. Pak J Surg 1991;7:57–60.
7. Khan RM. Childhood vesicolithiasis in the Hazara division NWFP, Pakistan. (Dissertation) Lahore: Punjab University, 1993.
8. Khand FD, Memon MS, Ansari AF *et al.* Morphological and chemical studies of urinary calculi. J Pak Med Assoc 1986;36:300–3.
9. Rizvi AM. Bilateral renal stones. (Dissertation) Karachi: College of Physicians and Surgeons of Pakistan, 1987.
10. Yoshida O, Okada Y, Horii Y *et al.* Descriptive epidemiology of urolithiasis in Japan. In: Walker V *et al.* editors. Urolithiasis. New York: Plenum Press, 1989:651–4.
11. Zafar MN, Hussain M, Mehdi H *et al.* Analysis of urinary calculi by infra red spectroscopy in a Pakistani population. (Abstract) First International Symposium of the Institute of Urology and Transplantation, 1994.
12. Hesse A, Nolde A, Hagmaier V *et al.* The Bonn urolithiasis post-episode care programme–new results. In: Ryall R *et al.*, editors. Urolithiasis 2. New York: Plenum Press, 1994:403–5.
13. Sperling O. Prevalence of uric acid urolithiasis in Israel and other parts of the world, in the last decade. Proceedings of the 13th Urolithiasis Symposium, Bonn, Vienna. Uro Res 1987;15:115.
14. Abolmelha MS, al Khadar AA. Urolithiasis in Saudi Arabia. J Urol 1990;35:31–4.
15. Borghi L, Feretti PP, Elia SF. Epidemiological studies of urinary tract stones in a Northern Italian city. Br J Urol 1990;65:231–5.
16. Schneider HJ. Epidemiology of urolithiasis. In: Schneider, editor. Urolithiasis, etiology and diagnosis. Berlin: Springer Verlag, 1985:137.
17. Ilievski P, Ilievska S, Nakovski R *et al.* Etiogenic factor for calcium oxalate lithiasis in southwestern Macedonia. In: Ryall R *et al.*, editors. Urolithiasis 2. New York: Plenum Press, 1994:483.
18. Atanasova S, Tabanska T, Donovski L *et al.* The surgical and spontaneous elimination of kidney calculi. Khirurgica-Sofia 1991;44:41–5.
19. Hussain M, Ali B, Lal M *et al.* Calculus renal failure, review of 360 cases. Abstracts, First International symposium of the Institute of Urology and Transplantation, 1994.
20. Naqvi S. Personal communication.
21. Takasaki E, Maeda K. A population study of urolithiasis. Tokyo J Med Sci 1977;4:88–92.
22. Holmgren K, Annuk M. Uric acid calculi in Estonia. (Abstract) 6th European Symposium on Urolithiasis, 1994.
23. Reis-Santos JM, Composition of urinary calculi in the South of Portugal. In: Ryall R *et al.*, editors. Urolithiasis 2. New York: Plenum Press, 1994:465.
24. Hwang TIS, Chang LS, Tazi T *et al.* Composition analysis of urinary tract calculi in Taiwan. Asian J Surg 1991;14:114–19.
25. Halabe A, Sperling O. Uric acid nephrolithiasis Miner Electrolyte Metab 1994;20:424–31.

2. Radiology in urolithiasis

SARWAT HUSSAIN

Radiology plays a pivotal role in the diagnosis of renal calculi. Plain abdominal films of the kidney, ureter and bladder (KUB) area help to identify the number, size, location and probable composition of radiopaque urinary calculi. Intravenous urography (IVU), or as it is sometimes called, intravenous pyelography, provides information on the status of the renal parenchyma, collecting system and the bladder. Percutaneous urological intervention further assists surgical management of calcular disease in many patients.

Stones composed of calcium oxalate or phosphate, magnesium ammonium phosphate, and cystine are radiopaque. Uric acid, 2,8-dihydroxy-adenine, xanthine, fibrin stones and stones composed of organic matter are non-opaque. Layers of calcium make a lucent calculus detectable on plain radiograph.

Contrast material

Water soluble tri iodinated salts of benzoic acid with sodium or meglumine as cations, are used in clinical urography as contrast agents. Iodine provides the radiopaque component. Excretion occurs mostly by glomerular filtration, with a little occurring by tubular secretion. Up to 2% is excreted by the liver and the colon.

The degree of concentration of contrast in the kidney is dependent on the concentration achieved in urine itself, dependent on dose administered, plasma concentration and the glomerular filtration rate of the iodine containing molecules. Beyond a maximum of 600 mg/ml in blood, the radiopacity of the urinary system will not increase proportionately, whilst the toxicity will increase sharply. Approximately 5% of patients show a transient rise in serum creatinine after IVU. Acute oliguric renal failure is rare. Patients with diabetes, multiple myeloma and pre-existing renal insufficiency are at particular risk for acute renal failure. Hypersensitivity reactions may occur and vary from mild urticaria to life threatening anaphylactic shock. Anaphylactoid reactions can occur on the first contact. Preparedness to deal with untoward effects of contrast administration can avert disasters.

Newer, non-ionic contrast media (Table 2.1) have one-half or less of the osmolality of conventional contrast. The iodine molecule is linked with uncharged benzene ring. It is believed that with these newer agents there is a reduced incidence of toxicity related to hyperosmolarity and minor to moderate hypersensitivity

J. Talati et al. (eds) The Management of Lithiasis, 11–20
© *1997 Kluwer Academic Publishers. Printed in Great Britain.*

Table 2.1

Trade Name	Generic	Concentration	Osmolality	I2 name Contents (mg/ml)
A. Conventional agents				
Ranografin	Maglumine/NA Diatrizoate	60	1420	288
Hypaque 50	Sodium ditrizoate	50	1550	300
Conray 60	Meglumine-10 Thalamate	60	1400	282
B. Low osmolality				
Omnipaque 300	IoHexol	64.7	709	300
Isovu	Ipamidol	76	796	370
Hexabrix	Ioxaglate Na and meglumine thalamate	58.9	600	320

reactions, but the issue is still controversial. The incidence of major reactions seems to be the same with all agents, and newer agents cost 10–20 times that of conventional contrast. Hence they are used selectively in patients with a history of contrast allergy or allergy to iodine or seafoods. The incidence of contrast nephropathy is 0–1% in a healthy population and up to 15% overall. Diabetes, multiple myeloma, hepatic disease, dehydration, multiple dosing, and pre-existing renal insufficiency, all increase the risk.

The plain film (KUB)

As 90% of calculi are radiopaque, a plain KUB X-ray and plain tomography will detect the majority of urinary tract stones (Figure 2.1). Opaque calculi may be obscured in a KUB film by various overlying shadows: calcified costal cartilages, bowel gas and vertebral processes may cause problems in differentiation from calculi. Additional films in oblique position (Figure 2.2), deep inspiration or expiration may be required. Calculi within the kidney will bear a constant relationship to the kidney ureters and bladder during respiratory manoeuvres.

Contrast medium administration and the intravenous urogram

The recommended dose of 25–35 g iodine for an average adult will produce satisfactory opacification on pyelography. Twelve hours of dehydration prior to IVU will improve the concentration on the preliminary films, but patients with multiple myeloma, diabetes mellitus and renal insufficiency must be hydrated before contrast studies.

The IVU has been the fundamental radiological examination, but is now being replaced by ultrasound. A preliminary KUB is essential as the contrast may obscure a radiopaque calculus (Figure 2.3), though lucent stones will appear as filling

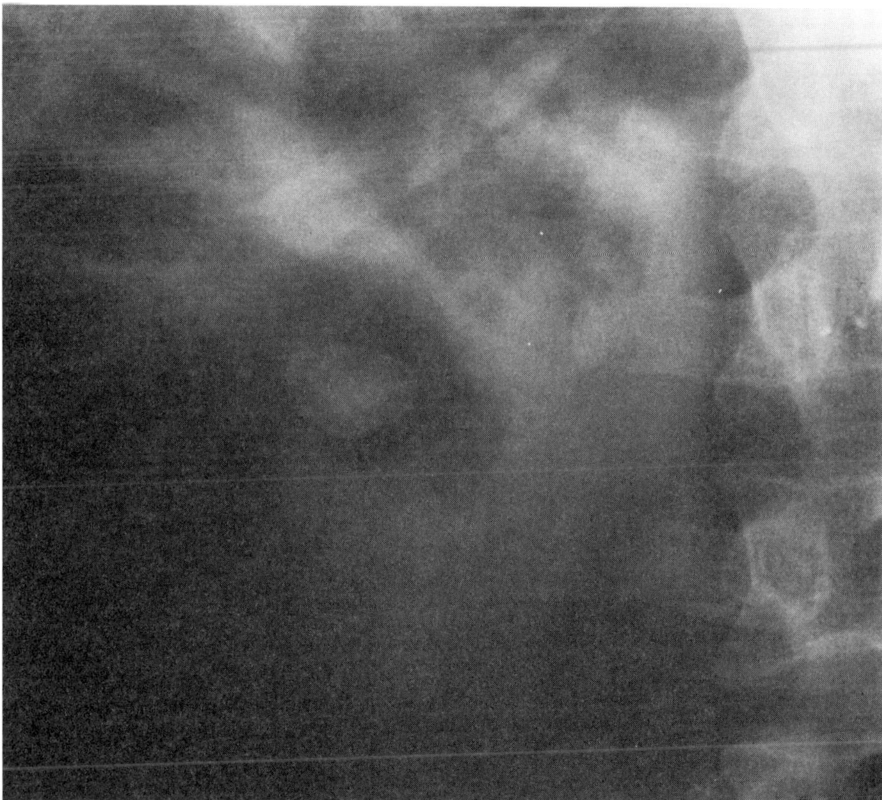

Figure 2.1 Plain film right renal area shows a laminated renal calculus. Layers of various opacities indicate that the calculus is located proximal to obstruction. Urogram (not shown here) demonstrated a stricture of the infundibulum of the calyx containing this calculus

defects within the collecting system. In addition to protocol films, later films may be necessary in patients with calcular obstruction or post-obstructive changes in the urinary system.

The three cardinal radiographic signs of obstruction are progressively dense nephrogram, delayed excretion of contrast, and stasis of contrast with dilatation of collecting system and ureters. The most constant finding in ureteric obstruction, on the delayed films, is the presence of a continuous column of opacified ureter up to the site of the calculus, usually with some proximal dilatation (Figure 2.4). Delayed films at 1, 2, 4 and 6 hours or later may be necessary to visualize the level of obstruction. Post-contrast delayed oblique films of the pelvic area may become necessary to confirm the intraureteric location of a calcular opacity, especially for those that overlie the sacrum, and where there is doubt that a phlebolith may be a ureteric stone (Figure 2.2). The lumen of the ureter distal to the stone is usually not visualized due to lack of good flow of the contrast beyond the stone.

An impacted stone at the uretero-vesical junction causes oedema that mimics a ureterocoele or bladder tumour. After passage of the stone the oedema rapidly sub-

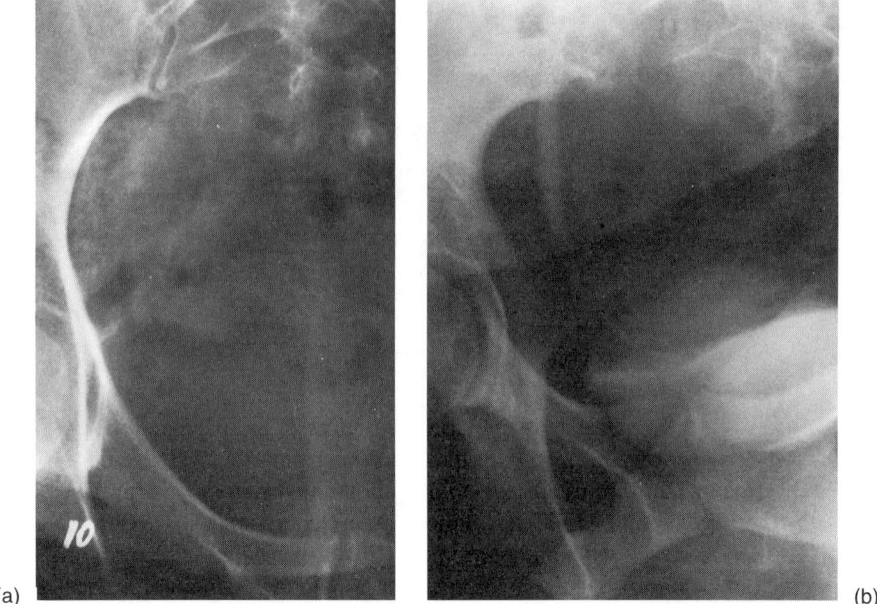

Figure 2.2 (a) Plain film of the right side of the pelvis shows two opacities that resemble phleboliths; (b) delayed (25-minute) oblique film from IVU shows that one of the opacities is located within the lower ureter

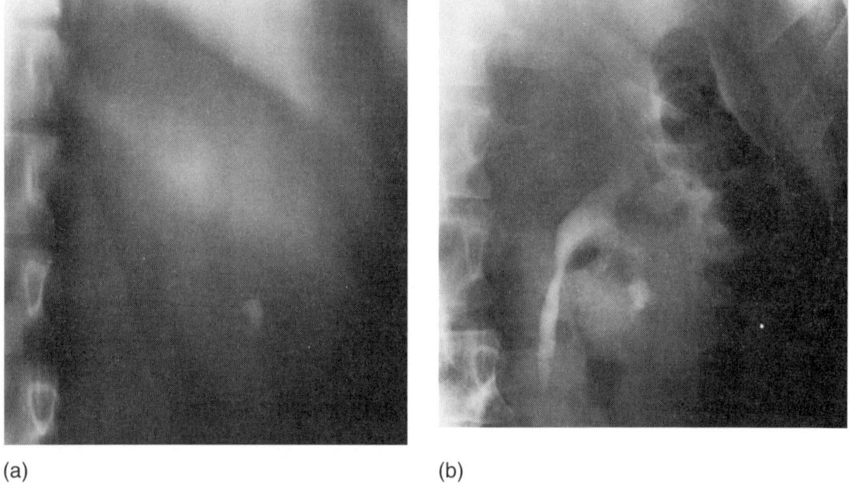

Figure 2.3 (a) Plain left renal tomogram; (b) fifteen-minute urogram film. Apart from the calculus, the left kidney is normal without evidence of obstruction

sides and thus can be correctly differentiated from significant other pathology. Mild ureteric obstruction may become apparent only on an erect film which shows a hold-up of the contrast column. Chronic ureteric obstruction leads to back pressure

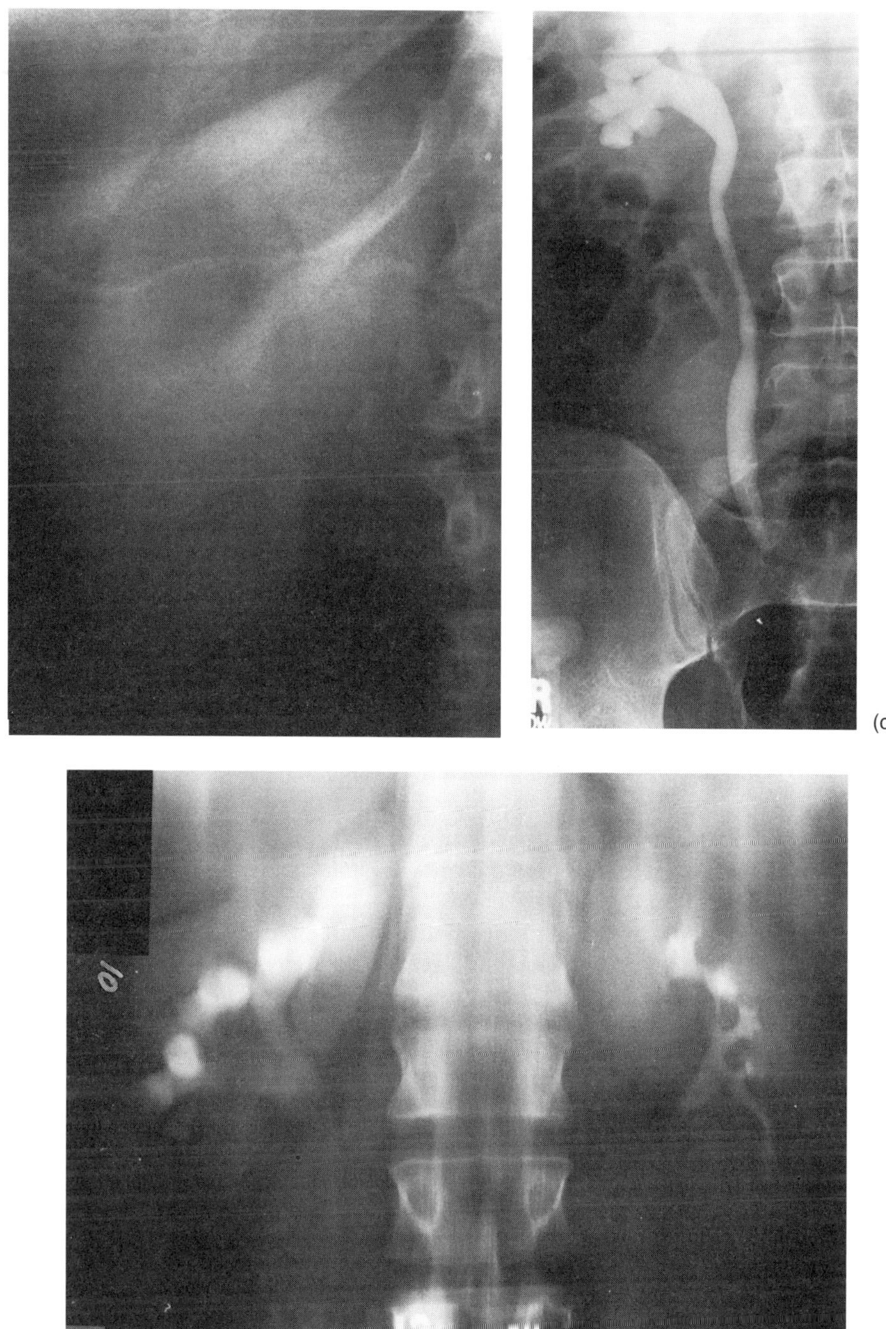

Figure 2.4 (a) Three-minute urogram film showing delayed pyelogram with dense nephrogram indicating obstruction; (b) tomogram of the renal area at 15 minutes after contrast demonstrates mild right hydronephrosis indicating ureteric obstruction; (c) 45-minute urogram film showing columnization of the right ureter down to the level of the obstructing lucent calculus

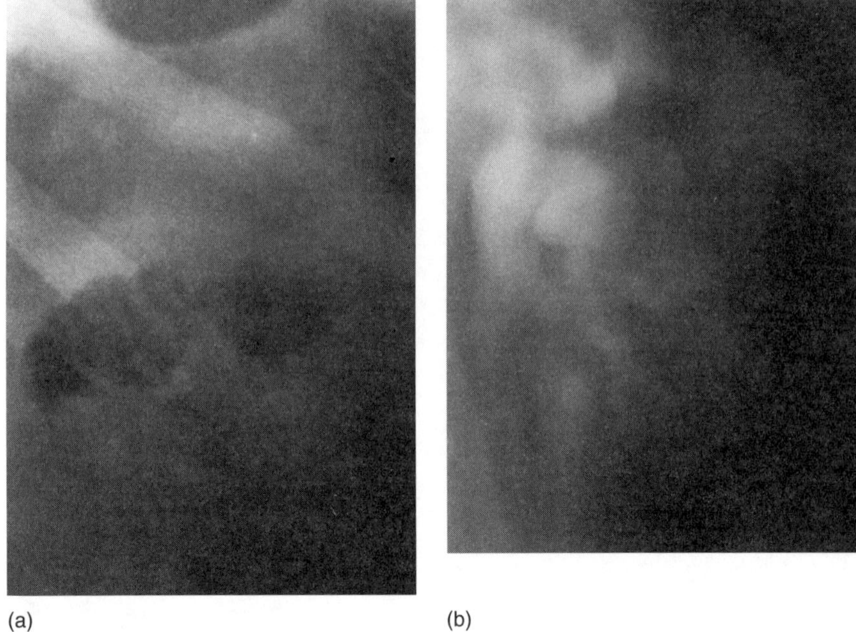

Figure 2.5 (a) Plain film of the left renal area; (b) 20-minute post-contrast tomogram of the left kidney shows non-obstructing calculi in the lower pole calyces. Note post-obstructive renal changes with blunting of calyces, mild thinning of the renal cortex from ureteric obstruction in the past

and atrophy of the renal cortex. In the absence of superadded infection there is uniform atrophy of the renal substance with dilatation of the collecting system (Figure 2.5). Kidneys atrophic from significant renal damage will opacify less than normal kidneys. Superadded infection may give rise to a picture of chronic pyelonephritis or a non-functioning kidney, either grossly hydronephrotic or markedly shrunken. A faintly opacified kidney may only be visible on thin section tomography, CT or MRI.

The IVU can detect calyceal or infundibular stricture, calyceal diverticula, pelvic-ureteral obstruction, ureterocoeles, bladder diverticula, bladder outflow obstruction, and ureteric stricture, all crucial to decisions about correct management.

Retrograde pyelography

This is an invasive procedure that involves the insertion of a radiopaque catheter, retrogradely through the ureteric orifice, at cystoscopy. Its main indication is the finding of a non-opacifying (non-functioning) kidney on urography with a delayed film. On retrograde opacification of the ureter, the site and cause of the obstruction can usually be determined. A non-opaque calculus causing the obstruction will show a smooth lower margin, whilst ureteral tumours will show irregular margins except in some polyps.

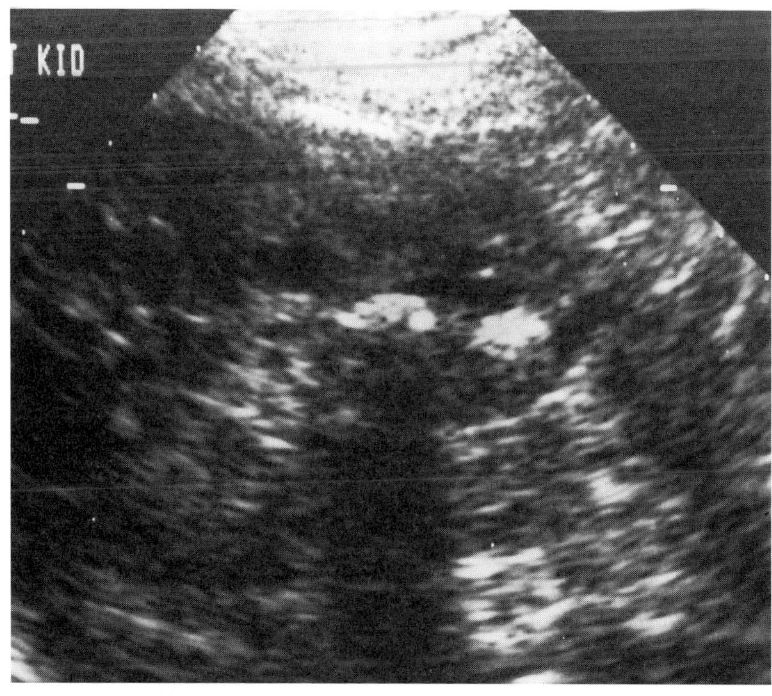

(a)

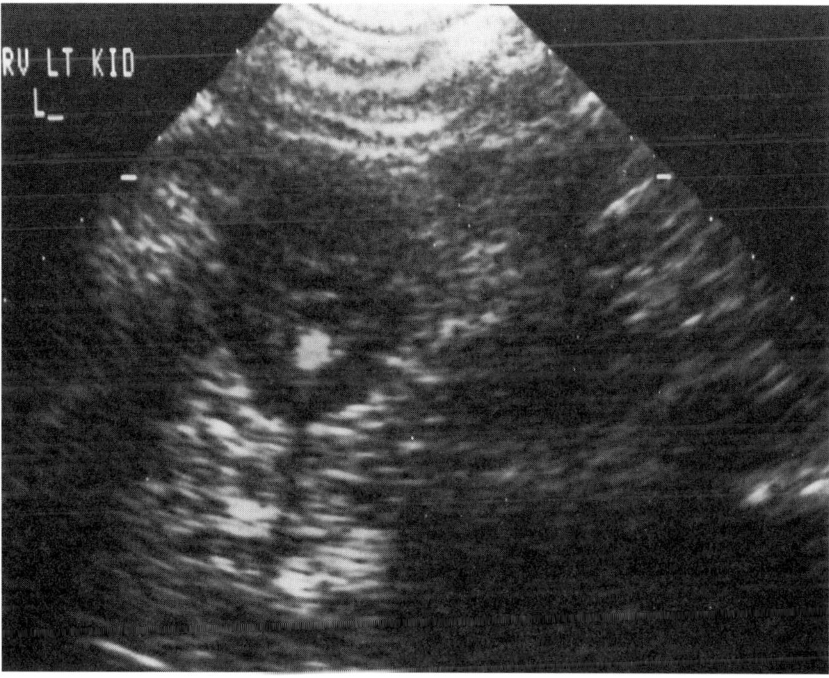

(b)

Figure 2.8 Sagittal (a) and coronal (b) sections show ecogenic foci of left lower renal pole, calyceal calculi with typical posterior acoustic shadowing

Antegrade pyelography

A thin needle can be entered percutaneously under ultrasound or fluoroscopic or CT guidance for percutaneous drainage of an obstructed kidney, especially when infected, or for performance of an antegrade pyelogram.

Computed tomography

Computed tomography (CT) is very sensitive in detecting non-opaque calculi and can differentiate them from tumour and blood clots. CT is generally not employed in the work-up of stones, but is used in the evaluation of acute and chronic sequelae of the stone disease.

Ultrasonography

Ultrasound can be used to establish the presence of a calculus, which appears as a sono-dense highly echogenic focus with posterior acoustic shadowing. Smaller stones that do not throw an acoustic shadow are difficult to differentiate from sinus fat, calyceal walls and vascular structures that are also echogenic. Ultrasonography is particularly important in the diagnosis of non-opaque renal calculi and can differentiate calculi from other causes of filling defect in the pelvis such as tumour and blood clot. Non-calcular filling defects are less echogenic and do not cause acoustic shadowing (Figure 2.6). Ultrasound is also helpful in differentiating the causes of a non-functioning kidney – hydronephrosis will suggest obstruction, and renal vein thrombosis can be detected. Colour flow Doppler differentiates hypervascular from non-vascular conditions of the kidney. Ultrasound is particularly helpful in the detection of vesical calculi.

Magnetic resonance urography

Magnetic resonance urography (MRU) does not require injection of iodinated contrast, or use of ionizing radiation. Heavily T2 weighted images or maximum intensity projection (MIP) images are taken to delineate fluid filled pelvi-calyceal systems, ureters and bladder (Figure 2.7). Renal parenchyma can be optimally evaluated in T1 weighted imaging. If needed, excretion of gadolinium-DTPA can provide valuable information on renal function. Currently the clinical application of MRU is mainly in patients with a history of anaphylactic reaction to contrast media, pregnant females and patients with renal failure where nephrotoxicity of iodinated compounds is to be avoided.

Isotope scanning

The main role of radionuclide scanning in urolithiasis is the quantitative assessment of renal function, which cannot be deduced from the IVU. Isotope scanning is

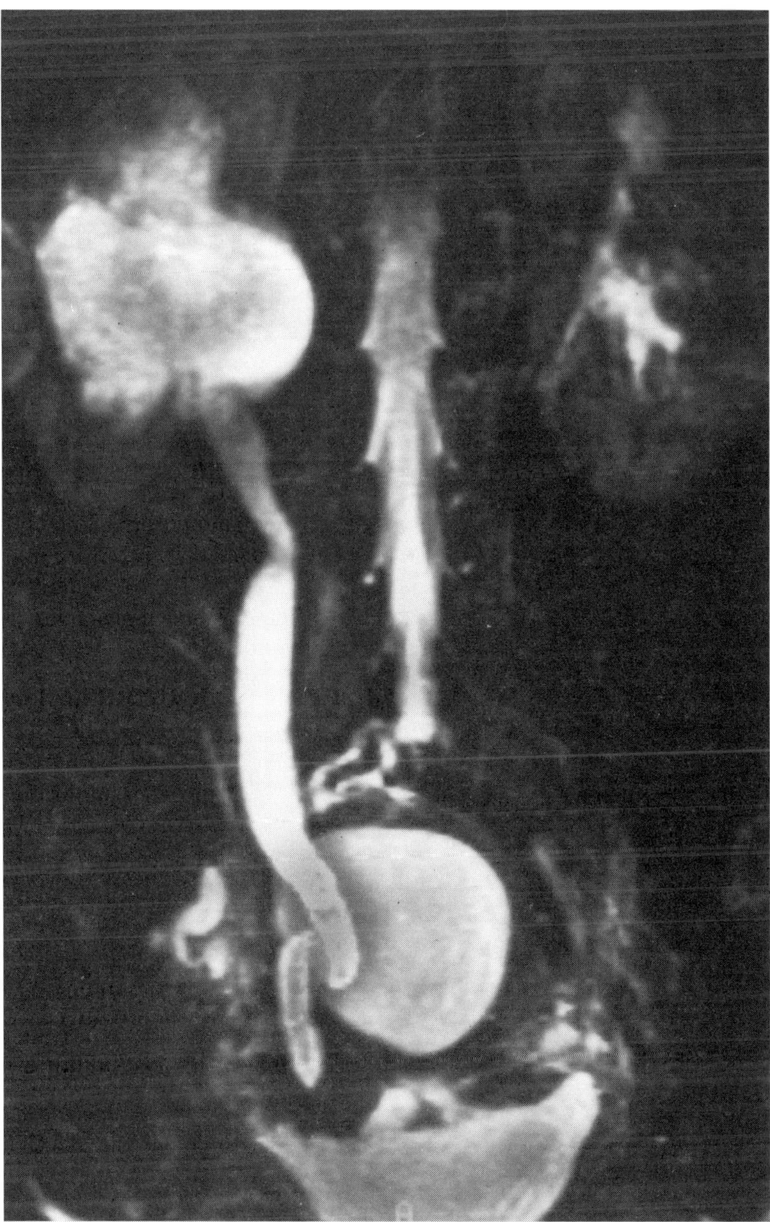

Figure 2.7 Coronal heavily T2 weighted maximum intensity projection (MIP) image of the abdomen, without any contrast medium. There is evidence of obstruction of the pelvic portion of the right ureter. Normal left kidney and ureter. Spinal subarachnoid space is also outlined. There is a fluid filled cyst in the pelvis above the bladder

inferior to other imaging modalities in depicting the anatomical details, but provides quantitative assessment of renal function in each kidney, and is important when choosing conservative surgery vs. nephrectomy.

Further reading

Keizur JJ, Das S. Current perspectives on intravascular contrast agents for radiological imaging. J Urol 1994;151:1470–8.

3. Epidemiology of urolithiasis in Pakistan

JAMSHEER TALATI, FARAKH KHAN, HERMIE DRAGO, ERNEST
LALL, NAEMUZ ZAFAR KHAN, ARDESHEER TALATI and JOOP
NOORDZIJ

Patterns of stone disease in impoverished nations vary from that in the first world.
The pattern in Pakistan, a developing nation emerging from the third world, forms
an interesting case study because of the coexistence of both first and third world
conditions.

Pakistan, an agricultural country, stretches from just above the Tropic of Cancer
to 36.75 degrees north. Large stretches of desert in the south in Sindh, fertile plains
irrigated by canals that have now caused much waterlogging and salinity in Punjab
in the middle, rugged barren mountains in the west and coniferous forests in the
north, lead to 10 of the world's 32 highest peaks (ranging in height from
7672–8611 m).

Gradual economic improvement has occurred from its birth as a nation in 1947
but the benefits of economic development have spread unequally. Prospects for a
decent income in Pakistan are bleak outside of cities. The GNP has risen from $170
in 1974 [1] to $400, but the population still struggles to survive, because wealth is
not equitably distributed, inflation (13–20%) crodes incomes, and the government
does not have resources to improve education or literacy (currently 28%, down
from 35% in 1990 [2]). If Pakistan had restricted its population growth to 1.5% per
annum (half of the current 3%), this GNP would have equalled $800 by 1994.

Incidence and hospitalization rates

Stone disease is a major problem in Pakistan. The incidence (per 100 000) in the
extreme north ranges from 2.4 in Chitral to 9.4 in Gilgit [3]. Across Pakistan, the
incidence ranges from 7.4 in the north [4], to 28 in the west [5], to 200 per 100 000
in the south [6]. A survey of operations (1985–1987) in 14 district general hospitals
and four hospitals attached to medical colleges [7], gives a minimal incidence of
8.3 per 100 000 for the whole of Punjab, 4.2 for the north and 16.4 for the south.
(In this study the authors divided the province by a line passing through the towns
of Sahiwal, Jhang, Sarghoda and Mianwalli, see Figure 3.1). It is conceded that
many hospitals were not surveyed and the figures regarding operations done for
stones were related to the entire population, hence the conclusion that this is the
minimal incidence.

J. Talati et al. (eds) The Management of Lithiasis, 21–33
© 1997 Kluwer Academic Publishers. Printed in Great Britain.

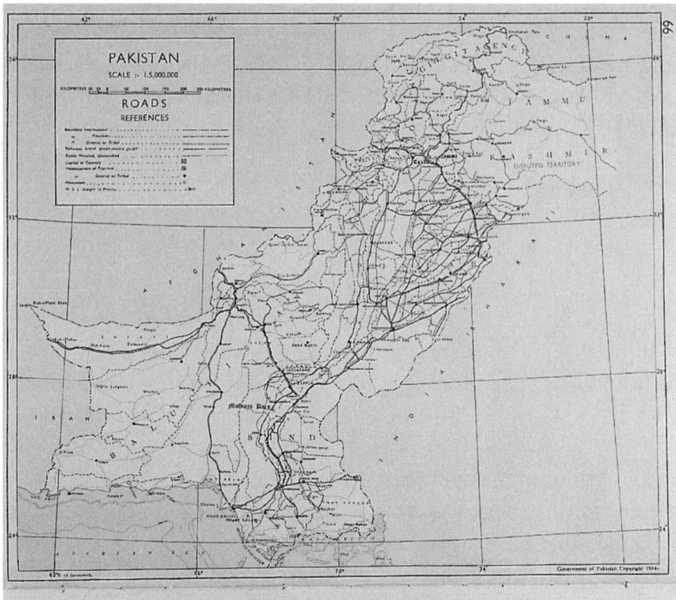

Figure 3.1 Map of Pakistan

Bladder stone disease has an incidence of 1.1, 0.6, and 0.2 per 100 000 in the districts of Abbotabad, Mansehra and Kohistan [8], and 1.2, 7.6 and 9 [4] in Hazara, Balochistan and Sindh.

Stone is the sixth most common condition requiring surgery in Pakistan [4,10]. Between 4–7% of a general hospital's operating output can be for stone disease [4, 6, 9]. In Balochistan, 9% of operations are for stone [5]. In Gilgit 3.8% of major and 1% of all operations are for stone [3] as against a rural average for the whole of Pakistan of 6.2%. In children under 11 years, 23% of operative procedures are for stone [4].

Eighteen per cent of a nephrourological unit's new outpatients are registered for stone disease [11] and 45% of the work of a urological unit in 1993 can be for stone disease [12]. In Sujjawal, in a rural area in Sindh, 34% of operations were done for stone disease [6]. In Thar, one of the regions included in Mirpurkhas district until recently, stones account for 0.35% of all outpatients seen (data courtesy Dr Ghulam Mohammed Memon). This is an underestimate, because the Thari (resident of Thar) is poor, and therefore roams peripatetically from village to village in search of work (which is mainly found in the cotton picking season). If there is sufficient rainfall, he returns to the Thar desert to cultivate a crop of *bajra* (millet), *jowar* (oats) and melons. Otherwise he continues to work as a labourer or domestic servant, moving from town to town. When he has enough money and accompanying relatives he visits the district hospital or other hospital nearest to his last working site, and has his operation. His stone disease therefore remains unrecorded in his own district.

In the Punjab, in a hospital for children, 1 in 73 hospital admissions in Islamabad, and 1 in 24 surgical paediatric admissions is for urinary tract stone [13]. In Chicago by comparison (1950–79), 1 in 6500–7400 paediatric patients were admitted for stone [14]. Operations for bladder stone at Taxila have continued to show a rise with 482 cases in the years 1982–90 compared to 85 cases in the 1922–31 period, a growth much more than that of the population (3.1%), but stone operations constitute much smaller proportions of total operations (5.2% in 1932–41 compared to 0.25% in 1982–1990) as the hospital laid greater emphasis on ophthalmic work (Ernest Lall, data from Christian Hospital Taxila).

Punjab has had a high incidence of bladder stone since very early recorded history. The problem must have been significant, as Ayur Veda, in the medical religious writings dated second millennium to 800 BC (Encyclopaedia Brittanica), describes perineal lithotomy and the suprapubic approach for bladder stone disease in children [15], and Susruta developed a lateral approach to bladder stones, during the golden age (800 BC to 1000 AD) of Indian medicine. Itinerant Vedic surgeons continued to practise this operation until the start of the twentieth century [15].

A report in 1863 notes removal of 554 bladder stones in six months. The records of the Punjab government document removal of around 2000 bladder stones each year between 1890 and 1913 [15].

McCarrison [16] reported a much higher incidence of stone formation in persons living around the Indus valley as compared to those in the south of India: 438 (per 100 000) in Dera Ghazi Khan in Punjab province, 266 in Hyderabad in Sindh province, and 156 in Sukkur, also in Sindh province (all of these are now part of Pakistan), as against 13 and 0.3 in Ahmednagar and Madras (in southern India) respectively [16]. The south is mainly Dravidian; the areas now in Pakistan have been subjected to repeated invasions form the north.

Changes in the frequency of bladder stones compared to upper urinary tract calculi – transition patterns

In the history of every country, bladder stones are first recorded as occurring most often in the young and middle-aged adult (phase 1). They then become more frequent in children (phase 2), and later as the country evolves, bladder stones are rarely seen except in the elderly with bladder outflow obstruction (phase 3). At the same time the incidence of kidney stones increases. Just appearing on the horizon is a new phase – phase 4 – with an increase in bladder stone due to congenital abnormalities and infection in children saved by miracles of technological support [17].

Within Pakistan, Balochistan is still in phase 1. Mirpurkhas was in phase one in the 1930s. In Kelantan province in Malaysia 69% of bladder stones are still seen in the young adult male without bladder outflow obstruction even today [18], also a phase 1 state.

Most developed countries are in phase 3. In Japan, only 0.8% of all stones were bladder stones in 1990 [19], whereas they contributed 5% [20] and 50% to the total stone population in 1979 and 1945 respectively. In Bristol, UK (1975) [21] and

24   *Jamsheer Talati* et al.

Table 3.1 Proportion of stones that are vesical in different countries at different phases of their development

High proportions		Moderate proportions		Low proportions	
50%	Japan 1945	15%	Turkey 1981–92	0.8%	Japan 1990
80%	Thailand 1953–59	15%	Taiwan	3%	Saudi Arabia
17%	Thailand 1993	5%	Japan 1979		
25%	Turkey 1970–81				
37%	Malaysia				

Canada (1971–80) [22], 9% and < 1% respectively, of children hospitalized for stone, had bladder stones, extremely uncommon since 1925 [21]. In 1993, in the USA, [23] almost all stones in children were found in the upper urinary tract.

The picture is changing in the West. In 1994, in units caring for babies saved by incubator care and surgery for congenital abnormalities, 30% of 270 paediatric stones were again vesical [17]. Infection is associated with these stones in a higher proportion (60%) of patients [17] than seen in 1975 when only 29% of stones were of infective aetiology [21] demonstrating the appearance of a new phase – phase 4.

Turkey, Egypt, Syria, Iran, Pakistan, India, and Indonesia are in various stages of moving from phase 2 to 3. In Turkey the proportion of bladder stone has decreased from 25% (1970–81) to 15% (1981–1992) [24]. In Singapore 66% of patients with bladder stone are over 65 years old [25]. In Taiwan, another Asian tiger, bladder stones account for only 15% of all urinary tract stones [26]. In Saudi Arabia, only 3% have bladder stones [27]. In Thailand, in 1953–59, 80% of stones were vesical; in 1993, only 17.3% were vesical [28].

Bladder stone disease in Pakistan

In 1934, every tenth to fifteenth patient operated in the Civil Hospital Mirpurkhas, in the province of Sindh, had a bladder stone (Drago, personal data). (Mirpurkhas was then the headquarters of Tharparkar district which encompassed the current Mirpurkhas, Thar and Sanghar districts.) Most patients were male adults. Children and old men constituted 5% (Dr Drago).

This was the era of bladder stone surgery in the middle-aged man and this is still the status in Quetta in the province of Balochistan, where 61% are seen in adults (20–39 years old) and only 3.7% are seen in children below 10 years of age [5], even in 1992.

In Sindh and Punjab, the picture has changed. In rural Sindh bladder stones remain common and constitute 73% of all (351) stone operations done in an 18-month period in Mirpurkhas, 75% in Sujjawal (see Table 3.2), and 63.5% in Taxila, in Punjab. Sixty-four per cent of bladder calculi at Mirpurkhas are now however seen in children aged under 10 years. In contrast, 85% of renal calculi are seen in adults aged over 45 years.

Whilst bladder stone disease continues to be the predominant stone in hospitals serving rural areas, it is now a disease of the young child (phase 2).

Table 3.2   Frequency of urological operations at the Taluka Hospital, Sujjawal (January–October, 1989)

Total operations	778
Urological operations	346
Bladder stones	199
Renal stones	53
Ureteric stones	7
Urethral stones	4

Modified from [6] with permission of publisher.

Bladder stones are slowly disappearing from urban areas except in Quetta where in 1992, 49% were in the upper urinary tract (40.8% in the kidney), and 51% in the lower urinary tract. Thirty years ago, every list in the teaching hospital in Lahore (the capital of the province Punjab) would contain a bladder stone case. Now these are rare. In 1990 only 15% of patients operated for stone in the general wards of a government hospital in Lahore, in Punjab, had bladder stones, 85% having upper urinary tract stones [29].

In Karachi, a sprawling metropolis variously rated as home for between 8 and 10 millions, the population has been stratified by ability to pay for medical treatment; interestingly the types of stones common in these divergent groups (those who can afford private treatment and those who cannot) were different. Bladder stones were the most common stone in free government hospitals serving the poor (Civil Hospital, Karachi) in 1971–75, though they were not as common as in the rural areas (56% were vesical, 29.5% renal, 10.5% ureteric, and 4% urethral, at the Civil Hospital, Karachi) [30]. In contrast, fee-for-service hospitals and hospitals which supported medical care through social security saw a different proportion of stones. At the Holy Family Hospital (1979–83), only 23.6% were bladder stones, 46.7% were renal, 23.6% ureteric and the rest urethral (J. Talati, unpublished data). In a social security funded hospital, where poor patients were given treatment through social security cover, in 1975, bladder stone remained the predominant stone (76%) in children, but only 29% of males and 7% of females had bladder stones requiring surgery [9]. At a later time, in a private hospital, only 19% were bladder stones, 36% and 43% being renal and ureteric, respectively (AKUMC statistics for 1988).

In patients from the Civil Hospital (1971–75), bladder calculi were the predominant stone in children, and again, the most common stone after 41 years of age – a stage where we see bladder stone of the child and bladder stone of the adult simultaneously.

The statistics have changed dramatically with the availability of the lithotriptor (see Table 3.4).

Aetiology of bladder calculi

Experimentally, bladder stones can be produced by feeding rats large quantities of uracil [31] or by inserting discs of Zn into the bladders of rats infected with

Ureaplasma urealyticum. The latter produces struvite stones which are quite different to the stones in human bladders.

Poverty and bladder calculi

In regions where bladder stones are more frequent, per capita income is low, and the diet is consequently low in calories and proteins. In the 1930s the Thari (the resident of Thar, a desert area in Sindh), ate *bajra* bread and *chilli* (red pepper) powder with whey, the by-product of the butter they produce for making *ghee* (clarified butter) for sale in the towns of Sindh, in order to get the money to buy the *bajra*. Addition of potatoes fried in *ghee* was a delicacy reserved for guests. Now the diet contains wheat, pulses, vegetables and *bajra*, with meat added occasionally. The Thari remains poor, and even today his diet contains little first-class protein.

In Abbotabad district, 88% of bladder calculi were seen in patients from villages. In this region, 45% of the general population earn Rs 101–250 (US$ 3.5–8 per month), and only 9% earn more than Rs 500 (US$ 17) [6]. The families of the vesical stone formers were even poorer, with 68% earning less than Rs 250 per month [8]. Mothers become pregnant whilst still lactating, and continued to breast feed during pregnancy.

Poverty limits education which restricts the individual to low paid jobs. Without education the individual cannot comprehend the need to space children, and the benefits of a small family. Large families have to be fed on small incomes. Nutrition suffers. Girls are married off at an early age. A pregnancy production line ensues. Child after child exhausts the mother. The breasts fail to deliver the milk the child needs. Weaning occurs early. Rice is substituted for milk. There is no cow to produce the milk so desperately needed. If available, powdered milk is fed in unhygienic unwashed unboiled bottles. Diarrhoea, dehydration and milk-deprivation combine to form the bladder stone. Bladder stone disease remains common in such a setting.

In Turkey, stone disease has a higher prevalence in patients with lower incomes (21 vs. 13%), and in patients who have had no education or education at the primary level only vs. those who are university graduates (19 vs. 9%) [24].

In Thailand, bladder stone disease was attributed to early weaning, lack of milk and low phosphorus levels [32] and this view appeared to be supported by the lowering of the incidence of bladder stones by pyrophosphate supplementation. However, bladder stone incidence has dramatically changed in other countries *pari passu* with an improvement in the GNP and without phosphate supplements.

Nutrition and dietary intake in stone formers and the general population in Pakistan compared to the West

Within Pakistan affluence determines the access to food. Food autarky has been attained; equitable distribution has not.

Table 3.3 Nutritional parameters in stone patients undergoing lithotripsy in a fee-for-service hospital

Height	164.9 ± 9.37 cm
Weight	66.0 ± 14.1 kg
Body mass index	24.4 ± 5.2
Triceps skin fold thickness	2.4 ± 0.99 cm*
Serum proteins	7.09 ± 0.49
Serum albumin	4.3 ± 3.6
Total WBC count	9.06 ± 2.5
Absolute lymphocyte count	2.3 ± 0.75

Data collected by A. Talati.

A survey of the nutritional status and dietary intake in an urban population in Karachi able to afford private tertiary hospital care (18 patients) showed the nutritional parameters and dietary intake detailed in Table 3.3.

It is obvious that in this tertiary setting, in the small number of randomly selected patients, there is no evidence of under-nutrition. The average calcium excretion in this group was 194.37 ± 131.3 mg/24 h. Their nutritional intake included an average milk intake of 0.855 ± 1.0 l per week, meat in 5.3 ± 4.6 meals per week; and pulses in 2.6 ± 3.1 meals per week. The protein intake is lower than that quoted by Rashid *et al.* [29] for a population from Lahore, where 20.9% of all stone patients consumed large amounts of proteins.

Distribution of food is inequitable. The relatively well fed patients coming to AKUMC have proportionately more renal stones than bladder stones (renal: bladder stone ratio of 13:1). In Sindh, 54% of children are chronically malnourished (as judged by height for age) and 25% acutely malnourished (weight for height) [33]. In a survey of 1878 children, 50% were reported to have had diarrhoea in the preceding two weeks [33]. In Thar, and Sujjawal, where nutrition is poor, the fish caught from the river is sold to obtain the money for vegetables to feed the

Table 3.4 Comparison of proportions of stones seen at various sites in different studies

	Renal	Ureteric	Bladder	Urethral	Up:low	Kid:ure
SITE (Paediatrics)	13.0	4	76	0.22	3.3	
SITE (Male)	48.0	23	29	2.5	2.1	
(Female)	73.0	20	7	13.3	3.7	
CHK (*n* = 400)	29.5	10.5	56.0	4	0.66	2.8
(1975)						
CHK (1990–94)	84.8	6.5	7.8	0.9	10.50	13.0
AKU 1992	62.0	31.0	7.0	0	13.30	2.01
(*n* = 625)						
Mirpurkhas	15.4	10.8	72.9	0.9	0.35	1.43
(*n* = 351)						
Sujjawal	20.7	2.7	75.1	1.5	0.3	7.67
(*n* = 265)						

SITE: Sindh Industrial Trading Estate Hospital; CHK: Civil Hospital Karachi; AKU: Aga Khan University Hospital; Mirpurkhas: data from Civil Hospital situated in a town, but serving a rural population; Sujjawal: data from Taluka level (subdistrict) hospital in a rural setting; Up:low, ratio of upper to lower urinary tract calculi; Kid:ure, ratio of renal to ureteric calculi.

family at bare subsistence levels. The resulting upper to lower tract stone ratio is 0.31 in this population.

Data from a Government of Pakistan National Nutritional Survey, 1985–87 indicates that the average Pakistani has a total calorie intake ranging from 1864 for Balochistan, to 2559 for NWFP (North West Frontier Province). In 1990, the average calorie intake has increased to 2380 [1]. Protein intake varies from 61 to 72 g per day; milk intake is poor in NWFP and Balochistan (44–60 ml per day as against 139 and 153 in Punjab and Sindh). Vegetable intake is extremely poor in Balochistan, and fruit intake low except in Punjab. There is a very high consumption of tea in Pakistan in office workers, though tea is taken with milk. Tea in excess of 4 cups can raise urinary oxalate levels significantly and when 20 g powdered tea is utilized, oxalate excretion can increase to 148 mg/24 h [34].

In France, 7% of men and 40% of women may have a higher than necessary calorie intake; 79% are overweight, protein intake is 87 ± 21 g per day, and calcium intake 934 ± 406 mg/day [35]. Concurrent with the increase in calorie and fat intake, the working week has shortened, travel by car become more common than travel by foot, bicycle or car, and energy expenditure and therefore calorie requirements have reduced. The calorie intake in the Netherlands today is lower than that in the 1950s and now averages 2105. Protein intake averages 94 g per day for the male and 76 for the female, and calcium intake 1075 mg per day in the male and 910 in the female (data courtesy Dr Noordzij).

Calorie intake in Europe in general, and North America is higher at around 3000 calories; proteins contribute 400 (animal proteins 150–272), fat 800–1200, and carbohydrate 1400–1900 calories [36]. The diet is rich in refined sugar and low in fibre (4 g as compared to 24 g for the Bantu in Africa). Sugar increases and fibre decreases calcium absorption.

In the East, in contrast, the natural diet is high in fibre, and low in refined carbohydrate. Unfortunately the East imitates the West as the world shrinks into one global community because of commercial ventures, and information technology. The use of carbonated water, increased use of refined sugar due to its easy availability, and reduction of dietary fibre follows. Altered diet habits may lead to hypercalciuria.

The effect of migration from village to town on nutrition

The doubling of the population from 1901 to 50, in the area that now constitutes Pakistan, and yet again from 1950 to 75 [2] has worsened economic plight and caused migration to towns, in attempts to improve personal income. In 1951, only 17% of Pakistan's population lived in urban areas, now 34% do so. Over-populated towns (Karachi contains 26% of the urban population of Pakistan) marginalize many who then remain poor. Migration to rich Middle-Eastern countries is possible only for a minority of individuals.

Migrated populations often change dietary practices. Increase of the minimum wage for low-paid unmarried workers, used to a simple life style, soon frees up cash for food. Unwilling or unable to cook, with the wife in the home town far away, the dietary pattern changes and protein intake increases. The intake of food differs in town and village. In Pakistan meat intake is higher in townsfolk. In northeast Thailand, villagers with renal stones had higher excretion of sodium, phosphorus and uric acid than healthy city dwellers or villagers [37]. Expatriates in Saudi Arabia are known to increase their stone-forming risk [38] because of increased meat intake, oxalate containing vegetables and dehydration.

Misleading perceptions from hospital statistics

An epidemiological study in Rochester showed that only 44% of patients require hospitalization for stone disease, and only 6.4% require surgical intervention [39]. Obviously, a number of ureteric calculi pass spontaneously and will remain unrecorded in hospital statistics. In third world countries the picture is compounded with the ease with which bladder stones are operated on in a hospital environment that does not allow investigation or management of renal calculi. Bladder calculi are diagnosed with ease. The child tugs at his penis, cries. The physician diagnoses this clinically, and can confirm it by sounding the bladder with metal bougies, without X-rays. The bladder stone gets operated on and so enters the hospital register. The renal stone remains undiagnosed and unrecorded. Additionally, unless the district hospital is close by, the patient will not be able to leave his farm to travel to the hospital as we have seen in the Thari.

Deductions about transitions based on data from hospitals may produce erroneous impressions perceived as transitions.

Effect of high technology on statistics

Even if there is a hospital close by, the patient may not want to visit the doctor. Tales of death at operation, the long scar and incapacitation at work, keep people away, an additional factor that results in fewer kidney operations for stone. Traditional thinking may keep patients away from doctors. In Hazara division in Pakistan, a survey showed that only 52% would consider consulting a doctor for illness; 32% would consult a Hakim or homoeopath, and 16% believed in cure by saints, visits to mazars (graves of saints) and Tavis (religious charm). Such (latter) patients would not attend hospital [6].

Hospital inpatient statistics in hospitals which are not supported by technology are even less representative of the true incidence and proportions of stone than are outpatient statistics. Without X-rays, the renal stone remains unrecorded.

Dramatic shifts in the relative proportions of stone occur when patient friendly devices such as the lithotriptor are installed. At the Civil Hospital, in Karachi, the percentage of renal stones has dramatically increased (see Table 3.5).

At the Aga Khan University Medical Center (AKUMC), in the period prior to the purchase of an extracorporeal lithotriptor (1985–87), only 19% of all stones were vesical; 43% were ureteric and 36% renal. This is a fee-for-service hospital, which in spite of enormous welfare funds is unable to serve the indigent. These figures parallel those from Germany before the advent of ESWL (1976), where 35.8%

Table 3.5   Stone treatment at the Civil Hospital, Karachi and Sindh Institute of Urology and Transplantation

		Renal	Ureteric	Bladder	Urethral
Pre-ESWL	(1972–80)	45%	4.3%	49.0%	1.7%
ESWL era	(1990–94)	84.8%	6.5%	7.8%	0.9%

Data courtesy of Dr Anwar Naqvi and Adib Rizvi, Sindh Institute of Urology and Transplantation, Karachi, Pakistan.

Table 3.6   Relative distribution of calculi in the urinary tract deduced from all interventional treatments including ESWL[a] at the Aga Khan University Medical Center

	Kidney	Ureter	Bladder	Urethra	Up:low[b]	Ren:ure[c]
1987	36.4	42.6	19.3	1.5	3.8	0.85
1989	65.9	26.8	6.2	1.1	12.7	2.46
1991	51.3	36.8	10.1	1.8	7.4	1.39

[a] Extracorporeal lithotriptor bought in November 1988.
[b] Up:low, proportion of upper to lower urinary tract stones.
[c] Ren:ure, proportion of renal to ureteric calculi.

were kidney stones, and 12% bladder stones [40], and are quite different from the figures at the Civil Hospital Karachi. After ESWL, because of rapid throughput, the proportions of upper to lower urinary tract stones rose further (see Table 3.6).

Just as the proportions of renal to vesical calculi change with the purchase of the lithotriptor, so also the proportions of renal stones detected in children and adults change when doctors have the appropriate technology to diagnose upper urinary tract stones. So far we have shown that renal stones are uncommon in Sujjawal. But the doctors there are overworked – a single surgeon serves 60 000 inhabitants – and do not have any technical support. The nearest IVP facility is across the river. In Taxila too, it is bladder stones that are receiving attention (see Figure 3.2). In a well supported children's hospital in the Pakistan Institute of Medical Sciences, not

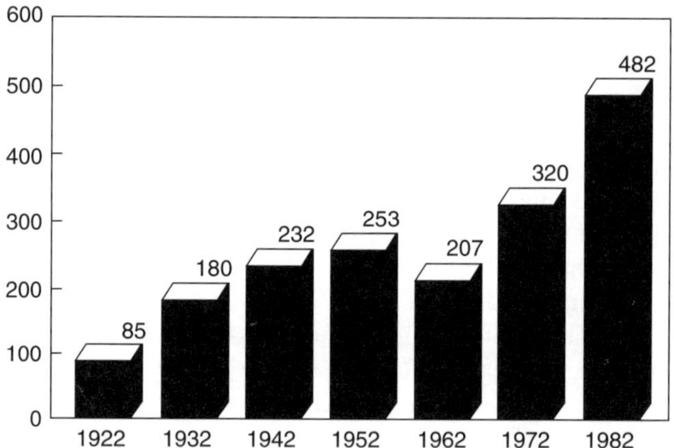

Figure 3.2 Seven decades of stone surgery: cystolithotomies at Taxila

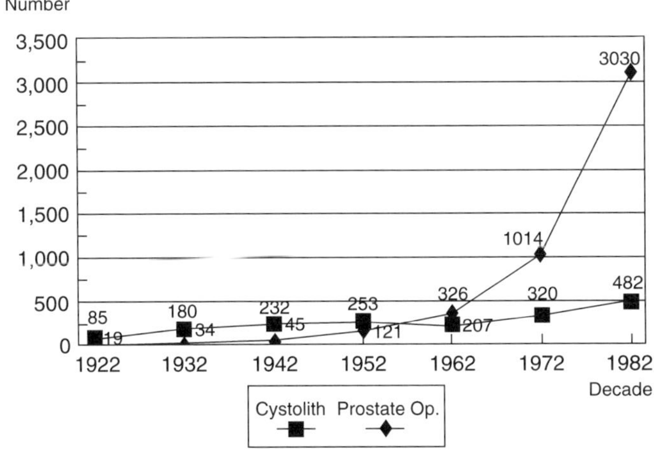

Figure 3.3 Seven decades of stones surgery cystolithotomy vs prostate operation at Taxila

many miles away from Taxila, 51.6% of stones in children are renal and 27.4% vesical; 6.3% patients have both renal and vesical stones, 8.4% ureteric and 6.3% urethral. The high proportion of renal stones is not due to the hospital attracting an affluent population. This does not support the hypothesis that it is mainly the vesical calculus that is seen in the poor. Much of their population is drawn from a vast poorly populated socioeconomically depressed hinterland. The poor state of health is reflected in the numbers who were anaemic (71% with Hb below 11 g/dl), and below the fifth centile for weight (55%). The average income was Rs 228 (< US$10) per month. Developmental abnormalities were seen in only 2 of the 46 patients studied and could not account for the higher incidence of renal stones. It is the better diagnostic and anaesthetic facilities, large number of ICU beds, and increased surgical expertise which contribute to the difference between what is operated on at Taxila and Islamabad.

Apart from the impact of availability of high technology, expertise in its use sways statistics. Increasing successes with the use of extracorporeal shock wave lithotripsy (ESWL) for renal stones, and then later with the ureteroscope and ESWL in the management of ureteric stones, shifted the proportions of renal to ureteric stones treated (see Table 3.6).

Technology affects statistics in yet another way: facilitation of other operations reduces the proportion of patients undergoing stone surgery. A review of operations done at the Taxila Hospital showed 5.2% of all operations in 1932–41 were cystolithotomies; seven decades later they constituted only 0.25% because of the rapid throughput of eye operations (personal data, Drs Ernest Lall and Jamsheer Talati). The percentage of bladder stones as a proportion of all urological operations has decreased from 14% in the second decade to 0.98% in the last, because of the increase in the numbers of transurethral resection of the prostate (TURPs). TURPs avoid abdominal incisions, and do not require blood, which is a scarce resource in peripheral hospitals. In peripheral hospitals, therefore, a TURP opens up the possibility of performing a large number of operations. Bladder stone surgery accounted for 100% of all stone surgeries in the first two decades. Subsequently, when operative facilities increased and renal and ureteric stone surgery was started, the contribution of bladder stone surgery fell to 63.5%.

Many of the statistics that have come down to us from previous generations even in the West have been records of hospital statistics. Thus the transitions seen in the West may also have been subject to these determinants in addition to factors such as nutrition, migration to towns, education, diet, economic advance, better roads to access hospitals, and greater availability of health cover.

References

1. Administrative Committee in Coordination, Subcommittee on Nutrition (ACC/SCN). Second report on the world nutrition situation Vol. II Chapter I, Country trends; Pakistan. Geneva: United Nations, March 1993.
2. Karim M. Population growth in Pakistan and its consequences: Some policy options. In: Talati J, Karim M, Qureshi AF, editors. A University's linkages for health and education in the developing world. Karachi: The Aga Khan University, 1994:33–8.
3. Rasmussen Z, Zaidi AKM. Review of existing data on the mortality and morbidity in Gilgit and Chitral districts. Karachi: Aga Khan University, 1988:119.
4. Blanchard RJW. Hospital surgery in rural Pakistan. In: Ahmed M *et al.*, editors. Surgery for all. Lahore: Ferozesons, 1992:49–59.
5. Pervez A. Urinary stone survey at Quetta division hospitals with reference to drinking water. (Dissertation). Lahore: Punjab University, 1992.
6. Talati J. Genitourinary surgery in Pakistan. In: Ahmed M *et al.*, editors. Surgery for all. Lahore: Ferozesons, 1992:352.
7. Khan FA, Khan JH. Stone survey of Punjab Hospitals. Pak Postgrad Med J 1990;1:7–13.
8. Khan RM. Childhood vesicolithiasis in Hazara division in NWFP, Pakistan. (Dissertation). Lahore: Punjab University, 1993.
9. Haziq ul Yakin. Urolithiasis in industrial workers. J Pak Med Assoc 1975;25:274–8.
10. Blanchard RJW. Epidemiology and spectrum of surgical care in the district hospitals of Pakistan. Am J Pub Health 1980;77:1439–45.
11. Farooqui S, Nasir NA, Naqvi AJ. Analysis of 1423 new patients referred to the nephrourology department of the JPMC, Karachi: A 5 year study. J Pak Med Assoc 1975;25:286–8.
12. Sheikh M. Quest for high technology, Abstract D9, 2nd Asian Congress of Urology, Bangkok, Asian Urological Association, 1994.
13. Khan MN, Islam S, Afzal S *et al.* Urolithiasis in children, a comparison of western and Pakistani data. Pak J Surg 1991;7:57–60.
14. Troup CW, Lawnicki CC, Bourne RB *et al.* Renal calculus in children. J Urol 1972;107:306.
15. Khan F. A history of calculous disease of the urinary tract. J Pak Med Assoc 1973;23:19–24.
16. McCarrison RA. Lecture of the causation of stone formation in India. Br Med J 1931;1:1009.
17. Diamond DA, Rickwood AM, Lee PH *et al.* Infection stones in children, a 27 year review. Urology 1994;43:527–7.
18. McAll G, Ghee LK, Edward R. Outflow obstruction and bladder stones in Kelantan Malaysia. Med J Malaysia 1989;44:52–7.
19. Katayama Y, Umekawa T, Ishikawa Y *et al.* Clinical studies in 32 cases of childhood urolithiasis. Nippon Hinyokika Gakkai Zaashi 1990;81:1379–83.
20. Yoshida O. Epidemiology of urolithiasis in Japan. Jap J Urol 1979;70:975–83.
21. Gaches CGC, Mitchell JP, Gordon IRS *et al.* The changing face of urinary lithiasis in childhood. J Pak Med Assoc 1975;25:282–6.
22. O'Reagen S, Homsy Y, Mongeau M. Urolithiasis in children. Can J Surg 1982;25:566–8.

23. Milliner DS, Murphy ME. Urolithiasis in the pediatric patient. Mayo Clinic Proc 1993;68:241–8.
24. Akinci M. Urolithiasis in Turkey: Epidemiological features and causal factors of stone formation. 7th Urolithiasis Conference, Australia, 1992.
25. Chia SJ. A review of ureteric colic – the outcome and value of initial investigations. (Abstract) Second Asian Congress of Urology, Bangkok, 1994:15.
26. Lin FS, Wang SS, Hsieh TS. Clinical analysis of urolithiasis in Poh Hi Hospital, of I Lan Taiwan, ROC – a comparative study with lithiasis in Japan. Hinyokika Kiyo 1992;381:349–55.
27. Abomelha MS, al Khader AA, Arnold J. Urolithiasis in Saudi Arabia. Urology 1990;35:31–4.
28. Aegugkatachit. Epidemiological studies of urinary tract stone in Thailand. First international symposium of the Institute of Urology and Transplantation, Karachi, 1994.
29. Rashid M, Ahmed W, Gardezi SAR *et al.* Composition and epidemiology of urolithiasis. Specialist 1992;9:219–26.
30. Rizvi SAH. Calculous disease – a survey of 400 patients. J Pak Med Assoc 1975;25:268–74.
31. Smith RA, Tebbels TS, Smith TE *et al.* Quantitation of uracil in rodent diet. Ann Biochem 1991;195:375–7.
32. Valyasevi A, Dhannamitta S, Wathanna-Kasetr S. Field preventive programme for bladder stones. In: Smith LH *et al.*, editors. Urolithiasis: clinical and basic research. New York: Plenum Press, 1981.
33. Shah SMA, Luby S. Prevalence of malnutrition in children in rural Sindh. (Abstract) 2nd National Symposium, The Aga Khan University, 1995;238.
34. Vathsala RK, Dhanalekshmy TG, Thomas NE *et al.* Coffee and tea consumption, risk for urolithiasis. In: Ryall R *et al.*, editors. Urolithiasis 2. New York: Plenum Press, 1994:431.
35. Mahe JL, Cledes J, Bigot JC *et al.* Results of dietary evaluation during calcium oxalate and calcium phosphate lithiasis. Nephrologie 1993;14:291–7.
36. Blacklock NJ. Epidemiology of renal lithiasis. In: Wickham JEA, editor. Urinary calculous disease. Edinburgh: Churchill Livingstone, 1979:21–40.
37. Sriboonlue P, Prasong Wattana V, Tung Sanga K *et al.* Measurement of the urinary state of saturation with respect to calcium oxalate and brushite in renal stone formers. J Med Assoc Thai 1990;73:684–9.
38. Roshni SV, Vathsala RK, Moorthy HK *et al.* Risk of urolithiasis in Gulf returned keralites. In: Ryall R *et al.*, editors. Urolithiasis II. New York: Plenum Publishers, 1994:479.
39. Johnson CM, Wilson DM, O'Fallow NM *et al.* Renal stone epidemiology, a 25 year study in Rochester, Minnesota. Kidney Int 1979;16:624.
40. Schneider HJ. Epidemiology of urolithiasis. In: Schneider HJ, editors. Urolithiasis: etiology and diagnosis. Berlin: Springer Verlag, 1979:137.

4. Urolithiasis in the Middle East: Epidemiology and pathogenesis

SALAH R. EL-FAQIH and IMTIAZ HUSSAIN

The pattern of urinary stone disease in the Middle-Eastern countries varies considerably in regard to prevalence, stone composition, site of stone formation, and the metabolic factors implicated in pathogenesis. The two main themes of primary upper and primary lower tract stones are determined by prevailing economic conditions and may be closely interwoven through different sections of society in the same country [1]. Urate containing bladder stones continue to be important in countries with predominantly agricultural based economies (such as Iraq, Iran, Turkey, Egypt and Sudan) [2] whilst oxalate containing upper tract stones prevail and indeed reach epidemic proportions in more affluent, oil rich states of the Arabian peninsula (Kuwait, United Arab Emirates and Saudi Arabia) [3, 4]. As nutritional standards improve in the countries with an agricultural based economy, the interplay of new factors brings about not just a diminishing incidence of bladder stone but an alarming increase of upper tract stone.

Epidemiology in the Middle East

As few reports of prevalence rates in the tropical and developing world are available, we have had to rely upon published hospital admission rates for comparative epidemiological study (Figure 4.1). These demonstrate that the pattern of stone disease in the Middle East is a transitional one with predominantly childhood endemic bladder stone in the agriculture dependent countries, similar to the pattern in south and south-east Asia [2, 5]; and overwhelmingly upper urinary tract distribution of stone, in adults in the economically advanced countries, identical to the picture in the industrialized Western world.

Looked at more closely, three prevalence patterns [1] can be distinguished:

- an upper belt of countries which includes Iran, Iraq, Turkey and Egypt, where bladder stones are still common;
- an intermediate group of countries such as Jordan and Syria where bladder stones have recently disappeared and upper tract stones are now predominant; and
- countries in the Arabian Peninsula such as Kuwait, the United Arab Emirates and Saudi Arabia where bladder stones are virtually unknown but where the occurrence of upper tract stones in both adults and children is of epidemic scale.

I. Talati et al. (eds) The Management of Lithiasis, 35–41.
© *1997 Kluwer Academic Publishers. Printed in Great Britain.*

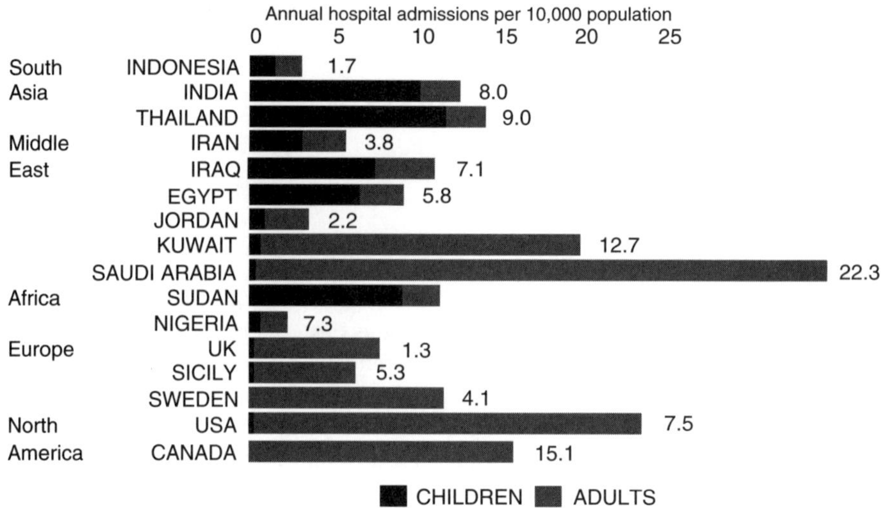

Figure 4.1 Annual rate of hospitalization for urinary stone per 10 000 population

In the last group, it has been estimated that 20% of men who reach the age of 60 years will have had at least one stone episode in their lives, the projected life-time risk being at least 50% higher than the highest corresponding figures in the West [1].

Stone composition

The spectrum of stone composition varies greatly from country to country and reflects the epidemiological pattern. Ammonium urate is the chief component of bladder stones in children, mainly boys, wherever these are endemic. In the Arabian Peninsula, where upper tract stones are overwhelmingly prevalent, the predominant constituent is calcium oxalate, often occurring in the 'pure' form (Figure 4.2). Of all calculi recovered for analysis, 11.5% are made up of uric acid or urates. It must be remembered, however, that a further number of uric acid stones will not be available for analysis on account of their disappearance with suc-

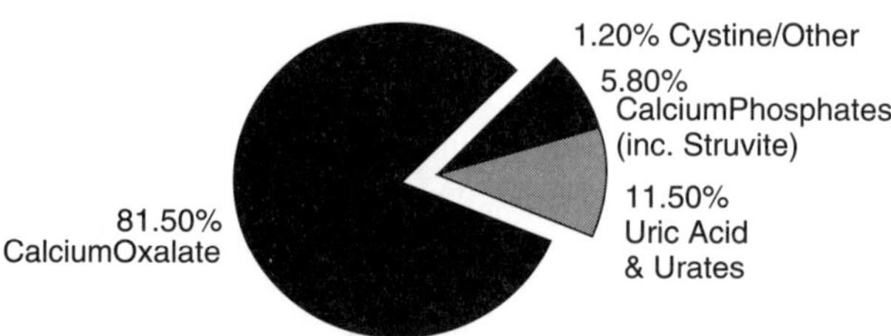

Figure 4.2 Stone composition (predominant content) in 514 urinary stones retrieved from patients treated at the King Khalid University Hospital, Riyadh, over a 12-month period, 1985–86

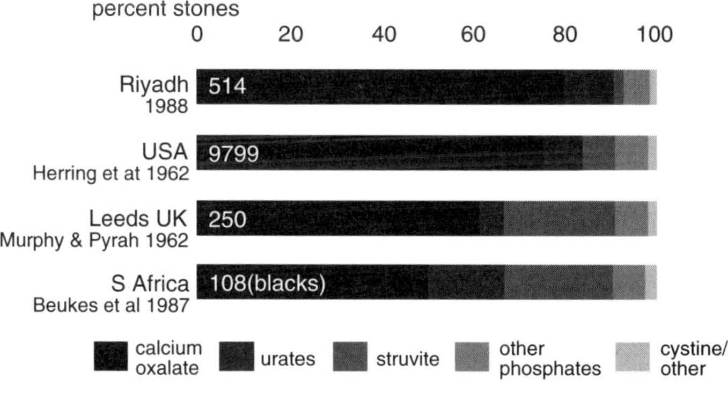

Figure 4.3 Geographical spectrum of urinary tract stone

cessful *in situ* dissolution therapy so that reports of proportionate stone composition based upon analysis of a series of retrievable stones generally underestimate the frequency of uric acid stones. Infection related struvite stones, and indeed all phosphate stones, account for little more than 5% of all urinary tract stones recovered in the region.

This stone spectrum is markedly different to that seen in Europe and North America [6, 7] (Figure 4.3) and also to that in some other areas of the tropical world [8]. Calcium oxalate stones still predominate in Western countries but the relative proportions are smaller on account of the larger numbers of infection stones in women. Phosphate stones also feature among the black subpopulation of South Africa who, in addition, show a much higher proportion of urate calculi than do the white population [8]. These variations largely reflect the wide variety of dietary and cultural differences that affect stone formation and are supported by evidence from metabolic investigation of selected stone formers.

Metabolic investigation of adult idiopathic stone formers

Dietary and metabolic studies of idiopathic renal stone formers in the Arabian Peninsula (Figure 4.4) correlate closely with the regional pattern of prevalence and stone composition outlined above and have revealed striking differences from studies in the West [3, 4, 9, 10]. Urine from men studied in the United Arab Emirates and Saudi Arabia has a lower volume, lower pH, lower calcium and citrate content, and much higher oxalate and uric acid content than urine from men in the West (Table 4.1). Thus, Middle-Eastern men generally have higher levels of urinary supersaturation with respect to calcium oxalate and uric acid but lower levels of supersaturation with respect to calcium phosphate, thus explaining the higher prevalence of urate stones and the low incidence of phosphate stone [1].

These differences in urine chemistry are, in turn, accounted for by the differences in dietary intakes of the main food substances that are known to influence the

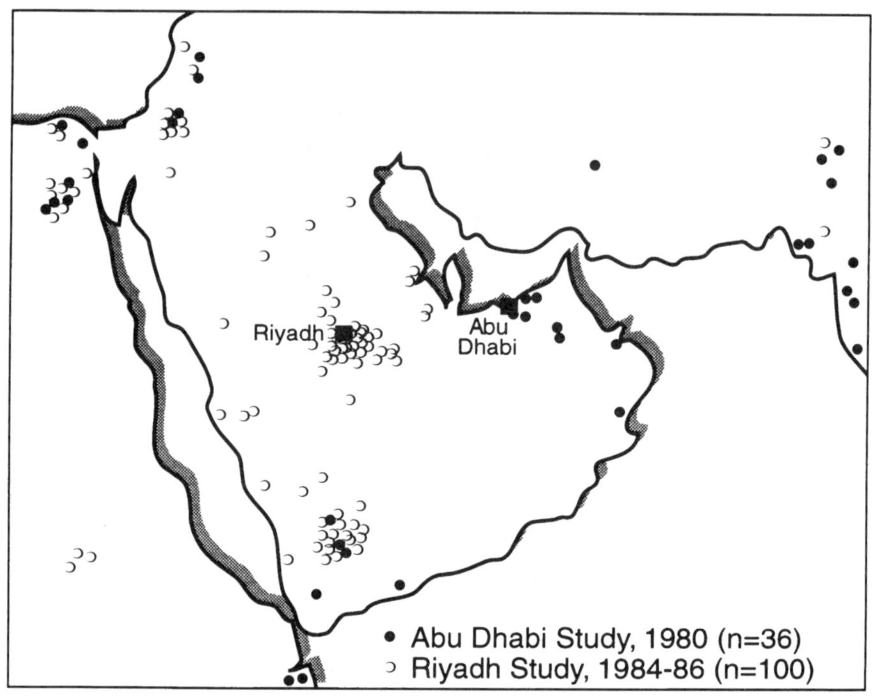

Figure 4.4 Origin of adult male patients with idiopathic calcium oxalate renal stone metabolically studied in controlled series in Abu Dhabi and Riyadh, 1980–86. Note that around 60% of patients were expatriate workers drawn from other areas of the Arabian Peninsula, the Middle East or the Indian subcontinent

Table 4.1 Comparison of 24-hour urine biochemistry in normal and stone-forming men (S-F) in the United Kingdom (UK), United Arab Emirates (UAE) and Saudi Arabia (KSA)

	UK		UAE		KSA	
	Normals	S-F	Normals	S-F	Normals	S-F
Urine volume (L)	1.60	1.76	1.44	1.68	1.25	1.56
Urine pH	6.04	6.00	5.90	5.70	5.82	5.68
Calcium (mmol)	6.0	8.8	4.2	5.2	3.2	4.6
Oxalate (mmol)	0.33	0.43	0.46	0.63	0.53	0.69
Uric acid (mmol)	2.9	3.3	4.6	4.7	4.7	4.8
Citrate (mmol)	3.3	3.1	–	–	1.0	–

From Robertson *et al.* [1] (reprinted by permission from Springer-Verlag).

excretion of stone-forming minerals in the urine [3, 4]. As shown in Table 4.2, male stone formers in the Arabian Peninsula are shown to have a considerably greater intake of animal protein and purines, mainly derived from a higher consumption of lamb and poultry, than their counterparts in the United Kingdom and the USA. Diets rich in animal protein have been shown to acidify urine, increase the excretion of stone-forming substances and decrease the excretion of citrate.

The extremely high oxalate intake results from consumption of certain oxalate rich vegetables popular in the Middle East (Table 4.3) and also from the habitual

Table 4.2   Daily dietary intake in male calcium stone formers in the United Kingdom (UK), United States of America (USA), United Arab Emirates (UAE) and Saudi Arabia (KSA)

	UK	USA	UAE	KSA
Animal protein (g)	61.0	85.0	High	87.0
Calcium (mmol)	24.5	25.0	23.0	13.0
Oxalate (mmol)	1.4	2.4	5.5	3.8
Purine (mg)	190.0	257.0	High	268.0
Oxalate: calcium (ratio)	0.06	0.10	0.24	0.29

From Robertson *et al.* [1] (reprinted by permission from Springer-Verlag).

Table 4.3   Oxalate contents of some foodstuffs popular in the Middle East

Foodstuff	Oxalate content (mg/100 mg)
Kusa (zucchini)	4.1
Kasbara (coriander leaves)	8.6
Jarjeer (watercress)	8.6
Kurath (leek-like)	12.4
Tea	12.5
Green peppers	16.0
Summer squash	22.0
Eggplant (aubergine)	24.0
Bagdunus (curly parsley)	46.0
Chocolate (plain)	117.0
Okra	146.0
Malooqia (spinach-like)	158.0
Sabanaq (spinach-like)	179.0
Peanuts	187.0
Pecan nuts	202.0
Salaq	309.0
Cashew nuts	318.0
Spinach	750.0

From Robertson *et al.* [10] (reprinted with permission of Plenum Publishers).

drinking of large quantities of tea without milk [4]. The intake of calcium is relatively low, on average being about two-thirds that recorded in Western subjects. In addition, absorption of calcium from a given oral load is unaccountably low, possibly related to the paradoxically low vitamin D levels recorded in the region [11]. The implication from this is that measures aimed at reducing stone recurrence in Western subjects are unlikely to show benefit in Middle-Eastern subjects.

In seeking to apply the above findings towards controlling stone recurrence, we embarked upon a series of controlled treatment trials to study the effect of adding calcium citrate supplementation to the diets of idiopathic stone formers [1]. In earlier trials, patients were allocated at random to a treatment group (Citracal, Mission Pharmacal, USA) or a placebo group and were metabolically investigated at intervals over two weeks whilst continuing with their free, home diets. Low-dose treatment (480 mg calcium/day) showed few significant changes in the urine biochemistry of the subjects and patients studied. However, higher dose supplementation (960 mg calcium/day) resulted in marked reduction in the oxalate excretion and the oxalate: calcium ratio in urine. There was a small increase in urinary calcium and a small but significant increase in urinary magnesium, presumably as a result of the increased throughput and reabsorption of calcium in the renal tubule. Both treatments failed to alkalinize the urine and there was no bad effect on the supersaturation of urine with respect to uric acid. A further treatment trial utilizing calcium carbonate (1000 mg elemental calcium/day) in conjunction with tri-potassium citrate (equivalent to 60 mEq sodium bicarbonate/day) showed substantial beneficial effects with respect to both oxalate and uric acid excretion.

The administration of calcium and citrate dietary supplements therefore offers considerable potential in the prevention of idiopathic stone recurrence in the given background of a hyperoxaluric and normocalciuric population of stone formers. The most probable mechanism for this reduction of oxalate excretion is through the binding or precipitation of oxalate in the intestine by the added calcium. Citrate supplementation has a twofold beneficial effect: first, by reducing the aciduria, a known promoting environment for uric acid precipitation; and second, by reducing ionic calcium concentration by promoting complexing of calcium by citrate [12].

Urinary lithiasis in children

Endemic, urate-containing bladder stones are associated with unsafe supplies of drinking water and with poor community hygiene and nutritional standards. These predispose to a high prevalence of chronic diarrhoeal diseases and the risk of forming ammonium urate stones. The dietary paucity of meat protein results in a low intake of phosphorus and thus, lower levels of urinary phosphate, which is normally required as a buffer. The consequent increased production of ammonia in conjunction with lower urine pH levels and the high uric acid excretion that is usual in children (due to rapid tissue turnover) results in urinary supersaturation of ammonium urate and the risk of stone formation [1]. The bladder affords the longest possible time for interaction, probably accounting for the site of stone formation, but as to why these should occur mainly in boys is a matter of conjecture.

In Saudi Arabia, where upper tract stones are equally common in children and adults, 17.6% of calculi are composed predominantly of uric acid or urates [13]. This contrasts strikingly with the reported range of 1.3–7.6% for urate-containing upper tract stones in children in the West [14]. The reasons for the higher prevalence of urate-containing renal stones in this age group in Saudi Arabia are not clear. Metabolic studies in these children have not revealed any overt abnormalities. Analysis of retrieved calculi has shown ammonium acid urate, uric acid, sodium urate (an exceedingly rare constituent of renal stones) and evidence of superimposed calcium phosphate and calcium oxalate.

Conclusions

The Middle East presents a varied pattern of urolithiasis, with urate-containing bladder stones in endemic regions and an overwhelmingly high prevalence of idiopathic renal stone in the Arabian Peninsula. Metabolic investigations of the latter population of stone formers have revealed low urine volumes, aciduria, increased concentrations of oxalate and uric acid, and a significantly lowered excretion of calcium. Dietary supplementation with calcium and citrate offers considerable potential in controlling stone recurrence, highlighting the fact that this is a hyperoxaluric and normocalciuric regional population of stone formers.

References

1. Robertson WG, Walker VR, Hughes H, Husain I, Faqih S. Renal stone disease in the Middle East. In: Hattano *et al.*, editors, Nephrology Vol. 1. Tokyo: Springer-Verlag, 1991:815–22.
2. Andersen DA. Historical and geographical differences in the pattern of incidence of urinary stones considered in relation to possible etiological factors. In: Hodgkinson A, Nordin BEC, editors. Proceedings of renal stone research symposium. 1969:7–31.
3. Husain I, Badsha SA, Al-Ali IH *et al.* A survey of urinary stone disease in Abu Dhabi. Emir Med J 1979;1:17–33.
4. Robertson WG, Nisa M, Husain I *et al.* The importance of diet in the aetiology of primary calcium and uric acid stone formation – the Arabian experience. In: Walker VR *et al.*, editors. Urolithiasis. New York: Plenum Press, 1989:735–9.
5. Sreenavasan G. Incidence of urinary stone in the various states of Mainland Malaysia. Med J Malaysia 1981;36:142–7.
6. Murphy BT, Pyrah LN. The composition, structure and mechanisms of the formation of urinary calculi. Brit J Urol 1962;34:129–59.
7. Herring LC. Observations on the analysis of ten thousand urinary calculi. J Urol 1962;88:545–62.
8. Beukes GJ, De Bruiyn H, Vermaark WJH. Effect of changes in epidemiological factors on the composition and racial distribution of renal calculi. Br J Urol 1987;6:387–92.
9. Al Ali IH, Husain I, Robertson WG *et al.* Metabolic aspects of calcium oxalate urolithiasis and the effect of allopurinol. Emir Med J 1980;3:293–9.
10. Robertson WG, Qunibi W, Husain I *et al.* The calculation of stone risk in the urine of Middle eastern men and western expatriates living in Saudi Arabia. In: Walker VR *et al.*, editors. Urolithiasis. New York: Plenum Press, 1989:669–71.
11. Walker VR, Bissada N, Qunibi W *et al.* Urinary calcium excretion in Saudi Arabia. In: Walker VR *et al.*, editors. Urolithiasis. New York: Plenum Press, 1989:717–19.
12. Harvey JA, Zobitz MM, Pak CYC. Calcium citrate: Reduced propensity for the crystallisation of calcium oxalate in the urine resulting from the induced hypercalciuria of calcium supplementation. J Clin Endocrinol Metab 1985;61:1223–5.
13. Al-Rasheed SA, El-Faqih SR, Hussain I *et al.* The etiological and clinical pattern of childhood urolithiasis in Saudi Arabia. (in press).
14. Polinsky MS, Kaiser BA, Baluarte HJ. Urolithiasis in childhood. Pediat Clin N Am 1987;34:683–710.

5. Epidemiology of urolithiasis in the Western world

KARIM HAMAWY, SARWAT HUSSAIN and YVONNE M. O'MEARA

Whereas bladder stones are rare in today's industrialized world, the incidence of upper urinary tract calculi has risen dramatically in the twentieth century, particularly in the temperate and economically developed countries such as the USA [1, 2] and Sweden [3] in the West, and Japan [4]. Urinary stone disease affects approximately 12% of the population in the United States at some point in their lives [5]. Sixty per cent suffer a recurrent stone within five years of the initial episode [6]. In the USA, it is expected that 2 million new symptomatic stones will be seen each year. It is estimated that Americans loose 14.7 million working days annually through urolithiasis [7] leading to an estimated 2 billion dollar loss in 1986 which has continued to increase [8].

The incidence and the types of calculi seen in the West are recorded in Tables 5.1 and 5.2. The majority (60–70%) are calcium oxalate or phosphate. Mostly idio-

Table 5.1   Incidence of stone disease as reported in various series from the West

USA	
Sierakowski *et al.* [5]	12% of the population of the USA will be affected at some point in their lives
Thun and Schobs [12]	18.5% age-adjusted prevalence in white males in Tennessee as against 7.7% in the rest of the country
Sierakowski *et al.* [13]	164 per 100 000 (represents a 41% increase over the figures quoted by Boyce, 1956 [25])
Johnson *et al.* [14]	80 per 100 000 in the 1950s for males 124 per 100 000 in the 1970s for males 36 per 100 000 for females (1950–74)
Curhan *et al.* [15]	340 per 100 000 for males 40–59 years
Sweden	
Almby *et al.* [16]	180 per 100 000
British Isles	
Power *et al.* [17]	34 per 100 000 for males 11 per 100 000 for females 93 per 100 000 for males 35–44 years
Rate of hospital discharges	
Mandel and Mandel [18]	7.9 per 1000 1974 9.97 per 1000 1974–83 7.58 per 1000 1983–86

J. Talati et al. (eds) The Management of Lithiasis, 43–49
© 1997 Kluwer Academic Publishers. Printed in Great Britain.

Table 5.2   Variations in composition of calculi in different countries

Stone type	USA [19]	UK [20]	Japan [21]	GDR [22]
Oxalate	68	60	60	71
Calcium phosphate	3	13	13	2
Struvite	13	15	22	5.1
Uric acid	5	8	2.2	14
Cystine	0.2	3	1	0.4
Other	10.8	1	1.8	7.5

In Israel (Herbstein *et al.*) [23] 33% are uric acid.
In the Soviet Union (Titinski) [24] up to 75% are uric acid.

pathic, a minority are due to hyperparathyroidism, renal tubular acidosis and hyperoxaluria. The remainder are composed of uric acid and struvite, cystine being uncommon, and accounting for only 1% of stones [9].

A variety of epidemiological factors have been suggested to explain the pathogenesis of stone disease. These include environmental influences such as geographic, climatic, socioeconomic factors and dietary and drinking patterns [10]; and intrinsic factors such as sex, age and genetic makeup, which may affect stone disease through inherited biochemical and anatomical factors [11].

Geographical and climatic variations

Within the United States the arid south-west, the south-east and the mountainous north-west are in the stone belt, and have a higher incidence [13, 25] of urinary calculi. The age-adjusted prevalence of stone disease is 18.5% in white males in Tennessee, compared with 7.7% in the rest of the country [12]. This geographical variation pertains only to calcium oxalate lithiasis, though some areas of the world such as Israel [23] and the Soviet Union [24], have a higher incidence of uric acid calculi (33 and 75% of the stones respectively), and one report from Nigeria has a higher incidence of struvite stones [26].

Some of the variations may be attributable to the climatic differences, higher temperature, increased sweating, urinary concentration and supersaturation [27]. Sun exposure does not affect stone formation in Nigerians [26], or residents of Ecuador and North Peru [28] who seldom form stones. In Kuwait, 74% of stone formers are expatriates [29]. Lack of adjustment to temperature appears to be an important factor, as shown by the higher incidence of stones in British and German army personnel stationed in North Africa in the Second World War as compared to their compatriots back home [30].

Heredity

Resnick [31] in 1968 proposed a polygenic defect with variable penetrance which may vary from one generation to the next. Genetic factors cause cystinuria, renal tubular acidosis (RTA), familial xanthinuria, 2, 8-dihydroxyadeninuria and oxalosis [10]. In the West, 25.7% of patients have a positive family history of stone [15] and stone recurrence is more common in patients with a family history of stone [32]. Familial clustering may result from a common diet. Robertson *et al.* [33] have shown a higher incidence of stone formation in wives of stone formers, and White *et al.* [34] have shown a higher calcium excretion in spouses of stone formers than in controls.

Sex and age

Stone formation is most common in the third to fifth decades. In men the peak age is 28 years for the first episode, but as stones tend to recur 5–10 years later, the most common age of occurrence is around 35–40 years of age [15, 35]. Stone disease is rare in patients older than 70 years. Men are affected five times as commonly as women, though struvite stones are twice as frequent in women. Stones affect Caucasians more than African–Americans [36] in a ratio of 3.6:1 for males and 4.6:1 for females [37]. The lower incidence in African–Americans may be because of the higher melanin content of their skin or a lower intake of animal protein. Differences in the incidence of stone disappear when the diets of Caucasians and Africans approximate each other [38].

Water intake and composition

Individuals drinking less than one litre of water per day are at risk for forming stone [39]. The effect of hard water on stone formation is disputed [40]. Power *et al.* [17] have failed to show variation in stone incidence from regions with a variable hardness.

Socioeconomic status

Stone disease is more common in socioeconomic groups with a higher income [17] and in industrialized cities compared to areas which rely on agriculture [41]. Affluence increases the dietary intake of calories. Physicians [42] and managerial staff [43] are at increased risk and Steg *et al.* [44] state that higher proportions of stones are seen in populations in sedentary occupations and who fail to exercise.

Nutrition

The influence of dietary factors on the pathogenesis of renal stones has been the subject of intense study and controversy [39, 45]. Economic affluence and a diet rich in proteins may increase the incidence of stone [39]. During the course of the twentieth century, hospital admissions or autopsy proven stone disease in Britain,

Germany, Norway and Italy have varied directly with the political and economic climate [39]. In the classical study by Schumann, a significant decline in the incidence of stones was documented during the First and Second World Wars with a rebound increase as the economic climate improved following the war years [6]. In the UK a direct correlation was noted between the number of hospital discharges for stone and the average per capita expenditure on food [46].

Ingestion of a diet high in certain foods results in greater excretion of lithogenic substances and enhances the urinary risk factors for stone formation. A high intake of animal protein has been associated with an increased incidence of stone [47]. The incidence of renal stones is threefold lower in vegetarians than in the general population [48]. A variety of mechanisms have been invoked to explain the effects of proteins. Metabolism of diet rich in purines increases urinary uric acid [49] and urinary calcium excretion [50]. The precise mechanism whereby increased dietary protein increases urinary calcium is not known. Increased protein consumption generates increased amounts of endogenous acid and therefore an increased net urinary acid excretion. This may inhibit tubule calcium reabsorption and/or increase skeletal demineralization. Increased urinary acid excretion also reduces urine pH and excretion of citrate, one of the most important inhibitors of stone formation.

The relationship between dietary calcium intake and stone formation is controversial. A recent prospective study by Curhan *et al.* in 49 976 men provides data on this relationship [15]. Dietary calcium was found to be inversely related to the risk of stone formation, whereas animal protein was directly associated with an increased risk. The incidence of stone formation over the follow-up period was almost 50% lower for those people with the highest calcium intake (1320 mg/day) compared to those with the lowest calcium intake (516 mg/day). With a lower calcium intake, less oxalate is complexed with calcium in the gut so that more oxalate is absorbed and excreted in the urine. It is well-known that small increases in oxalate concentration substantially increase calcium oxalate supersaturation and thereby the tendency to stone formation. However, urinary oxalate was not measured in this study.

Other dietary factors play a role in urolithiasis. A high dietary oxalate to calcium ratio [51] as well as a low magnesium to calcium ratio [52] have been proposed as factors that contribute to increased stone formation. Dietary fat, carbohydrate and sodium intake have also been implicated in the pathophysiology of stone formation [45]. A consumption of large amounts of caffeine may contribute to increased calcium oxalate stone formation [53, 54]. Alcohol consumption has been linked to increased calcium stone formation [55, 56]. Beer may contain a significant amount of oxalate and guanosine, the latter being metabolized to uric acid. Consumption of a high fibre diet protects against stone formation [51] as fibre may complex with calcium in the gut and so prevent its absorption. Much is controversial, and Curhan *et al.* [15] found no link between dietary sodium, magnesium, phosphate, sucrose or fibre on stone incidence.

The pathogenesis of urinary stone is multifactorial. A variety of epidemiological risk factors appear to interact with individual traits to trigger stone formation.

References

1. Backman U, Danielson BG, Ljunghall S. Etiology, management and treatment. In: Backman, Danielson, Ljunghall, editors. Renal stones. Stockholm: Almquist and Wiksell, 1985:7.
2. Coe F, Favus MJ. Nephrolithiasis. In: Brenner, Rector, editors, The kidney, 4th edition. Philadelphia: Saunders, 1993:1728.
3. Norlin A, Lindell B, Granberg PO *et al.* Urolithiasis: a study of its frequency. Scand J Urol Nephrol 1976;10:150–3.
4. Yoshida O, Okada Y. Epidemiology of urolithiasis in Japan: A chronological and geological study. Urol Int 1990;45:104.
5. Sierakowski R, Finlayson B, Landes R. Stone incidence as related to water hardness in different geographical regions of the United States. Urol Res 1978b;7:157.
6. Schneider HJ. Epidemiology of urolithiasis. In: Schneider HJ, editor. Urolithiasis. Berlin: Springer-Verlag, 1985:137.
7. Davis GK, Cummings NB, Finlayson B *et al.* Urolithiasis. In: Geochemistry and the environment. Washington: Natl Acad Sci, 1978:133.
8. Lingeman JE, Saywell RM Jr, Woods JR *et al.* Cost analysis of extracorporeal shock wave lithotripsy relative to other surgical and non-surgical treatment alternatives for urolithiasis. Med Care 1986;24:1151.
9. Buck C. The epidemiology, formation, composition and medical management of idiopathic stone disease. Curr Op Urol 1993;3:316.
10. Drach G. Urinary lithiasis: Etiology, diagnosis and medical management. In: Walsh, Retik, Stamey, Vaughan, editors. Campbell's urology, 6th edition. Philadelphia: Saunders, 1992:2085.
11. Anderson DA. Environmental factors in the etiology of urolithiasis in urinary calculi. In: Cifuentes, Rapado, Hodgkinson, editors. Urinary calculi: Proceedings of an international symposium on renal stone research. New York: Karger, 1973:130.
12. Thun MJ, Schobr S. Urolithiasis in Tennessee: An occupational window into a regional problem. Am J Publ Health 1991;81:587.
13. Sierakowski R, Finlayson D, Landes R. Stone incidence as related to water hardness in different geographical regions of the United States. Urol Res 1978b;7:157.
14. Johnson CM, Wilson DM, O'Fallon WM. Renal stone epidemiology: A 25 year study in Rochester. Kid Int 1979;16:624.
15. Curhan G, Willet W, Rimm E *et al.* Calcium and the risk of symptomatic kidney stones. New Engl J Med 1993;328:833.
16. Almby B, Meirik O, Schonbeck J. Incidence, morbidity and complications of renal and ureteral calculi in a well-defined geographical area. Scan J Urol Nephrol 1975;9:249.
17. Power C, Barker JP, Blacklock NJ. Incidence of renal stones in 18 British towns: A collaborative study. Br J Urol 1987;59:105.
18. Mandel NS, Mandel GS. Urinary tract stone disease in the United States veteran population. II. Geographical analysis of variations in composition. J Urol 1989;142:1516.
19. Keefe WE, Smith MJV. Fourth International Symposium, Urol Res Williamsburg, USA, 1981.
20. Westbury EJ. Some observations on the quantitative analysis of over 1000 urinary calculi. Br J Urol 1974;46:215.
21. Takasaki E, Maeda K. A population study of urolithiasis. Tokyo J Med Sci 1977;4:88.
22. Schneider HJ, Schuler G, Janetzky HZ. Psychosomatic parameters in urolithiasis and their relation to sex and type of calculus – study using a modified complaint questionnaire.Urol Nephrol 1980;73:523.
23. Herbstein FH, Kleeberg J, Shalitin Y. Chemical and x-ray diffraction analysis of urinary stones in Israel. Isr J Med Sci 1974;10:1493.
24. Titinski OL. On the pathogenesis of stone formation in stone-eliminating patients. Eur Urol 1979;4:22.
25. Boyce WH, Garvey FK, Strawcutter HE. Incidence of urinary calculi among patients in general hospitals 1948–1952. J Am Med Assoc 1956;161:1437.
26. Mbonu O, Attah C, Ikeakor I. Urolithiasis in an African population. Int Urol Nephrol 1984;16:291.

27. Toor M, Massry S, Katz AL, Gamon J. The effect of fluid intake on acidification of urine. Clin Sci 1964;27:159.
28. Pyrah LN. Epidemiology of urolithiasis. In: Renal calculus. Berlin, Heidelberg, New York: Springer, 1979:3.
29. Salem SN. Die häufigkeit von nierenkoliken und harnsteinen in Kuwait. Eine epidemiologische untersuchung. Lab Med J 1969:747.
30. Frank M, Lazebnik J, de Vries A. Uric acid lithiasis, a study of six hundred and twenty-two patients. Urol Int 1970;25:32.
31. Resnich ML, Pridgen DB, Goodman HO. Genetic predisposition to formation of calcium oxalate renal calculi. N Engl J Med 1968;278:1313.
32. Ljunghall S, Danielson BG, Fellstrom G *et al.* Family history of renal stones in recurrent stone formers. Br J Urol 1985;57:370.
33. Robertson WG, Peacock M, Baker M *et al.* Studies in the prevalence and epidemiology of urinary stone disease in men in Leeds. Br J Urol 1983;55:595.
34. White RW, Cohen RD, Vince FP *et al.* Minerals in the urine of stone formers and their spouses. In: Hodgkinson, Nordin, editors. Renal stone research symposium. London: Churchill, 1969:289.
35. Prince CC, Scardino PC, Wolan TC. The effect of temperature, humidity and dehydration on the formation of renal calculi. J Urol 1956;75:209.
36. Sarmina I, Resnick ML. Urinary lithiasis in the black world. An epidemiologic study and review of the literature. J Urol 1987;138:15.
37. Schey HM, Corbett WT, Resnick MI. Prevalence rate of renal stone disease in Forsyth County, North Carolina during 1977. J Urol 1979;122:288.
38. Manson JC, Miles BJ, Belville WD. Urolithiasis and race: Another viewpoint. J Urol 1985;134:501.
39. Goldfarb S. Dietary factors in the pathogenesis and prophylaxis of calcium nephrolithiasis. Kid Int 1988;34:544.
40. Rose GA, Westbury EJ. The influence of calcium content of water, intake of vegetables and fruit and other food factors upon the incidence of renal calculi. Urol Res 1975;3:61.
41. Mates J. External factors in the genesis of urolithiasis. In: Hodgkinson, Nordin, editors. Renal stone research symposium, London: Churchill, 1969:59.
42. Scott R. The incidence of renal colic in the medical profession in the West of Scotland. Health Bull (Edinb) 1971;29:72.
43. Sutor DJ, Wooley SE, Illingworth JJ. A geographical and historical survey of the composition of urinary stones. Br J Urol 1974;46:393.
44. Steg A, Landier JF, Teyssier P. Congrès Société Internationale d'Urologie, Paris, Kongressbericht, 1979;I:S163.
45. Schwille PO, Herrmann U. Environmental factors in the pathophysiology of recurrent idiopathic calcium urolithiasis with emphasis on nutrition. Urol Res 1992;20:72.
46. Robertson WG. Epidemiology of urinary stone disease. Urol Res 1990;181:S3.
47. Robertson WG, Peacock M, Heyburn PJ *et al.* Symposium in urolithiasis, a risk factor model for stone formation: Application to the study of epidemiological factors in the genesis of kidney stones. In: Smith, Robertson, Finlayson, editors, Urolithiasis. New York: Plenum Press, 1981:303.
48. Robertson WG, Peacock M, Marshall DH. Prevalence of urinary stone disease in vegetarians. Euro Urol 1982;8:334.
49. Coe F, Davalach AG. Hypercalciuria and hyperuricosuria in patients with calcium nephrolithiasis. New Engl J Med 1974;291:1344.
50. Breslau NA, Brinkley K, Hill N. Relation of animal protein-rich diet to kidney stone formation and calcium metabolism. J Clin Endocrin Metab 1988;66:140.
51. Robertson WG, Peacock M, Heyburn PJ. Epidemiologic risk factors in calcium stone formation. Fortschr Urol Nephrol 1979;14:105.
52. Schwille PO, Scholz D, Schwille K *et al.* Citrate in urine and serum and associated variables in subgroups of urolithiasis. Nephron 1982;31:194.
53. Larson L, Tiselius HG. Hyperoxaluria. Miner Elect Metab 1987;13:242.

54. Massey LK, Sutton RAL. Effect of caffeine consumption on urinary calcium, magnesium, oxalate and citrate in calcium stone formers. In: Ryall R *et al.*, editors. Urolithiasis. New York: Plenum Press, 1994:383.
55. Fellstroem B, Danielson BG, Karlstroem B *et al.* Dietary habits in renal stone patients compared with healthy subjects. Brit J Urol 1989;63:575.
56. Zechner O, Scheiber V. Alcohol as an epidemiological risk in urolithiasis. In: Smith, Robertson, Finlayson, editors. Urolithiasis; clinical and basic research. New York: Plenum Press, 1981:315.

6. Metabolic and dietary risk factors for urolithiasis

ROGER A.L. SUTTON and JAMSHEER TALATI

Risk factors are different for the various chemical types of urinary calculus, which include uric acid, cystine, struvite, and calcium oxalate/phosphate. Rational stone prophylaxis requires the identification of stone type. In the developing world, even more than in the West, results of the analysis of previous renal stones are usually not available. However, as in the West, the predominant stone type in Pakistan and throughout most of the world is calcium oxalate, with or without calcium phosphate. If the stones are radiopaque, and there is no particular reason to suspect any other stone type, it is usually safe to assume that the stone consists of calcium salts. In the patient with a calcium stone (proved or presumed) it is important to rule out specific underlying causes which may be amenable to treatment, including primary hyperparathyroidism, renal tubular acidosis, enteric hyperoxaluria, etc.

Primary hyperparathyroidism appears to be responsible for a smaller proportion of stone disease in Pakistan than is usually quoted for the West. In our series, 1.25% of stones proved to be due to underlying primary hyperparathyroidism. The clinical presentation of primary hyperparathyroidism is different in Pakistan from the West. The disease tends to be much more florid, with overt parathyroid bone disease (osteitis fibrosa cystica) often coexisting with stone disease. Although the precision of serum calcium determination may not always be as good as in the developed world, there appears to be a greater incidence of normocalcaemia than is the case in primary hyperparathyroidism in the West. An unequivocally normal serum calcium level (allowing for the serum albumin) reliably excludes primary hyperparathyroidism in the West. It is possible that vitamin D deficiency, which is much more common in South Asia than in North America, may alter the clinical and biochemical manifestations of primary hyperparathyroidism. Vitamin D deficiency in this region results from cultural avoidance of the sun, coupled with low dietary vitamin D intakes related to the absence of vitamin D supplementation of dairy products.

Overt renal tubular acidosis (RTA) with hypokalaemia and other obvious manifestations is rare among South Asian stone formers. It is reported to be more frequent in north-east Thailand, where severe hypokalaemia and renal stones are common manifestations. The incidence of incomplete RTA in Pakistan is not known, but unexplained hypocitraturia is frequent (see below). A low urine citrate may be a useful marker for the identification of incomplete distal RTA. Other specific causes of calcium stones, such as enteric hyperoxaluria, are infrequent in

J. Talati et al (eds) The Management of Lithiasis, 51–56
© *1997 Kluwer Academic Publishers. Printed in Great Britain.*

Pakistan, as they are in the West. Most calcium stones are not associated with any of these underlying disorders, and may be termed 'idiopathic'. The known risk factors for idiopathic calcium oxalate stones (with or without a component of calcium phosphate) are low urine volume, high urine calcium, oxalate or uric acid, low urine citrate, and possibly low urinary magnesium excretion.

Urine volume

A low urine flow rate is likely to be a major contributor to the high prevalence of stones in this region. In a group of urban controls, it averaged 1316 ± 481.7 Most of Pakistan is desert, supplied almost exclusively with water from the river Indus and its tributaries, which arise in the Himalayas. The climate is extremely hot and dry. Other reasons for a low urine volume include the scarcity of potable drinking water. Much of the population does not have immediate access to potable water, which may well limit the consumption compared with Western countries. In Lahore, 50% of stone patients drank less than 1 litre of liquids per 24 hours. In addition there is a very high incidence of diarrhoeal disease, which further limits the urine flow rate, at least intermittently.

The composition of drinking water varies markedly across the country, depending on the nature of the rock and soil from which the water drains, and depending on whether the water for drinking is obtained from rivers or wells. Certain areas (in Baluchistan) have extremely hard water, with in excess of 300 parts per million of calcium (0.3 mg per litre), but the importance of this in relation to the risk of stone is unclear. Where dietary calcium intakes are otherwise low, it is possible that this additional calcium in the drinking water could serve to bind dietary oxalate, and actually be beneficial in terms of overall stone risk as suggested by Curhan. Conversely, in a patient taking a generous calcium intake, the extra calcium derived from several litres per day of very hard water could contribute to high urinary calcium values, and therefore increase stone risk.

In Punjab, 61% of stone patients obtain their drinking water from subsoil sources, and 39% from canals, rivers or aqueducts as the ultimate source. Although increased soil salinity is a widespread problem in the irrigated areas of Pakistan, owing to problems with the construction or maintenance of irrigation channels, it is unclear whether this leads to an important increase in the sodium content of the drinking water, sufficient to have a significant impact on the total daily sodium intake.

Urinary calcium

Hypercalciuria is the commonest identified risk factor for idiopathic calcium stones in the West. There has been debate as to how best to define hypercalciuria. Reasonably well accepted values for the upper limit of normal for 24-hour urinary calcium in the West are 300 mg in men and 250 mg in women. So defined,

13.3–19% of stone patients (seen at the AKUMC) were hypercalciuric. However, there are differences in normal values between different developed countries; for example, 400 mg has been suggested as an upper limit for normal males in the United Kingdom. Mean urinary calcium values (and calcium: creatinine ratios) in normal adults in Pakistan are substantially lower than in the developed world. Mean excretion rates between 110 and 166 mg per day have been reported in normal subjects in different studies in Pakistan (Table 6.1) and the calcium: creatinine ratio is 0.087 ± 0.051. Mean values for stone patients ranged from 130 to 188 mg per day (Table 6.2). These data suggest that, if the normal range is defined as the mean, plus or minus two standard deviations, the normal range would be lower in Pakistan than that quoted in the West, and more patients would be labelled as being hypercalciuric. As the limit of the normal calcium:creatinine ratio is 0.19 in our population, 56% of our patients would be considered hypercalciuric in spite of low total calcium excretions. Presumably the ultimate determinant of stone risk is the calcium concentration in the final urine. This depends on urine volume as well as renal calcium excretion. In Pakistan, normal urinary calcium concentrations measured 9.5 ± 5.4 mg/dl in a population with a calcium excretion of 110 ± 67.5 mg/dl. It is worth noting that 19% of our patients have calcium excretion below 50 mg/24 hours, and 8% of patients are hypocalciuric.

Reasons for the lower mean urinary calcium excretion in Pakistan compared with developed countries may include a lower dietary calcium intake (since the con-

Table 6.1   Twenty-four-hour excretion rates in the normal population/controls (mg/24 h)

	Rizvi (1975) [1]	Talati (1990)	Khand (1994) [2]
Ca	166.1 ± 26.5	110 ± 67.5	138.8 ± 17
Oxalate		20.7 ± 11.7	23.4 ± 1.65
P	332.3 ± 44.3	521.3 ± 253.3	405.8 ± 51.7
Citrate			608.9 ± 54.4
Mg			95.3 ± 7.3
Uric acid		381.5 ± 202	

Table 6.2   Twenty-four-hour urinary excretion rates in stone patients (mg/24 h)

	Rizvi (1975) [1]	Talati (1990)	Meer (1994)	Khand (1994) [2]
Ca	161.3 ± 26.5	187.5 ± 104.2	167 ± 123	138.8 ± 17
Oxalate		17.1 ± 9.26		28.7 ± 2.3
P	332.3 ± 44.3	689.5 ± 296.9		846 ± 71
Citrate			127.9 ± 112.2	377 ± 41.2
Mg				102.6 ± 9.2
Uric acid		456.9 ± 190.3		

sumption of dairy products is generally only moderate, though in some regions of Pakistan, milk based drinks (Lassi) are heavily consumed) together with a low nutritional vitamin D status. The latter may appear paradoxical, but is also seen in similarly sunny regions such as Saudi Arabia. As mentioned above, the low vitamin D status in this region probably results from the combination of a cultural avoidance of skin exposure to direct sunlight, coupled with a low dietary vitamin D intake. Poor intestinal absorption of ingested calcium consequent upon the vitamin D status would not only tend to lower the urinary calcium excretion, but would also diminish the intestinal absorption of oxalate, since non-absorbed calcium in the gut lumen would precipitate dietary oxalate to render it non-adsorbable. Thus it is possible that widespread vitamin D supplementation in this subcontinent might lead to a significant increase in the urinary excretion of both calcium and oxalate, and therefore a further increase in the prevalence of stones.

Uric acid

Hyperuricosuria is a risk factor for calcium oxalate stones, though the mechanism of this effect is controversial. In the West, this variety of hyperuricosuria appears to be predominantly dietary, and relates to a high purine intake. Much of the population of Pakistan can only afford the very infrequent intake of purine rich food such as meat, fish and poultry. However, the affluent minority are often very heavy meat eaters, and in this group hyperuricosuria would be expected to be more common. The mean 24-hour urinary uric acid in our calcium stone formers was 457 ± 190 mg in 24 hours as compared with the mean in normal control subjects of 382 ± 202 mg/24 hours, and 6.1% excreted more than 800 mg uric acid in 24 hours (11% excreted more than 700 mg/24 hours). The urinary uric acid concentration was 33.5 ± 21.6 mg/dl; in 43% patients it was more than 30 mg/dl. The contribution of hyperuricaemia to idiopathic calcium stones is uncertain. Four per cent of our patients were hyperuricaemic (more than 8 mg/dl).

Urinary oxalate

The contribution of mild hyperoxaluria to idiopathic calcium stones is of considerable current interest, as is the pathogenesis of this condition. This topic is dealt with in more detail in a separate chapter. In parts of India, a very high incidence of hyperoxaluria has been reported among stone formers, and it is believed to relate to the intake of high oxalate containing green leafy vegetables. Earlier studies in Karachi, Pakistan, suggested that hyperoxaluria (based on Western values for the upper normal limit) was uncommon in idiopathic calcium stone formers. However, in more recent studies, the incidence appears to be similar to the West, in the order of 20%. A wide array of different vegetables and fruits is consumed in Pakistan, and it is not clear which are the major sources of bioavailable dietary oxalate. It has recently been appreciated that the molar ratio of oxalate to calcium may be an independent predictor of stone risk, in addition to the absolute values of calcium and oxalate. The tendency to low urinary calcium excretions, coupled with normal or slightly increased urinary oxalate excretions, may engender an unfavourable oxalate to calcium ratio in this population. Where mild hyperoxaluria is found, particularly in combination with low urinary calcium excretion, modest dietary calcium supplementation may well prove to be effective therapy for stone prevention as has been observed by Robertson in Saudi Arabia.

Citrate

A low urine citrate is common among idiopathic calcium stone formers in Pakistan. It appears to be the most common identifiable metabolic risk factor, more frequent than hypercalciuria. As with calcium, there is a problem with the definition of the normal range for urinary citrate. Even in the West, normal values have not generally been based on studies of large groups of normal subjects. Rather, an arbitrary value of 320 mg per day has been used to define the lower limit of normal. Using this value, 50% of our local stone formers and 75% of controls have hypocitraturia. Urinary citrate excretion rates were lower (127.9 ± 112.2 mg/24 hours) in patients than in controls (247 ± 193 mg/24 hours). These patients do not have overt renal tubular acidosis. The cause of their hypocitraturia is uncertain, and is under current investigation. The major known determinant of urinary citrate excretion is acid–base balance. Hypocitraturia is associated with a low net intestinal alkali absorption, which in turn results from a diet high in meat protein and low in vegetables. This type of diet is frequent in the affluent urban Pakistani, but not in the impoverished rural Pakistani. It is possible that incomplete renal tubular acidosis could be a significant contributor to this apparently idiopathic hypocitraturia. In the West a small group of patients with apparently renal hypocitraturia, not due to incomplete renal tubular acidosis, has been defined. Citrate exerts its inhibitory effect upon calcium oxalate stone formation in several ways, including the complexing of calcium, and the inhibition of crystal agglomeration. It is likely that any increase in urinary citrate excretion would diminish the risk of recurrent calcium oxalate stone formation. Any form of ingested alkali elevates the urinary citrate excretion, providing the potential for an inexpensive method of prevention of recurrent calcium oxalate stones. It is possible that oral alkali therapy may prove to be the most useful form of long-term stone prophylaxis in this part of the world.

Urine pH

Data are limited on urine pH in Pakistan, in comparison with developed countries. However, urine pH is not an important independent determinant of calcium oxalate stone formation. The solubility of calcium oxalate is affected little by changes in pH within the physiological range.

Dietary protein

The ingestion of protein, particularly meat protein, adversely influences most of the known risk factors for calcium oxalate stone formation. An increased intake of meat protein is associated with an increased urinary excretion of calcium, oxalate, and uric acid, and a decreased urinary excretion of citrate. As already indicated, a high meat protein intake is a luxury confined to the affluent minority in Pakistan. It is unlikely that high meat protein intake contributes to the generally high incidence of urinary calculi in rural Pakistan. It is notoriously difficult to dissuade those who can afford a high meat protein intake from doing so.

Other inhibitors

In addition to the risk factors mentioned, there is a growing list of macromolecular inhibitors, which are believed to operate against the formation of renal calculi in normal people. These include nephrocalcin, uropontin, crystal matrix protein and Tamm–Horsfall protein. There is preliminary evidence that molecular abnormalities in some of these macromolecular inhibitors, presumably inherited, may contribute to calcium oxalate stone formation in some patients in the West. There are as yet no data to indicate whether these specific inhibitor abnormalities play a significant role in the causation of stones in the developing world.

It has long been suspected that abnormalities in the stone matrix or in the properties of the urothelium, the surface lining of the lower urinary tract, might be the cause of stone formation in some patients. Again, there are no data for or against this hypothesis in patients in this part of the world.

Of interest, however, is the remarkably high familial incidence of stones in Pakistan, despite the absence of the traditional Western risk factors. It will therefore be of interest to search for inherited defects among this large group of stone patients.

References

1. Rizvi SAH. Calculous disease, a survey of 400 patients. J Pak Med Assoc 1975;25:268–274.
2. Khand FD, Ansari AF, Khand TU *et al.* Is hypocitraturia associated with phosphaturia a potential cause of calcium urolithiasis in first time stone formers? J Pak Med Assoc 1994;44:179–181.

7. Oxalate and urolithiasis

ROGER A.L. SUTTON

Oxalate and nephrolithiasis

The importance of oxalic acid in medicine derives from the extreme insolubility of its calcium salt in water, at around 12 mg or 0.13 mM per litre, which is affected little by pH above 5, but increases as the pH falls below 5 [1]. Because calcium and oxalate require to be excreted in substantial quantities by the kidneys, averaging 4–5 mM and 0.3 mM per day respectively in the adult, urinary supersaturation with calcium oxalate is the norm. Complex and elaborate mechanisms exist to prevent the formation, growth and agglomeration of crystals in the urinary tract, processes which are believed to be precursors of stone formation.

Calcium oxalate is the major constituent of over 70% of upper urinary tract stones. In calcium-containing stones, oxalate is most commonly the major anion, with varying amounts of calcium phosphate. Pure calcium oxalate stones are common, whereas predominantly calcium phosphate stones are less frequent (< 10%). It has generally been assumed that the determination of the relative amounts of oxalate versus phosphate in idiopathic calcium stones is of little clinical value. Gault *et al.* [2], using a semiquantitative infrared analytical method [3], have recently addressed this issue in detail, and found that phosphate stones (oxalate: phosphate ratio < 1) are commoner in females, tend to be larger than predominantly oxalate stones (oxalate: phosphate > 10), and in about 25% of patients are associated with a defect in urinary acidification. These patients did not have complete distal renal tubular acidosis, and most did not have hypocitraturia. It is unclear whether these patients should receive different therapy from the commoner idiopathic calcium oxalate stone former [4]. Aside from these idiopathic calcium phosphate stone formers, calcium phosphate stones are usual in complete distal renal tubular acidosis (RTA), and are common (though less so than calcium oxalate) in primary hyperparathyroidism [5].

Sources of urinary oxalate

It is generally stated that in normal man, some 40% of urinary oxalate is derived from serine and glycine via glyoxylate, 40% from ascorbic acid via as yet uncertain metabolic intermediates, and 5–10% from dietary oxalate. An average (Western)

J. Talati et al. (eds) The Management of Lithiasis, 57–68
© *1997 Kluwer Academic Publishers. Printed in Great Britain.*

dietary oxalate intake is probably about 100 mg [1] but data on the bioavailability and content of oxalate in foods is poor. Whether the food oxalate is present as soluble potassium or ammonium oxalate or insoluble calcium oxalate is probably important, and generally unknown. Oxalate intakes in some parts of the world have been reported to be as high as 2000 mg/day [6]. It is possible that humans, like other animals, may adapt to high oxalate intakes. The fractional intestinal absorption of ingested oxalate in health is generally less than 10%; the sum of absorbed plus faecal oxalate is much less than dietary oxalate, as a result of oxalate degradation by bacteria in the gut lumen. Although oxalate absorption is normally less than 10%, many factors are known to enhance absorption, including low calcium diets and intestinal disease with malabsorption (see below).

Endogenous production of oxalate from serine and glycine occurs via glyoxylate. Oxalate may also be derived from other amino acids including hydroxyproline and tryptophan, as well as from sugars and other precursors, but the amounts from these sources are thought to be small.

It is believed that ascorbic acid usually contributes about 40% of normal urinary oxalate. It was formerly suspected that high ascorbic acid intakes caused hyperoxaluria, but this is no longer believed to be the case (see below).

Renal handling of oxalate

Earlier studies suggested that there was net tubular secretion of oxalate [7]. However, recent studies in man, using newer methods to measure plasma oxalate levels – a notoriously difficult analytical challenge – have suggested fractional excretions of less than 100%, or net tubular reabsorption, in the majority of normal subjects [4, 8, 9].

Oxalate crystal and stone formation

As noted, urine is typically supersaturated with calcium oxalate, and calcium oxalate crystals are commonly observed in the urine of healthy subjects. Increased crystalluria, and especially larger crystals and crystal masses, are typical of idiopathic calcium oxalate nephrolithiasis [ICON] [10].

Recognized risk factors for so-called ICON (those patients in whom underlying disorders such as primary hyperparathyroidism or enteric hyperoxaluria have been excluded) include low urine volume, hyperoxaluria, hypercalciuria, hypocitraturia and hyperuricosuria. In studying these risk factors, Robertson *et al.* noted that low urine volume and hyperoxaluria appeared to be the most potent risk factors [11]. For a given degree of supersaturation, the largest mass of crystals forms when the molar ratio of calcium to oxalate is 1 [12]. As noted above, the molar ratio is normally greater than 10:1. This is probably one reason why an increase in urinary oxalate is more harmful than a similar increase in urinary calcium [12–14]. In addition to insoluble calcium oxalate, soluble calcium oxalate complexes form. In response to an increase in calcium, they result in a disproportionate depletion of free oxalate, whereas in response to an increase in oxalate, only minor changes occur in free calcium [14]. For these reasons, it is now considered that small increases in oxalate above normal, and probably even increases in oxalate within the normal range, may substantially increase stone risk [12]. Oxalate excretion varies during the day, increasing postprandially, as well as with the seasons, and a single snapshot view of 24-hour urinary oxalate may be quite inadequate to assess the potential contribution of urinary oxalate concentration to crystal or stone formation.

Urine contains a variety of substances that exert inhibitory effects on calcium oxalate crystal formation, growth and agglomeration, as well as some promoter substances. Inhibitors include small molecular weight substances such as magnesium (which complexes oxalate) and citrate (which inhibits growth and aggregation of calcium oxalate crystals), as well as high molecular weight substances including nephrocalcin, uropontin and Tamm–Horsfall protein [15]. Citrate has been recognized as a potential 'inhibitor' for decades, and was believed to act mainly by forming soluble complexes with calcium; however recent studies by Kok *et al.* have demonstrated a very potent action of citrate as an inhibitor of the agglomeration of calcium oxalate monohydrate crystals [16]. It is possible that agglomeration is a key step in the initiation of stone formation, since single crystals are sufficiently small to readily traverse the renal tubules. Low urine citrate is a well-established risk factor, and occurs in conditions causing intracellular acidosis (e.g. diarrhoea, acetazolamide ingestion and RTA) as well as in a small proportion of ICON patients in whom it may result from a defect in intestinal alkali or citrate absorption [17]. In addition, dietary factors such as excesses of protein or salt reduce urinary citrate and reduce the normal inhibition of agglomeration of calcium oxalate crystals [18]. Low citrate excretion is readily corrected by the administration of oral alkali, such as potassium citrate [19].

Nephrocalcin is produced in the proximal tubule, and its major role may be to prevent crystal formation in the thin loop of Henle, while Tamm–Horsfall protein arises in the thick ascending limb, and its inhibitory actions may be exerted in the collecting duct where the urine again becomes concentrated. Some data have been presented suggesting that molecular defects in these inhibitors may occur in some stone patients [20, 21]. Such defects could account for familial ICON in some of the many patients in whom none of the usual chemical risk factors are present.

In addition to agglomeration, it has recently been appreciated that specific interactions occur between calcium oxalate (and other) crystals and the lining epitheliums of the renal tubule and collecting system. Riese *et al.* [22, 23] have studied the attachment of calcium oxalate crystals to the surface of cultured epithelial cells, while Lieske and Toback [24] have demonstrated internalization of crystals in cultured cells that is modified by a variety of factors; for example, it is inhibited by Tamm–Horsfall protein. If these interactions are indeed important early events in the process of initiation of stone formation, it is of course possible that disturbances such as enhanced crystal adhesion to the epithelium could underlie some cases of ICON.

Causes of hyperoxaluria

As already emphasized, even minor increases in urinary oxalate may substantially increase the risk of calcium oxalate stones. It has been customary to classify hyperoxaluria as severe (greater than 1 mmol/day), including primary (genetic) hyperoxaluria and enteric hyperoxaluria, or mild (0.5–1 mmol/day).

Primary (genetic) hyperoxaluria

Type I, the commoner variety of this rare disorder, is of particular interest because of recent advances in the understanding of the nature of the genetic defect [25–27]. It is an autosomal recessive disorder, in which the defect is in the hepatic peroxisomal enzyme alanine glyoxylate aminotransferase (AGT) which normally transaminates glyoxylate to glycine. In its absence (or deficiency), glyoxylate accumulates and is converted into oxalate, as well as glycolate, both of which are excreted in increased amounts. The gene for this enzyme has now been cloned and sequenced [28], but before this was achieved it was appreciated that some families with the disease had no catalytic enzyme activity. Some of these patients had immunoreactive AGT protein in the peroxisomes. About one-third of patients had catalytic activity which, in some, exceeded that of asymptomatic obligate heterozygotes. However, in these patients the enzyme proved to be in the wrong intracellular compartment, i.e. the mitochondria. AGT in the mitochondria is ineffective, since the peroxisome is probably the main site of glyoxylate production in the liver. In some species (but not in man) the normal location of the enzyme is in the mitochondria. The location has switched several times during evolution. Danpure has suggested that the mitochondrial location is appropriate in carnivores, where the enzyme has a role in gluconeogenesis, while in herbivores the peroxisomal location is more appropriate for the detoxification of glyoxylate. In man, however, this mistargeting to the mitochondria is a result of an abnormality in the AGT gene which produces a mitochondrial targeting sequence that is, surprisingly, not analogous to the mitochondrial targeting sequence in carnivores such as rat. In man the N–terminal sequence that produces mitochondrial targeting in the rat is not translated; the abnormally targeted enzyme results from the combination of a Pro-11-Leu polymorphism (normally present in about 15% of normals, resulting on its own in mitochondrial targeting of about 5% of the enzyme) together with a Gly-170-Arg mutation that results in 90% mistargeting to mitochondria [26]. For a while, diagnosis *in utero* required a foetal liver biopsy, but now that the gene has been cloned, diagnosis can be made from DNA from other sources such as leukocytes.

The disease varies in severity but typically causes calcium oxalate stones in childhood and renal failure by age 20 [27]. Patients may, however, present in later life [29]. Treatment with pyridoxine, which is converted to pyridoxal-5-phosphate, the cofactor for AGT, reduces oxalate production in some patients [30], and other therapies including magnesium and phosphate can markedly delay the progression of the disease [31]. As renal failure develops, plasma oxalate levels rise rapidly, and widespread oxalosis develops. Renal transplantation should be done before this occurs. In some patients combined liver and kidney transplantation has been performed – this restores the missing enzyme, but should also not be delayed until severe oxalosis has supervened, since mortality is then high [31].

Type II primary hyperoxaluria is rarer and less well characterized. Urinary glycolate excretion is normal, and L-glycerate is increased. This disorder was attributed to deficiency of d-glyceric dehydrogenase, but in a recent report [32] glyoxylate reductase was also deficient, which would reduce the conversion of glyoxylate to glycolate in the cell cytosol.

A third genetic variety, in which neither glycolate nor L-glycerate are increased, has been called type III or absorptive hyperoxaluria. A patient reported by Yendt and Cohanim [33] had hypercalciuria and hypermagnesuria as well as hyperoxaluria, and hydrochlorothiazide abolished the hyperoxaluria.

Enteric hyperoxaluria

Enteric hyperoxaluria, the association of hyperoxaluria with small bowel disease or resection, was first recognized in 1970 and has recently been extensively reviewed [31, 34]. The hyperoxaluria is frequently severe, in excess of 1 mmol/day and is believed to originate from hyperabsorption of dietary oxalate [35]. This results from preferential binding of dietary calcium by non-absorbed fatty acids in the gut lumen, so that oxalate fails to be rendered non-absorbable by conversion to insoluble calcium oxalate. Most of the absorption of the oxalate probably occurs in the colon, which is rendered abnormally permeable to oxalate by non-absorbed bile salts that are delivered from the ileum. It is possible that a lack of oxalate-degrading bacteria in the colon could also contribute to the hyperoxaluria [36]. The condition is seen with extensive inflammatory bowel disease, small bowel resection or bypass. It is not seen in patients who have an ileostomy, or have had a colectomy. It can cause very intractable calcium oxalate stone formation, and even oxalosis and renal failure. The pathogenesis of the stones is multifactorial and includes hyperoxaluria, low urine volume, low urine pH and citrate (secondary to diarrhoeal loss of bicarbonate), low urine magnesium and low urinary ionic strength (which reduces calcium oxalate solubility). Treatment may include dietary oxalate restriction, increased fluid intake, dietary calcium supplements, potassium citrate, low fat diet, parenteral magnesium salts, and/or cholestyramine (to bind bile salts) [31]. However, none of these treatments has been proved to be effective in randomized prospective studies [34]. In extreme cases, secondary to bowel bypass for obesity, this complication may require reversal of the bypass.

Mild idiopathic hyperoxaluria

Urinary oxalate excretion above the upper limit of normal has been observed in 15–50% of ICON patients [31]. Hyperoxaluria may be the most important risk factor for these stones [12], and it is probably worth instituting measures to reduce urinary oxalate in the ICON patient even when urinary oxalate is not increased above the upper normal limit.

Suggested mechanisms for the production of mild idiopathic hyperoxaluria have included:

1. Increased dietary oxalate or oxalate precursors, such as protein, ascorbic acid or sugar alcohols.
2. Decreased dietary calcium, or increased intestinal calcium absorption, promoting oxalate absorption.
3. Primary enhancement of intestinal oxalate absorption; isolated, or part of a more generalized oxalate transport abnormality.
4. Mild forms of primary hyperoxaluria and vitamin B_6 deficiency.
5. Defect in renal oxalate handling.

Increased dietary intake of oxalate or its metabolic precursors
It is generally held that under normal circumstances less than 10% of ingested oxalate is absorbed. However, some authorities have felt this to be an underestimate [37]. It would seem prudent to advise all calcium oxalate stone formers to moderate their dietary oxalate intake, and this can be achieved, at least in Western countries, with fairly simple dietary advice [38]. There are seasonal variations in urinary oxalate which may relate to seasonal variations in the consumption of oxalate containing vegetable foods, as well as to other factors such as varying intake and production of vitamin D [35] (see below). Several circumstances can lead to an increase in fractional oxalate absorption, of which low dietary calcium is potentially the most important (see below). Oxalate can be generated in the body from a variety of precursors. Glycine and serine (via glyoxylate) and ascorbate are normally the major sources as reviewed above. Oxalate can also be derived from dietary glycolate, and other amino acids including hydroxyproline and aromatic amino acids such as tryptophan. These are believed to be minor sources [1, 31]. However, increased protein intake may contribute to hyperoxaluria. Yendt and Cohanim found that, in ICON, both oxalate and glycolate were mildly increased in the urine [39]. There was no correlation between oxalate and glycolate, but glycolate correlated with urinary uric acid and with dietary protein.

There is evidence that glycolate, which is present especially in foods of vegetable origin, is well absorbed and at least partially converted into oxalate [40].

It is unclear what proportion of urinary oxalate normally arises from glycollic aldehyde via glycolate, and hence represents two carbon fragments transferred in the transketolase reaction, which is linked to the oxidative pathway of carbohydrate metabolism [41]. Xylitol, an artificial sweetening agent and parenteral carbohydrate source, has been associated with calcium oxalate crystal deposition in tissues. It appears that normally little conversion to oxalate occurs, but in the presence of severe illness and tissue anoxia, much greater glycolate production may occur, and some of it may be oxidized to oxalate [42]. Nguyen *et al.* [43] have recently examined the effects of single 20-g oral doses of glucose, maltisorb, sorbitol and xylitol on urine composition. Both xylitol and glucose increased urinary calcium, but only xylitol increased oxalate (by about 50%). It is not known whether xylitol ingestion contributes to renal stone disease.

The contribution of ingested ascorbic acid to oxaluria is controversial. Because ascorbic acid can be non-enzymatically converted to oxalate, particularly in alkaline media, and this reaction can occur in urine after voiding, it is necessary to take appropriate precautions to ensure that apparent increases in urinary oxalate actually reflect *in vivo* conversion of ascorbic acid to oxalate. Recent studies, in which appropriate precautions were taken, suggest that intakes of up to 4 g/day ascorbic acid may not significantly increase urinary oxalate [44, 45]. However, it is still possible that a subset of patients may respond with greater conversion to oxalate, and therefore increase their risk of stone recurrence by taking megadoses of vitamin C. Cowley *et al.* [46] have presented data suggesting that calcium stone formers may have impaired intestinal absorption of hydroxycarboxylic acids (including citrate and ascorbate). They also found that, in tests employing single oral loads of hydroxycarboxylic acids, citrate inhibited ascorbate absorption, and increased urinary oxalate excretion after an ascorbate load both in normal subjects and in stone formers.

Decreased dietary calcium or enhanced intestinal calcium absorption
There is abundant evidence that the amount of calcium in the gut lumen available to complex with oxalate is an important determinant of oxalate absorption. Robertson and Hughes have calculated 'free' dietary oxalate, based on dietary oxalate minus the amount of oxalate bound by non-absorbed dietary calcium reaching the colon, and have found a striking relationship between free dietary oxalate and urinary oxalate [12]. Several studies [47–50] have shown that reducing dietary calcium increases urinary oxalate, while increasing ingested calcium reduces urinary oxalate. This relationship is important in the pathophysiology and management of enteric hyperoxaluria [31]. Several investigators have noted that ICON patients show a positive correlation between urinary oxalate and calcium. This has been attributed to enhanced intestinal calcium absorption reducing available luminal calcium and thus enhancing oxalate absorption. The oxalate excretion enhancing effect of reduced dietary calcium is exaggerated in individuals with intestinal calcium hyperabsorption [49]. Vitamin D administration increases calcium absorption and has been noted to be associated with an increase in urinary oxalate excretion [35, 51], presumably as a result of a similar mechanism. The possibility exists that dietary calcium restriction might increase oxalate absorption and excretion, and even increase risk of calcium oxalate stones. Such a phenomenon may contribute to the high incidence of calcium oxalate stones in Saudi Arabia [12, 52, 53]. We have also identified ICON patients with hyperoxaluria in whom liberalization of calcium intake corrected the hyperoxaluria, with little or no change in urinary calcium excretion [54]. Such a mechanism may underlie the recent observation that a high calcium intake decreased the risk of symptomatic kidney stones in a large population study [55]. Finally, the low incidence of stones associated with calcium supplement ingestion among postmenopausal women may relate in part to the offsetting of any resultant increase of urinary calcium by a fall in urinary oxalate [56]. In conclusion, in terms of the general problem of ICON, the ratio of calcium

to oxalate in the diet as well as the chemical form of the oxalate in the food are probably of great importance, and require further study.

Enhanced intestinal oxalate absorption
There is little evidence to suggest that a primary oxalate transport defect underlies ICON. However, Borsatti has presented a large amount of data suggesting that an underlying defect in cellular oxalate transport may be common among these patients. This has been reviewed in detail [57]. The initial observation was made on erythrocytes [58]; those from calcium oxalate stone formers showed greatly enhanced oxalate self-exchange compared with erythrocytes of normal subjects. This was decreased with a thiazide diuretic, and appeared to have a hereditary (autosomal dominant) basis. Subsequently, the same authors provided data suggesting that the anion transporter band 3 protein might be responsible, and that this might be related to a defect in glycosaminoglycan production [57]. It is possible that such a generalized oxalate transport defect could contribute to enhanced intestinal oxalate absorption (causing intermittent hyperoxaluria) and/or enhanced renal tubular oxalate secretion. These very original observations require further research. Hereditary hyperoxaluria type III represents another form of enhanced intestinal oxalate absorption apparently related to, and perhaps secondary to, enhanced intestinal calcium absorption [33].

Mild forms of primary hyperoxaluria, mild metabolic hyperoxaluria and pyridoxine deficiency
Now that the gene for the enzyme AGT which is deficient in type I primary hyperoxaluria has been cloned and sequenced [32], it will be possible to determine whether some patients with apparent ICON actually have a genetically determined abnormality of AGT. It is known that a few patients with type I primary hyperoxaluria are atypical and present later in life with rather mild disease [25, 27, 29]. Preliminary data presented at the 1993 Oxalate Gordon Conference by Milliner *et al.* [59], in which the polymorphism of the AGT gene responsible for the Pro-11-Leu mutation was examined in calcium oxalate urolithiasis, indicate that the frequency of this genetic abnormality is not increased in these patients. In due course the gene for type II primary oxaluria will need to be similarly studied.

Pyridoxal phosphate is a cofactor for AGT, and pyridoxine deficiency has been shown to cause hyperoxaluria in experimental animals. However it does not appear to be an important contributor to human ICON.

The term 'mild metabolic hyperoxaluria' [60] describes a small subset of patients with recurrent calcium oxalate stone formation and mildly increased urinary oxalate and glycolate excretion in whom pyridoxine therapy may or may not cause a complete remission. Edwards and Rose [61] have recently reported the finding of impaired conversion of pyridoxine to pyridoxal-5-phosphate in mild metabolic hyperoxaluria, which was more severe in those individuals that responded only partially to pyridoxine than in those with a good response. Conversion was normal in type I primary hyperoxaluria. Thus mild metabolic hyperoxaluria may result from impaired conversion of pyridoxine to pyridoxal-5-phosphate. Pyridoxine has not been found to be useful therapy in the general population of ICON patients, but may be useful in a small subset of patients.

Abnormal renal oxalate handling
In order to undertake detailed studies of renal oxalate handling (except by means of isotopically labelled oxalate) it is necessary to have an accurate estimate of the plasma oxalate concentration. This had not been possible until recently, when enzyme and ion chromatographic methods have been described, and give consistent results for plasma oxalate concentration in the range 1–3 μmol/l [14, 15]. Using these methods, two groups have reported that the fractional urinary excretion of oxalate is higher in ICON with mild hyperoxaluria than in normal subjects [3, 8]. The observation of Borsatti [57] would be consistent with such a finding. However, it seems unlikely that a primary abnormality of renal oxalate handling (e.g. increased tubular oxalate secretion) would cause sustained hyperoxaluria. Rather, it would be expected to cause a reduction in the plasma oxalate level for a given daily excreted load. Hatch has examined renal oxalate handling in 35 patients with mild idiopathic hyperoxaluria [4]. In 22 patients, oxalate clearance was decreased relative to creatinine, and serum oxalate was increased. In these patients hyperoxaluria was felt to be absorptive. In 13 patients in whom hyperoxaluria was present during fasting, renal clearance was normal and the hyperoxaluria was felt to arise from increased endogenous production. There was no evidence for a renal oxalate leak in these patients. Now that the methodology for examining renal oxalate transport in man is becoming available, further studies comparing normal subjects and hyperoxaluric stone formers need to be undertaken.

Conclusions and future directions

The understanding of oxalate metabolism had been retarded for decades by the lack of reliable analytical methods. There is now a choice of accurate and reproducible methods for the measurement of urinary oxalate; the enzyme kit methods are currently the most widely used [14]. However, there continues to be problems with the measurement of oxalate [62]. Urinary glycolate, which is of some value in differentiating the many causes of hyperoxaluria, can also be reliably measured [63–65], but the assay is not widely available. Measurement of plasma oxalate and glycolate is also becoming more feasible [63] but remains technically demanding.

There have been exciting advances in our understanding of oxalate metabolism in recent years, but there is still much to be learned regarding the origin of urinary oxalate, particularly in recurrent calcium oxalate stone formers. It is not yet clear whether the best hope for large-scale prevention of these stones lies in the manipulation of the urinary content of the stone constituents oxalate and calcium, or whether it will prove more practical to use approaches that modify the urinary content of small molecular weight inhibitors such as citrate, or even high molecular weight inhibitors. Perhaps a combination of both approaches will prove to be most effective in the management of ICON.

References

1. Hodgkinson A, Oxalic acid in biology and medicine. New York: Academic Press, 1977.
2. Gault MT, Chafe K, Morgan TM *et al.* Comparison of patients with idiopathic calcium phosphate and calcium oxalate stones. Medicine 1991;70:345–59.
3. Gault MT, Ahmed M, Kalva J *et al.* Infrared analysis of stones. Clin Chem Acta 1980;104:349–59.
4. Hatch M, Oxalate status in stone-formers. Two distinct hyperoxaluric entities. Urol Res 1993;21:55–9.
5. Halabe A, Sutton RAL. Primary hyperparathyroidism as a cause of calcium nephrolithiasis. In: Coe FL, Favus MJ, editors. Disorders of bone and mineral metabolism. New York: Raven Press, 1991: 671–81.
6. Singh PP, Kothari LK, Sharma DC *et al.* Nutritional value of foods in relation to their oxalic acid content. Am J Clin Nutr 1972;25:1147–52.
7. Prenen JAC, Boer P, Mees D *et al.* Renal clearance of [^{14}C]oxalate: Comparison of constant infusion with single-injection techniques. Clin Sci 1982;263:47–51.
8. Wilson DM, Smith LH, Erickson SB *et al.* Renal oxalate handling in normal subjects and patients with idiopathic renal lithiasis: Primary and secondary hyperoxaluria. In: Walker VR, Sutton RAL, Cameron ECB *et al.*, editors. Urolithiasis. New York: Plenum Press, 1989:453–5.
9. Schwille PO, Manoharan M, Rumenapf G *et al.* Oxalate measurement in the picomol range by ion chromatography: Values in fasting plasma and urine of controls and patients with idiopathic calcium urolithiasis. J Clin Chem Clin Biochem 1989;27:87–96.
10. Robertson WG, Peacock M. Calcium oxalate crystalluria and inhibitors of crystallization in recurrent renal stone formers. Clin Sci 1972;43:499–506.
11. Robertson WG, Peacock M, Heyburn PJ *et al.* Risk factors in calcium stone disease of the urinary tract. Brit J Urol 1978;50:449–54.
12. Robertson WG, Hughes H. Importance of mild hyperoxaluria in the pathogenesis of urolithiasis – New evidence from studies in the Arabian Peninsula. Scanning Microscopy 1993;7:391–402.
13. Robertson WG, Peacock M. The cause of idiopathic calcium stone disease: Hypercalcuria or hyperoxaluria? Nephron 1980;26:105–10.
14. Hallson PC, Kasidas GP. Hyperoxaluria in calcium oxalate urolithiasis. In: Wickham JEA, Buck AC, editors. Renal tract stone. Metabolic basis and clinical practice. Edinburgh: Churchill Livingstone, 1990.
15. Coe FL, Parks JH, Nakagawa Y. Inhibitors and promoters of calcium oxalate crystallization. In: Coe FL, Favus MJ, editors. Disorders of bone and mineral metabolism, New York: Raven Press, 1991: 671–81.
16. Kok DJ, Papapoulos SE, Bijvoet OLM. Crystal agglomeration is a major element in calcium oxalate urinary stone formation. Kidney Int 1990;37:51–6.
17. Sakhaee K, Williams RH, Oh MS *et al.* Alkali absorption and citrate excretion in calcium nephrolithiasis. J Bone Min Res 1993;8:789–94.
18. Kok DJ, Iestraj Doorenbos CJ, Papapoulos SE. The effects of dietary excesses of animal protein and sodium on the composition and crystallization kinetics of calcium oxalate monohydrate in the urines of healthy man. J Clin Endoc Metab 1990;71:861–7.
19. Pak CYC. Citrate and renal calculi: New insights and future directions. Am J Kidney Dis 1991;17:420–5.
20. Coe FL, Parks JH, Nakagawa Y. Inhibitors and promoters of calcium oxalate crystallization. In: Coe FL, Favus MJ, editors. Disorders of bone and mineral metabolism. New York: Raven Press, 1991: 671–81.
21. Hess B, Nakagawa Y, Parks JH *et al.* Molecular abnormality of Tamm–Horsfall glycoprotein in calcium oxalate nephrolithiasis. Am J Physiol 1991;260:F569–78.
22. Riese RJ, Riese JW, Kleinman JG *et al.* Specificity in calcium oxalate adherence to papillary epithelial cells in culture. Am J Physiol 1988;255:F1025–32.
23. Riese RJ, Mandel NS, Wiessner JH *et al.* Cell polarity and calcium oxalate crystal adherence to culture collecting duct cells. Am J Physiol 1992;262:F177–184.

24. Lieske JC, Toback FG. Regulation of renal epithelial cell endocytosis of COM crystals. Am J Physiol 1993;264:F800–7.

25. Danpure CJ. Molecular and clinical heterogeneity in primary hyperoxaluria type I. Am J Kidney Dis 1991;17:366–9.

26. Danpure CJ. Primary hyperoxaluria type I and peroxisome-to-mitochondrion mistargeting of alanine:glyoxylate aminotransferase. Biochimie 1993;75:309–15.

27. Scheinman JI. Primary hyperoxaluria: Therapeutic strategies for the 90s. Kidney Int 1991;40:389–99.

28. Takada Y, Kaneko N, Esumi H *et al.* Human peroxisomal L-alanine:glyoxylate aminotransferase. Evolutionary loss of mitochondrial targeting signal by point mutation of the initiation codon. Biochem J 1990;268:517–20.

29. Irish AB, Doust B. Late presentation and development of nephrocalcinosis in primary hyperoxaluria. Aust NZ J Med 1992;22:48–50.

30. Yendt ER, Cohanim M. Response to a physiologic pyridoxine in type I primary hyperoxaluria. N Engl J Med 1985;312:953–7.

31. Smith LH. Hyperoxaluric states. In: Coe FL, Favus MJ, editors. Disorders of bone and mineral metabolism. New York: Raven Press, 1991:671–81.

32. Mistry J, Danpure CJ, Chalmers RA. Hepatic D-glycerate dehydrogenase and glyoxylate reductase deficiency in primary hyperoxaluria type 2. Biochem Soc Trans 1988;16:626–7.

33. Yendt ER, Cohanim M. Absorptive hyperoxaluria: A new clinical entity – successful treatment with hydrochlorothiazide. Clin Invest Med 1986;9:44–50.

34. McLeod RS, Churchill DN. Urolithiasis complicating inflammatory bowel disease. J Urol 1992;148:974–8.

35. Erickson SB, Cooper K, Broadus AE *et al.* Oxalate absorption and postprandial urine supersaturation in an experimental human model of absorptive hypercalcuria. Clin Sci 1984;67:131–8.

36. Allison MJ, Dawson KA, Mayberry WR *et al. Oxalobacter formigenes* gen. nov., sp. nov.: Oxalate-degrading anaerobes that inhabit the gastrointestinal tract. Arch Microbiol 1985;141:1–7.

37. Rose GA. Urinary stones. Clinical and laboratory aspects. Lancaster: MTP Press, 1982.

38. Massey LK, Roman-Smith H, Sutton RAL. Effect of dietary oxalate and calcium on urinary oxalate and risk of calcium oxalate kidney stone. J Am Dietetic Assoc 1993;93:901–06.

39. Yendt ER, Cohanim M. Hyperoxaluria in idiopathic oxalate nephrolithiasis. In: Leklem JE, Reynolds RD, editors. Clinical and physiological applications of vitamin B-6. New York: Alan R. Liss, 1988:229–44.

40. Harris KS, Richardson KE. Glycolate in the diet and its conversion to urinary oxalate in the rat. Invest Urol 1980;18:106–9.

41. Watts RWE, Hyperoxaluric states. In: Wickham JE, Buck AC, editors. Renal tract stone. Metabolic basis and clinical practice. Edinburgh: Churchill Livingstone, 1990:387–400.

42. Conyers RAJ, Basis R, Rofe AM. The relation of clinical catastrophes, endogenous oxalate production, and urolithiasis. Clin Chem 1990;36:1717–30.

43. Nguyen N, Dumoulin G, Henriet MT *et al.* Carbohydrate metabolism and urinary excretion of calcium and oxalate after ingestion of polyol sweeteners. J Clin Endoc Metab 1993;77:388–92.

44. Liedtke RR, Wilson DM, Moyer TP *et al.* Analysis of an immobilized oxalate-oxidase method in urine: Problems solved and methods compared. In: Walker VR, Sutton RAL, Cameron ECB *et al.*, editors. Urolithiasis. New York: Plenum Press, 1989:535–8.

45. Fituri N, Allavi N, Bentley M *et al.* Urinary and plasma oxalate during ingestion of pure ascorbic acid: A re-evaluation. Eur Urol 1983;9:312–15.

46. Cowley DM, Mcwhinney BC, Brown JM *et al.* Chemical factors important to calcium nephrolithiasis: Evidence for impaired hydroxycarboxylic acid absorption causing hyperoxaluria. Clin Chem 1987;33:243–7.

47. Zerembski PM, Hodgkinson A. Some factors influencing the urinary excretion of oxalic acid in man. Clin Chim Acta 1969,25.1–10.

48. Marshall RW, Cochran M, Hodgkinson A. Relationships between calcium and oxalic acid intake in the diet and their excretion in the urine of normal and renal-stone forming subjects. Clin Sci 1972,43.91–9.

49. Jaeger P, Portmann L, Jacquet A *et al.* Influence of the calcium content of the diet on the incidence of mild hyperoxaluria in idiopathic renal stone formers. Am J Nephrol 1985;5:40–4.

50. Smith LH. Diet and hyperoxaluria in the syndrome of idiopathic calcium oxalate urolithiasis. Am J Kidney Dis 1991;17:370–5.

51. Giannini S, Nobile M, Castrignano R *et al.* Possible link between vitamin D and hyperoxaluria in patients with renal stone disease. Clin Sci 1993;84:51–4.

52. Abdel Halim RE, Al-Hadramy MS, Hussein M *et al.* The prevalence of urolithiasis in the western region of Saudi Arabia: A population study. In: Walker VR, Sutton RAL, Cameron ECB *et al.*, editors. Urolithiasis. New York: Plenum Press, 1989:711–12.

53. Barkworth SA, Louis S, Walker VR *et al.* Stone type and urine composition in the Middle East with particular reference to Saudi Arabia. In: Walker VR, Sutton RAL, Cameron ECB *et al.*, editors. Urolithiasis. New York: Plenum Press, 1989:715.

54. Walker VR, Sutton, RAL, Chan S. Case report: Hyperoxaluria and dietary calcium. New York: Plenum Publishing, in press.

55. Curhan GC, Willett WC, Rimm EB *et al.* A prospective study of dietary calcium and other nutrients and the risk of symptomatic kidney stones. N Engl J Med 1993;328:833–8.

56. Ringe JD. The risk of nephrolithiasis with oral calcium supplementation. Calcif Tissue 1991;48:69–73.

57. Borsatti A. Calcium oxalate nephrolithiasis: Defective oxalate transport. Kidney Int 1991;39:1283–98.

58. Baggio B, Gambaro G, Marchini F *et al.* An inheritable anomaly of red-cell oxalate transport in 'primary' calcium nephrolithiasis correctable with diuretics. N Engl J Med 1986;314:599–604.

59. Milliner DS, Allsop J, Wilson DM *et al.* 'C154 fi T polymorphism in the AGT gene in patients with calcium oxalate urolithiasis. Abstracts, Gordon Conference on Oxalate, 1993.

60. Gill HS, Rose GA. Mild metabolic hyperoxaluria and its response to pyridoxine. Urol Int 1986;41:393–6.

61. Edwards P, Rose GA. Metabolism of pyridoxine in mild metabolic hyperoxaluria and primary hyperoxaluria (type I). Urol Int 1991;47:113–17.

62. Samuell CT. Experiences with an external quality assessment scheme for urinary oxalate. In: Rose GA, editor. Oxalate metabolism in relation to urinary stone. London: Springer-Verlag, 1988:27–44.

63. Hagen L, Walker V, Sutton RAL. Plasma and urinary oxalate and glycolate in healthy subjects. Clin Chem 1993;39:134–6.

64. Wandzilak TR, Hagen LE, Hughes H *et al.* Quantitation of glycolate in urine by ion-chromatography. Kidney Int 1991;39:765–70.

65. Marangella M, Petrarulo M, Vitale C *et al.* Plasma and urine glycolate assays for differentiating the hyperoxaluria syndromes. J Urol 1992;148:986–89.

8. Familial clustering and sex incidence of urolithiasis

JAMSHEER TALATI

The sex distribution of upper urinary tract stone disease

Upper urinary tract stone disease is a predominantly male disease. It is seen 1.2–3.3 [1] times more frequently in the male than female – in some countries (e.g. Saudi Arabia) as much as 5 times more frequently in the male [2]. In Pakistan at the Aga Khan University Medical Centre (AKUMC), the sex ratio in patients with upper urinary tract stone is 2.8:1.

In America, the sex ratio in patients with calcium oxalate stones in the white and Asian populations favours the male, but is reversed in Hispanic and Black communities living in Chicago [3], in whom stones are commoner in females. In Scotland, a ratio of 1.03:1 (males:females) was noted in a prevalence study scanning a population of 7000 [4]. Others have noted a ratio of 0.7:1 in young females [5]. A recent review of paediatric lithiasis at the Mayo Clinic has shown a male:female ratio of 0.955:1 [6].

A distinctive sex ratio was seen for each type of stone in one study from Australia – 2.8:1 for oxalate, 3.7:1 for uric acid and 1.4:1 for calcium phosphate, favouring males [5].

Is the high sex ratio in adults in Pakistan and Saudi Arabia because women do not come forward for treatment? Is it because social security financial cover for medical treatment does not give free treatment to women? This was so in the 1960s in Pakistan, but not now. Women get free treatment for any illness if their husband is covered by industrial social security benefits. It is possible that the sex difference is because of the higher excretion of citrate – a potent inhibitor – in females.

Sex distribution in bladder stone disease

Bladder stones are seen 8–10 times more frequently in Pakistani male children than in females (data from Thar, Mirpurkhas and AKUMC). In contrast, in Spain, male children are affected only twice as commonly as females [7]. The male preponderance in paediatric bladder lithiasis is not due to preferential treatment meted out to the male child – the sex ratios in rural areas are the same as in towns where there is better access to hospitals.

J. Talati et al. (eds) The Management of Lithiasis, 69–75
© 1997 Kluwer Academic Publishers. Printed in Great Britain.

Table 8.1 Number of patients who have at least one relative affected by stone disease

	Percentage with positive family history					
	Karachi	Karachi (Controls)	Malaysia[a]	Czechs [18]	Leeds [19] (Controls)	Germany [1]
n	100	100				169
At least one member affected by stone disease	52	18	33	23.6 (7.8)	14.8 (9.1)	29
Three generations affected	41					
Grandparents affected	8	0	0			2.8
Parents affected	21	6	14	5.9 (2.1)		16.9
Father	14	5	8		5.2 (3.0)	
Mother	9	1	5.3		2.6 (2.1)	
Siblings affected	22			8.6 (3.4)	1.8 (1.4)	
Brothers affected	16	3	7			
Sisters affected	7	3	8			
Offspring of patients	4	0	3.5	3.0 (0.6)	0.9 (0.5)	
Maternal aunts, uncles and cousins	14	2	7			
Paternal aunts, uncles and cousins	11	7	5.3			
Spouse	6	2				

[a] Hussain T. *et al.* (AKUMC study in Malaysia).
Figures in brackets denote frequency (as %) in controls.

Hereditary and familial factors that increase the risk for stone formation

A number of distinctive genetic disorders predispose to stone disease. Most, such as Lesch–Nyhan syndrome, Dent's syndrome, and type I and II hyperoxaluria are rare. Other examples are cystinuria, xanthinuria and familial hypercalciuria; and hyperparathyroidism in families of patients with idiopathic familial hypocalciuric hypercalcaemia.

Holmes *et al.* [8] have suggested that co-dominant alleles may determine calcium excretion rates. A colony of genetic hypercalciuric rats has been developed by close in-breeding [9]. Such rats show an increase in the vitamin D receptor in the intestines [10], but these rats do not produce stones. Hypercalciuria of the absorptive type has been noted in several members of kindred of stone formers [11]. Pedigree analysis suggests autosomal dominant inheritance [11–13].

In Dent's syndrome, a microdeletion of DXs255 on Xp11.22 has been identified [14]. In Lesch-Nyhan syndrome an X-linked defect of the enzyme HGPRT involved in purine metabolism results in excess production of uric acid [15].

Possible genetic transmission in 'idiopathic' calcium oxalate lithiasis

In a study conducted in Karachi at the AKUMC, 52% of stone patients (vs. 18% of controls) had at least one other first-degree relative with a history of stone disease (Tables 8.1 and 8.2). In our study on Malaysian patients, in Kelantan province, 33% had a first degree relative with stone (data collected by S. T. Hussain). In the West, 13–30 % [1] give a family history. In Portugal, 32% of patients and 17% of controls have a family history of stone [16]. In Italy, the first degree relatives of 34% of stone patients and 14% of controls have stone [17].

Table 8.2 Percentage of relatives affected by stone

	Pakistan controls	Pakistan patients	Malaysia patients
Brother	1.2 (50)	6.0*	3
Sister	1.5 (30)	2.6*	4
% of sons (of patients) affected by stone	0	1.6	2
% of daughters (of patients) affected by stone	0	1.4	0
% of sons of all stone formers	5.5	27.4***	25
% of daughters of all stone formers	6.6	14.1	16
Paternal aunts	0.93	0	0
Paternal uncles	1.22	4.00	1
Paternal cousin	0.21	0.22	0
Maternal aunts	0.35	0.83	0
Maternal uncles	0.42	4.00	3
Maternal cousin	0.07	0.30	1

In families where:

* A brother has stone disease then 26.15% of brothers are affected

** A sister has stone disease then 28% of sisters are affected

***A father and son are affected then 36.2% of all sons are affected by stone; when father and daughter affected then 26.31% of all daughters are affected.

Table 8.3   Consanguinity

In Schneider's report (Russia)	between parents of paediatric stone formers	43%
Hussain (Malaysia) (AKUMC study)	between parents of stone formers	18%
	between interviewed patients	15.7%
	between 2 stone-forming patients	3.5%
	between 2 stone-forming parents	1.8%
Talati (Karachi, Pakistan)	consang. marriage between parents	16%

The higher familial incidence in Pakistan could be because we have larger families, and consanguineous marriages are common (often quoted as up to 60% of all marriages). However in the group studied by us, only 16% were the product of a consanguineous marriage (Table 8.3).

The familial incidence is distinct for each type of stone: 30% for cystine lithiasis, 24% for oxalate stones, 24% for mixed and unidentified stones and 14–16% for uric acid stones and phosphate stones [18]. Trinchieri *et al.* [21] noted a 25% rate of positive family history in families affected by calcium stones and 43% in families affected by urate stones as against 11% in controls without stones.

The high rate of involvement of first degree relatives suggests that genetic factors may be responsible. The low incidence of stone disease in Negroes (less than 1% as compared to 12% in white males and 5% in white females) [22] appears to support this. However, when the diet of the Bantu African approximates that in the West, a higher incidence of stone results [23] and this may indicate the influence of environmental factors. In our series, 7% of stone patient's spouses also had stone disease, possibly because the spouses share the same dietary fare.

In our study in Kelantan, most of the stones were seen in the Malays as compared to the Chinese. This should not be interpreted as a racial predisposition, because in Singapore [24], most of the stone formers are Chinese. The frequency of stone in the communities simply reflects the population demographics (see Figure 8.1 and Table 8.4).

Earlier studies by us in Edinburgh (1967) and Karachi had failed to show any correlation of stone incidence with blood groups. The percentage distribution of ABO blood groups in stone patients was different in Edinburgh and Pakistan, but simply reflected the frequency distribution of blood groups in the respective country (Table 8.5).

Table 8.4   Proportions of Chinese and Malays affected by stone in Malaysia and Singapore

	Chinese		Indians		Malays		Others	
	%pop	%SF	%pop	%SF	%pop	%SF	%pop	%SF
MALAYSIA Hussain & Talati	18.5	8.8	7.7	7.0	72.4	80.7	0.4	3.5
SINGAPORE Foo *et al.* [24]	76.9	85.4	6.4	2.1	14.6	8.5	2.1	1.3

%pop: Contribution of ethnic groups to the total population.
%SF: Contribution of ethnic group to the stone-forming population.

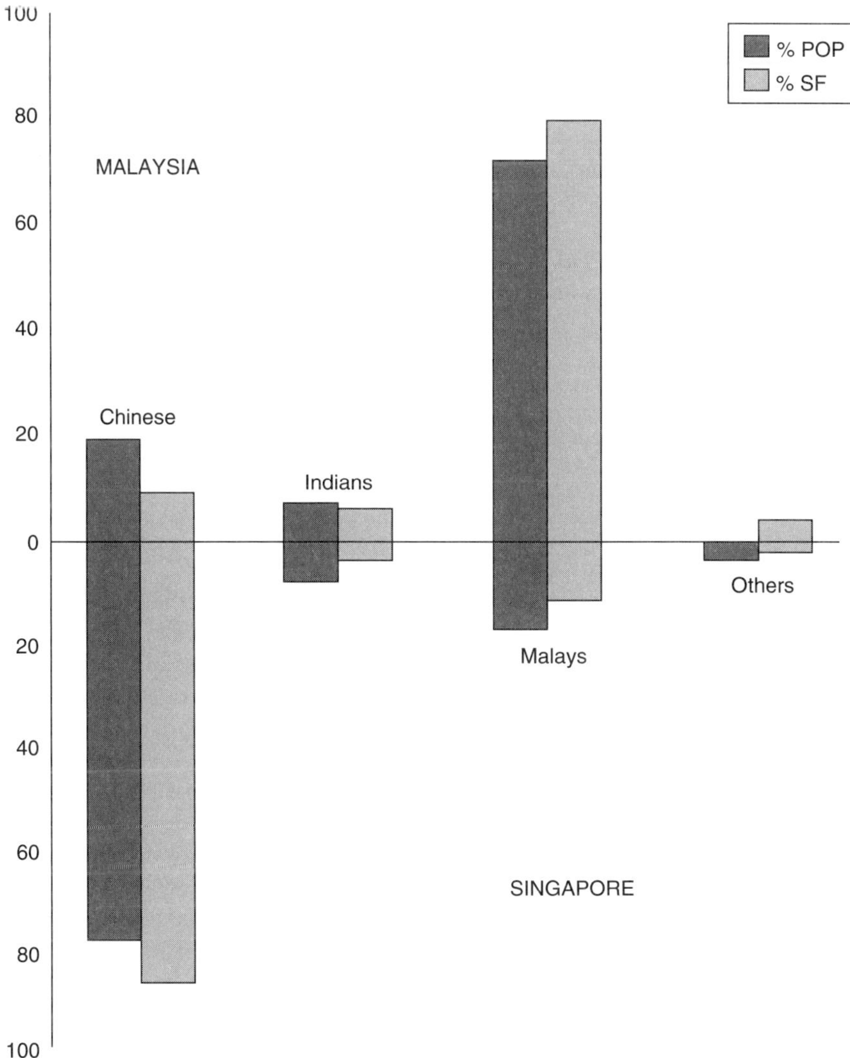

Figure 8.1 Porportions of Chinese and Malays affected by stone in Malaysia and Singapore.

Conclusion

Whilst there is sufficient evidence to indicate that genetic factors may be playing a part in stone formation, there is lack of clarity as to whether inheritance is autosomal or sex linked.

Whatever the genetic background, environmental risk factors (such as hypercalciuria) also play an important part. In Pakistan, generations of intra tribal marriages, as discussed by Khoury *et al.* for other diseases [25], precede the

Table 8.5   Blood groups in Pakistani and Edinburgh stone patients compared to controls

Blood group	Stone patients Pakistan			Controls[c]	Stone patients Edinburgh[d]	Controls UK[e]
	HFH[a] (*n* = 369)	AKUMC[b] (*n* = 146)		(*n* = 51257)	(*n* = 136)	
A	17.6	Rh+	19.8	20.5	37.5	42.0
		Rh–	0.0	1.3		
B	36.7	Rh+	28.8	33.9	9.6	9.0
		Rh–	1.3	2.3		
AB	6.6	Rh+	14.3	7.9	2.2	3.0
		Rh–	0.0	0.5		
O	39.1	Rh+	33.5	30.9	50.7	46.0
		Rh–	1.3	2.7		

[a] 369 patients studied at Holy Family Hospital in 1970s.
[b] November 1985–July 1988 frequency of blood groups among patients with renal calculi treated at AKUH. Blood groups known in 53% (146) of 275 patients.
[c] Data from a 10-year study of 34 675 donors at AKUMC (courtesy Dr M. Khursheed).
[e] Data from 1967.
[d] Race R.R., Sanger R. Blood Groups in Man, 6th Ed. Blackwell Scientific Publications: Oxford [27].

consanguineous marriage of the parents of the proband. This setting favours an increase of the frequency of a single or a set of gene(s) causing stones [26]. In such a setting, stone formation may occur in the absence of environmental factors such as a high calcium diet. In the West, a wider gene pool and fewer consanguineous marriages decrease gene frequency; environmental factors such as the high intake of milk and consequent hypercalciuria become important.

This superimposition of environmental risk factors on genetic predisposition would influence the ratios of individuals with and without stone disease, thus making deductions about the type of inheritance from pedigree analysis more difficult.

If genetic causes are conclusively shown to play a major role in the genesis of stone disease, efforts must be made to reduce the tight inbreeding seen in some of our communities.

Acknowledgements

Data for family history in Pakistan were collected by Dr Gul Rukh Ahmed and Liaquat Ali Khan, and for family history in Malaysia by S. Tahir Hussain.

References

1. Schneider HJ. Epidemiology of urolithiasis. In: Schneider HJ, editor. Urolithiasis etiology and diagnosis. Berlin: Springer-Verlag, 1985.
2. Abomelha MS, al Khader AA, Arnold J. Urolithiasis in Saudi Arabia. Urology 1990;35:31–4.
3. Michaels EK, Nakagawa Y, Miura N *et al.* Racial variation in gender frequency of calcium urolithiasis. J Urol 1994;152:2228–31.

4. Scott R. Prevalence of calcified upper urinary tract stone disease in a random population survey. Report of a combined study of general practitioners and hospital staff. Br J Urol 1987;59:111–17.

5. Baker PW, Coyle P, Bais R *et al.* Influence of season age and sex in renal stone formation in South Australia. Med J Aust 1993;159:390–2.

6. Milliner DS, Murphy ME. Urolithiasis in the pediatric patient. Mayo Clin Proc 1993;68:241–8.

7. Moreno Villares JM, Muley Alonso R, Espino Hernandez M *et al.* Urolithiasis in childhood. An Esp Pediat 1991;35:13–16.

8. Holmes RP, Goodman HO, Assimos DG. Genetic influences on urinary calcium excretion. In: Ryall R *et al.*, editors. Urolithiasis 2. New York: Plenum Press, 1994;3–8.

9. Bushinsky DA, Kim M, Sessler NE *et al.* Increased urinary saturation and kidney calcium content in genetic hypercalciuric rats. Kidney Int 1994;45:58–65.

10. Li XQ, Tembe V, Horwitz GM. Increased intestinal vitamin D receptor in genetic hypercalciuric rats. A cause of intestinal hyperabsorption. J Clin Invest 1993;91:661–7.

11. Harangi F, Mehes K. Family investigations in idiopathic hypercalciuria. Eur J Pediat 1993;152:64–8.

12. Favus MJ. Familial forms of hypercalciuria. J Urol 1989;141:719–22.

13. Kaul P, Sidhu H, Vaidyanathan S *et al.* Study of urinary calcium excretion after oral calcium load in stone formers, their spouses and first degree relatives. Urol Int 1994;52:93–7.

14. Pook MA, Wrong O, Wooding C. Dent's disease, a renal Fanconi syndrome with nephrocalcinosis and kidney stones is associated with microdeletion involving DXs255 and maps to Xp11.22. Hum Mol Genet 1993;2:2129–34.

15. Kenney JJ. Renal sonography in longstanding Lesch Nyhan syndrome. Clin Radiol 1991;43:39–41.

16. Reis Santos JM. Studies on the prevalence of renal stone disease in Portugal. Abstracts of 5th European Urolithiasis meeting, Manchester, 1994.

17. Borghi L, Ferretti PP, Elia GP *et al.* Epidemiological study of urinary tract stones in a northern Italian city. Br J Urol 1990;65:231–5.

18. Kruzek V, Vondrova M. Familial incidence of urolithiasis in Czechoslovakia. Abstracts of 13th Urolithiasis Symposium. Urol Res 1987;15:115.

19. Robertson WG, Peacock M, Baker M *et al.* Epidemiological studies on urinary stone disease in Leeds. In: Rayall RL, Brockis JG, Marshall VR *et al.*, editors. Urinary stone disease. Edinburgh: Churchill–Livingstone, 1984:8–9.

20. Power C, Nelson M. Diet and renal stone, a case control study. In: Ryall R, editor. Urinary stone disease. London: Livingstone, 1984:32.

21. Trinchieri A, Mandressi A, Luongo P *et al.* Recurrence and family history of renal stone disease. In: Liniari F *et al.*, editors. Contr Nephrol Basel: Karger, 1987;58:31–3.

22. Meyers AM, Whally N, Zakolsky WJ *et al.* Chemical composition of the urine in normal black and white population. In: Ryall R *et al.*, editors. Urolithiasis 2. New York: Plenum Press, 1994:422.

23. Charlton CAC. A urinary detergent and urolithiasis. Br J Urol 1989;63:561–4.

24. Foo KT, Tung KH, Tan EC *et al.* The pattern of urinary stone disease in a surgical department in Singapore. In: Ryall RL, Brockis JG, Marshall VR *et al.*, editors. Urinary stone. London: Livingstone, 1984:80.

25. Khoury MJ, Adams MJ, Flanders WD. An epidemiological approach to ecogenetics. Am J Hum Genet 1988;42:89–95.

26. Klug WS, Cummings MR. The genetics of populations. In: Concepts of genetics. Toronto/London: Merril Publishing Company, 1983.

27. Race RR, Sanger R. Blood groups in man. 6th ed. Oxford and Edinburgh: Blackwell Scientific Publications, 1975.

28. Brown EM, Pollack M, Siedman CE *et al.* Calcium-ion-sensing cell surface receptors. New Engl J Med 1995;333:234–9.

Section II
Choices in the Management of Urinary Tract Calculi

9. Decisions! Decisions!

JAMSHEER TALATI

With the explosive advance of technology it is now possible to treat almost any type of stone. The concerned physician will however be interested in treating the patient, rather than the stone, avoiding unnecessary therapy, timing therapy to avoid complications, and ensuring compliance. A number of decisions have to be made and the physician may have to ask him/herself the following questions:

- Does the patient need interventional therapy?
- Is treatment required immediately or after a period of observation?
- If intervention is required, what is the best mode of treatment?
- What factors in the patient's world will modify his acceptance of offered treatment?

To be effective in management of stones, the urologist has to keep abreast of the developments in all fields – pharmacology, biochemistry, technology, sociology and communication – in order to communicate effectively and counsel the patient. The physician should be cognizant of ethical issues and aware of the potentials of different forms of technology and the hazards involved in their use; awareness of their own limitations in using the technology is also necessary. The relative costs of the various options will also require consideration.

The need for treatment

The need for treatment is obvious in a patient with anuria: he requires urgent therapy, otherwise the outcome will be death. Decisions about patients with small, non-obstructing ureteric stones and asymptomatic calyceal and staghorn calculi are not as easy. Here decisions are helped by knowledge of the natural history of the stone e.g. 60% of ureteric stones will pass spontaneously [1]. Such a patient may be simply observed to allow natural events to take their course. The degree of co-operation expected from the patient during follow-up will also influence management decisions. If the patient is unlikely to comply with requests for repeated visits to the hospital, he is at risk from possible ureteric obstruction and its disastrous consequences, if the stone is not expelled.

Asymptomatic small renal calculi have the potential for causing ureteral obstruction. But how often does this occur? Reviewing the course of 107 calculi, Glowacki et al. [2] noted that 68% remained asymptomatic, 16% passed spontaneously and

J. Talati et al. (eds) The Management of Lithiasis, 79–83
© *1997 Kluwer Academic Publishers. Printed in Great Britain.*

16% needed removal. The probabilities of the symptomatic events at 1, 2, 3, 4 and 5 years were 7.8, 20.4, 33.8, 40.6 and 48.5% [3] if the calculus remained asymptomatic for six months; colic occurs once per 100 patient months, spontaneous passage of calculi once in 50 patient-months and the need for stone removal once in 238 patient-months [3]. Management of asymptomatic calyceal and staghorn calculi is discussed in Chapters 16 and 18.

Knowledge of the natural history of urinary calculi should not lull a physician into advising conservative management until he/she has considered whether a trial of conservative management would result in a higher complication rate, alter the success rate of operation or extracorporeal shock wave lithotripsy (ESWL), or make it more difficult. Delaying treatment may allow a ureteric stone previously at a site suitable for ESWL to descend into a position out of reach of an ultrasound monitored lithotriptor – it may then cause severe obstruction.

The most difficult decisions for physicians are ones that involve a wait and watch policy; but these are important decisions. In poor countries with limited financial resources, every unnecessary treatment for stone may take away the ability to treat another patient desperately in need of therapy. The potential to treat almost anyone given the advances in screening, urological skills and armamentarium, does not absolve us of the responsibility of critically deciding the best treatment for a patient, and weighing costs and risks against benefit.

The patient's viewpoint

Discussing treatment plans with the patient and family brings to light many additional issues: allergies, untoward events during previous anaesthetic use or IVP, and susceptibility to wound infections, may suddenly come to the patient's mind as the plan is discussed. The patient's fears are sometimes expressed; these may be detected by the alert physician from facial expressions.

The patient may request a form of therapy other than what is recommended, due to: logistics (he cannot leave his farm at harvest time, he cannot come from far off for repeated treatments, or he may have to attend an important business meeting or conference); hidden fears about anaesthesia or pain; or his perception of safety and harmfulness of different procedures. In Pakistan, information gained by word of mouth about how a friend or relative fared after a procedure often determines the choice of the doctor, and at times the procedure!

Patient insistence on a particular form of treatment and bias against another needs to be considered with empathy. If a patient refuses lithotripsy, because of complications he has heard about from others, the physician can present the unit's experience based on data gained from audit, and explain the probabilities of such an event, showing that the patient does not come in a category in which one expects such complications. The physician can explain measures such as stenting, used to reduce complications. The physician has a responsibility to present data impartially and accurately, for example, the irritating symptoms of stenting should be explained. Stating results from audit data helps the patient understand that he is dealing with an experienced, conscientious and safe physician. The physician will also need to explain that the risks are not all or none; there is a gradient ranging from safe to harmful. Risks should however never be minimized when discussing outcomes. Patients may demand therapy when none is needed (for a small stone for example), because they are due to retire and fear progression of stone size and complications requiring treatment at a time when the firm for which they are working will no longer support them financially. Insurance cover similarly induces patients to demand use of available technology because they feel they have paid insurance, and therefore should get some return – described as 'sunk costs'. The patient may wish treatment of a small stone fearing it will cause colic on a holiday trip, or when busy with an important project, or at harvest time.

The physician must spend time to try and understand these issues and help the patient rationalize these concerns.

Dilemmas of practice in a poor country

It is important that the choice of procedure, and the decision to treat or not treat the patient, should be based on sound, logical deductive thinking, free from any pressures such as the surgeon's ego, the inability of the patient to pay, the need to increase revenues for financial gain, or the need to pay back a banker's loan.

Lithotriptors tend to be used just because they are available, and because the liberal use of all information media to 'advertise' advances in medicine subtly alters public opinion and creates a demand for their use. At other times machines are not used when they should be: it is all too easy to operate on a ureteric stone because a country is too poor to afford a lithotriptor or ureteroscope. This is one form of inequity that physicians should struggle to resolve.

Costs have not been mentioned in the above decision-making process, but they must be considered. Issues concerning the delivery of costly technology at affordable cost to all are addressed below.

The physician's expertise in the context of the available armamentarium

The urologist should reach a decision after considering how the particular procedure fares in his hands. One should not worry about the fact that in the West, only 2% patients require open surgery for stones. The porportions of open to closed procedures will change when both technological equipment and expertise are available. In Japan, in the Hara genitourinary hospital [4], between 1976 and 1980, the majority of stones were treated by open surgery, whereas in the 1986–91 period only 8.2% of 4150 stones were so treated. Similarly, at the Aga Khan University Medical Centre, with increasing experience, only 24% of our stones are treated by procedures other than ESWL; and only 7% of renal, 2% of ureteric and 9% of bladder stones require surgery (data pertain to January to June 1995). Even when all technology and expertise is available, multiple complex technological procedures should not be chosen just so that the audit looks good, or to satisfy the surgeon's ego. In the absence of expertise, the morbidity from a succession of minimally invasive procedures on a single patient may be greater than that from a single open procedure [5].

Alternate medicines for stone

There is little scientific information on traditional cures for urinary tract stone. It is therefore difficult to include the use of such drugs as an option when planning therapy. Takusha and Kagosou [6], commercially available medicines from Japan, and Veerathardi Kashayanm [7] have been noted to inhibit crystallization *in vitro*. Musa (*Paradisiaca Linn* cultivar) stem juice has been found to be effective in preventing stone formation in the rat, and dissolving preformed stones [8].

Case study

The following case presents the conflicts that frequently arise between a reasoned decision and the patient's wishes. Effective resolution is not always reached.

A busy businessman from a town 400 miles from the base hospital presented for treatment of a 5-mm spindle shaped stone in the lower left ureter, just above the ischial spine. It was not causing any pain or obstruction to the ureter. The physician questioned the need to treat it. A survey of world literature revealed that:

- though 60% of all calculi pass spontaneously, 71% of lower ureteric calculi will do so [1];
- 93% of calculi < 4 mm long will pass within 6 weeks of onset of pain, as against only 50% of those 4–7 mm long [9] (this calculus is 5 mm long); and
- stones < 10 mm which move down the ureter within 6 weeks, will pass spontaneously [10].

The physician's decision to treat conservatively, but monitor progress, was justified. However, stone movement is notoriously capricious [9], and the physician therefore intended to monitor stone movement closely. At this point, the physician's knowledge of the levels of health consciousness of our population, and the intensity of the patient's involvement in his business, cautioned her. Conservative management requires conscientious follow-up and patient compliance. Compliance in third world countries is low, often because of inability to pay for repeat X-ray and the physician's next visit [11], but at times simply from lack of awareness of the need for attention to health issues and ignorance. Many patients think their stone has passed because there is no pain. As in this case, patients are sometimes too busy to be bothered about a stone. Failure to attend follow-up puts the patient at risk for hydronephrosis, silent renal atrophy and renal failure. In such circumstances, an aggressive interventional approach is acceptable. A decision to extract this stone endoscopically was made.

What were the modifying factors in the patient's world that influenced this decision? He was completing the construction of an extension to his factory, and it was not possible for him to return to the hospital in a month's time, and after that he would be in Germany. He is obese and smokes 40 cigarettes a day – evidence that he is careless about his health and focuses on work alone.

What were the patient's wishes? He refused all interventions other than medication. Had he been an airline pilot, or flight attendant, or a soldier about to be sent overseas or to a front line, his employer would have refused to deploy his services unless he was stone-free, and he would have had no other option but to comply.

Here, the final decision was to treat the patient conservatively. An ultrasound and Scout film abdomen (KUB) surveillance was suggested. He was to fax the reports of his investigations, but he failed to comply. When faxed, he did not reply. When contacted by phone, his wife said, 'he must have passed the stone as he is pain free and working as usual'. A KUB X-ray was requested. This was done, and fortunately, the patient had passed the stone.

The following chapters in this section discuss operations, machines and choices in the management of renal ureteric bladder and urethral calculi. Calculi in children are discussed in Chapter 46. Choices when treating high-risk patients and choices in management that reduce the frequency of second treatments are discussed in Section III.

References

1. Morse RM, Resnick MI. Ureteral calculi. Natural history in an era of advanced technology. J Urol 1991;145:263–5.
2. Glowaci LS, Beecroft ML, Cook RJ. Natural history of asymptomatic urolithiasis. J Urol 1992;147:319–21.
3. Churchill DM, Beecroft ML, Taylor DW. Prognosis of asymptomatic urolithiasis. Urol Res 1988;16:238.
4. Hara S, Omae H, Shinozake M *et al.* Statistics of operations at the Hara genitourinary Hospital, 1971–91. Hinyokika Kiyo 1992;38:603–11.
5. Whitfield HN. Management of complex renal calculi. Abstracts of Symposium of Sindh Institute of Urology and Transplantation, 1994 P–6.
6. Yosiaka T, Utsonomiya M, Yamaguchi S *et al.* The effect of Kanpou medicines on the growth and aggregation of calcium oxalate calculi *in vitro*. In: Urolithiasis 2. Ryall R *et al.*, editors. New York and London: Plenum Publishers, 1992:240.
7. Aravindakshan C, Bai NJ, Nair CPR *et al.* Verathardiin urolithiasis. Urolithiasis 2. In: Ryall R *et al.*, editors. New York and London: Plenum Publishers, 1992:664.
8. Prasad KV, Bharathi K, Srinavasan KK. Evaluation of Musa stem juice for antilithiatic activity in albino rats. Indian J Pharmacol 1993;37:337–41.
9. O'Flynn JD. Clinical management of ureteral calculi. In Roth RA, Finlayson B, editors. Stones: Clinical management of urolithiasis; urology. Baltimore and London: William Wilkins, 1983.443–4.
10. Ibrahim AIA, Shetty SD, Awad RM *et al.* Prognostic factors in the conservative management of ureteric stones. Br J Urol 1991;67:358–61.
11. Talati J, Khan LA, Noordzig JW *et al.* The scope and place of ultrasound monitored lithotripsy in a multimodality setting and the effects of experiential audit evoked changes on the management of ureteral calculi. Br J Urol 1994;73:480–6.

10. Advantages and hazards of open surgery

JAMSHEER TALATI

In Pakistan, many patients refuse open surgery because they are afraid they will die during or after an operation, or that they will not awaken after anaesthesia. They dread pain, and the number of days off work. Mass media communication via satellite television, and working expatriates in the affluent Middle East provide information on the latest modes of therapy to all strata of the population of the third world. With their knowledge of technological advances, many refuse operation and demand extracorporeal shock wave lithotripsy (ESWL). There is an unprecedented demand for technology before it is even available in the town, province or country. Illiteracy is no longer an impediment to the aquisition of knowledge.

Advantages of open surgery

Carefully selected open surgery can still be the best treatment option as in patients with obstruction due to ureteropelvic junction (UPJ) stenosis or ureteral stricture distal to the stone; for certain types of staghorn calculi, large ureteral and bladder calculi; and for the very obese, open surgery can be the ideal option. It is often the least expensive modality, and requires no instruments other than those found in any major operating room. As specialized expensive equipment is not needed, maintenance is not a problem, and large fees do not have to be paid in foreign exchange for repair and preventive maintenance. Most instruments can be made efficiently at low cost in the country – Pakistan is a leading manufacturer of quality surgical instruments – thus saving foreign exchange.

For bulky staghorns, simultaneous bilateral transperitoneal pyelolithotomies can be undertaken through a midline incision, allowing rapid resolution of a complex problem affecting both renal units. Bilateral simultaneous operation saves operating room time as both kidneys are tackled through one incision, and closure also takes less time. Costs go down as a consequence of reduced operating room time utilization. Additionally, postoperative hospitalization is reduced as convalescence for each kidney operation is telescoped, again reducing costs. The transperitoneal approach is to be avoided in a patient with infected urine. It is also not ideal for the obese patient in whom peri-renal fat makes renal manipulation difficult, and in whom bilateral flank incisions may be a better choice.

Large ureteric stones greater than 10 mm in length may best be treated by ureterolithotomy if overlying the iliac vessels. Large stones in the paediatric

J. Talati et al. (eds) The Management of Lithiasis, 85–88
© 1997 Kluwer Academic Publishers. Printed in Great Britain.

bladder are best removed by surgery. Two-layer watertight closure of the bladder reduces the risk of leakage. Catgut can be used as effectively as vicryl and costs less ($0.3 per suture, compared with $1.3 for a vicryl suture). Meticulous suture technique rather than the suture material ensures fistula-free healing.

Very large stones (greater than 3 cm) composed of calcium oxalate monohydrate in the adult bladder, or those with a jackstone appearance, are hard and take an unduly prolonged time to fragment when using transurethral modalities. Treatment by ESWL requires spacing over a number of sessions. Hence these stones are best treated by surgery, combined with treatment of any bladder outflow obstruction as from prostatic hyperplasia.

For simple single stones, surgery is definitive, clearing all calculi at the time of operation. Although these stones are easily treated by ESWL, repeated shock wave application and prolonged follow-up are required for clearance. Patient attendance for post-ESWL follow-up increases outpatient volume. In contrast, after operation, the patient may need only a single postoperative visit for removal of sutures.

Disadvantages

Stones can be left behind after open surgery, in spite of diligent preoperative X-rays. These need to be confirmed by postoperative X-rays in the radiology department, once abdominal distension has subsided. Most portable X-ray machines are of 100 mA, and cannot reproduce the fine quality X-rays from machines in the department which are of 400 mA. Problems arise when the patient has uric acid calculi which cannot be visualized preoperatively, except by ultrasound which often is not available. Complex stones however leave residuals after any method of treatment.

Open surgery presents other hazards for the patient. Wound infection, incisional hernia, fistulae, risk of contracting viral diseases and malaria, are all disadvantages, as is the need for operating room and anaesthesia time, and a hospital bed.

Transmission of viral diseases to the operating team during open surgery can have disastrous results. In Baluchistan, Pakistan, various haemorrhagic virus infections transmitted through needle prick injuries during surgery have been the sporadic but repeated cause of death of young surgeons. Hepatitis B and C are very common in India and Pakistan. Screening before surgery is necessary but expensive, and adds to costs. Today, the risk of AIDS becomes pertinent, as it is becoming more common, even in Pakistan. Double gloving for the surgical team may give some protection. Physicians should be immunized against viral hepatitis, though this is costly.

Blood transfusions if improperly screened can transmit multi-drug resistant malaria, hepatitis and now AIDS, to the patient. Anatrophic nephrolithotomy and multiple nephrotomies may require large transfusions. Blood transfusion, required in 4.6% of patients with stones less than 2 cm, increases to 26.2% in patients with larger stones [1]. A policy of combining surgery for the pelvic and major calyceal components of complex stones with ESWL for the more peripheral difficult-to-approach calyceal calculi reduces blood loss.

In order to avoid blood-borne infections, patients can be asked to donate their own blood. Up to three pints of blood can be drawn, over the 7–10 days prior to surgery. Administration of iron supplements ensures a rapid build-up of haemoglobin levels prior to surgery. This is cost-effective and eliminates the need for hepatitis and AIDS screening of donated blood.

The mortality of open operations on the kidney in third world countries – where operations are done for complex stones in less than ideal circumstances with limited blood transfusion services, and ill-monitored anaesthesia – is higher than in the West, where mortality for open surgery is 0.9% and percutaneous nephrolithotomy (PCNL) 0.7%. ESWL has no direct mortality. There has been no stone open operation related mortality at the Aga Khan University Medical Center (AKUMC) in the last ten years.

Operations involve the anaesthesia team, and use of operating rooms and hospital beds. A larger team is needed than in lithotripsy and operating room time is blocked for 2–3 hours per case. In open surgery, in-patient hospitalization averages 6 days, most patients being fit for discharge on the fourth postoperative day. Arrone *et al.* [2] have shown that the mean hospital stay for PCNL and ESWL is 8.7 and 2.9 days respectively. We perform ESWL as a day care procedure in 85% of patients. Many are incapacitated by the long incision required by open surgery and require longer admission. The return to work is delayed. The average stay for PCNL is similar to that for open surgery but patients can return to work in a short time. By contrast ureteroscopy (URS) can be done as ESWL is done, on an ambulatory basis.

How often is open surgery needed?

With the striving for improvement in stone management with minimal patient discomfort and rapid return to routine life activities, open surgery is performed for only 2–5% [3, 4] of stones in the West. In one series of 893 procedures, only 23 were ureterolithotomies, 8 anatrophic nephrolithotomies, 3 pyelolithotomies, and 2 partial nephrectomies. Of the ureterolithotomies, 16 were after unsuccessful ureteroscopy [3]. Boyle *et al.* [4], analysing 2474 procedures, noted that 65% were treated by ESWL, 18% by ureteroscopies, 15% by PCNL and 2% by open surgery.

In the Philippines, 64% of private and 57% of non-private patients had surgery when the renal stone could have been removed by other means. This was because of the non-availability of ESWL to all sectors. Thirty-seven per cent of private but only 11% of non-private patients underwent ESWL; it is believed that economic factors were the most important determinant [5].

At the Holy Family Hospital (personal data), between 1979 and 1983, at a time when ureteroscopes, and C arm imaging were not available, we 'operated' on 283 patients with urinary stone. The 213 available records showed that 33.8% had pyelolithotomy, 7.4% nephrolithotomy, 2.3% nephrectomy, 3.2% partial nephrectomy, 15.7% ureterotomy, 7.9% Dormia basket aided extraction, 19.0% cystolithotomy, 4.6% litholapaxy, and 6.1% extraction of a urethral calculus.

Table 10.1 Proportion of 170 patients (95 with renal calculi, 27 with ureteric and 8 with vesical calculi) treated on the lithotriptor in the first half of 1995 at AKUMC

Renal calculi (n = 102)	
ESWL	93%
Pyelolithotomy	7%
Ureteric calculi (n = 46)	
ESWL	59%
Ureterolithotomy	2%
Ureteroscopy	39%
Vesical calculi (n = 22)	
ESWL	36%
Cystolithotomy	9%
Litholapaxy	55%

At AKUMC, ESWL was available in November 1988. In the 2.5 years from July 1988 to December 1990, 843 patients underwent ESWL, 631 had operations or endoscopic extraction. In 1995 (January to June), 24% had treatment by methods other than ESWL. In 1989, of all procedures for stone other than ESWL, 50% had open surgery (20% pyelolithotomy, 1% nephrectomy, 25% ureterolithotomy, 4% cystolithotomy) and 50% endoscopic extraction. Endoscopic procedures performed were: PCNL in 9%, URS in 31%, transurethral removal or litholapaxy in 10%. In 1995 (January to June), only 24% of patients required treatment other than ESWL and only 7% of renal stones required pyelolithotomy, 2% of ureteric stones required ureterolithotomy, and 9% of bladder stones required cystolithotomy.

These proportions will continually change as experience, expertise and judgement develop. These figures show progression towards endoscopic procedures and away from open procedures, as time allowed sequential purchase of technological innovations and extension of surgical skills.

References

1. Charig CR, Webb DR, Payer SR *et al.* Comparison of treatment of renal calculi by open surgery, percutaneous nephrolithotomy and extracorporeal shockwave lithotripsy. Br Med J 1986; 292:879–82.
2. Arrone LJ, Braham RL, Rielhe R. Cost effectiveness of ESWL. Urology 1988;31:225–30.
3. Assimos D, Boyce WH, Harrison LH *et al.* Role of open surgery since ESWL. J Urol 1989;142:263–7.
4. Boyle E, Segura J, Patterson D *et al.* Role of open surgery in stone disease. J Urol 1987;137:243A.
5. Arada E. Quest for high technology. The Asian regional effect in Philippines. Abstract D12, in the 2nd Asian Congress in Urology, 1993. Asian Urological Association, 1993:D12.

11. Choices, limitations, hazards and value of technology in the treatment of lithiasis

JAMSHEER TALATI

Modern technology has provided two major advances in stone therapy: the production of endoscopes through which stones can be destroyed by a variety of fragmenting modalities; and the extracorporeal lithotriptor, where shock waves produced outside the body, are focused on to the stones to destroy them without any obvious porthole of entry.

Endoscope assisted lithotripsy, lithotomy and nephrectomy

The ureteroscope allows endoscopic removal of ureteral calculi; the nephroscope allows percutaneous removal of renal calculi; and the laparoscope has been used for pyelolithotomy and stone related nephrectomy.

Endoscopic management (compared to open surgery) reduces morbidity and allows a rapid return to work. Major complications can occur: haemorrhage, perforation of the pelvis or ureter, and stricture. Endoscopic fragmentation requires X-ray monitoring and exposure of the patient to radiation is an additional hazard.

A large variety of fragmenting modalities can be introduced through endoscopes. Ultrasound probes either drill the stone (lithotriesis) or fragment it by mini-shock waves. Lithotriesis requires pressure applied against the stone. Fragmenting modalities using ultrasound is less prone to causing perforations (of the bladder, ureter or pelvis) than electro-hydraulic lithotripsy (EHL) probes, but pressure on the stone without counter pressure from a Dormia basket ensnaring the stone in the ureter, may lead to expulsion of the stone through an erosion in the ureter. The probes are much thicker than the electro-hydraulic probes, and cannot be introduced through 7Fr scopes. Electro-hydraulic lithotripsy (EHL) produces a shock wave through a spark discharged across the gap of a coaxial cable. Care must be taken to ensure that the electrode does not jump off the stone during the application of the shock wave, and so perforate the ureter or pelvis (during percutaneous pyelolithotony). This can be done by drilling a hole into large stones by ultrasound lithotriesis, and placing the EHL probe in this cavity to 'anchor' it and avoid the jump out effect. The repeated hammer like impacts of an electro-mechanical impacter can fragment stones, as can the ultrasound vibrations produced in the special fine steel probes of the lithoclast. The laser produces vaporization of the stone transmitted through a fine fibre, but remains very costly.

1 Talati et al. (eds) The Management of Lithiasis, 89–93
© *1997 Kluwer Academic Publishers. Printed in Great Britain.*

The ureteroscope has the potential for damaging the ureter with consequent sepsis and stricture. The smaller ureteroscope (7Fr) should be used to reduce trauma. These also have other advantages – ureteral dilatation is not required and hence the integity of the ureteric orifice in maintained; introduction and manoeuvring is facilitated, and success rates increase. The lithoclast and laser can be used through these scopes.

Extracorporeal shock wave lithotripsy

Extracorporeal shock wave lithotripsy (ESWL) allows fragmentation of stones within the body by focused shock waves produced outside the body. Lithotriptors are equipped with a shock wave generator, a focusing mechanism, and a monitoring mechanism which allows the operator to visualize stone fragmentation. Lithotriptors vary in their energy source (electromagnetic, electro-hydraulic or piezo-electric) and system for monitoring stone destruction (ultrasound or radiological). The piezo-electric machines and the Dornier MPL 9000 are ultrasound monitored. Piezo-electric shock wave lithotriptors usually have a small focus and an ultrasound monitor; in general they produce less tissue damage. The Dornier MPL 9000 produces shock waves electro-hydraulically but has a very small focus. The HM4 (Dornier) monitors fragmentation radiologically, and the Lithostar (Siemen) and MPL X have both modalities. Each combination method has advantages and disadvantages, some of which are more important in ureteric stones.

Radiologically monitored lithotriptors (RML)

Although RML have the ability to visualize stones in all sections of the urinary tract, ancillary measures are required to visualize radiolucent stones, and biliary stones in the gallbladder cannot be treated. Before treatment with RML, non-opaque stones need to be opacified by coating them with solutions containing barium, strontium, ytterbium or gadolinium (all still experimental) through a retrograde ureteric catheter. Alternatively, stones can be demonstrated as filling defects by intermittent or continuous retrograde instillation of radiocontrast through flushing double J (DJ) stents or ureteral catheters.

Whilst stones in any section of the ureter can be localized, there may be difficulty in localizing stones near the spine. This can be overcome by placing the patient prone.

The disadvantage of RML is the risk of irradiation to the patient, which forces the operator to minimize fluoroscopic imaging. Hence the image is obtained at intervals, fragmentation cannot be monitored continuously, and it cannot be ensured that the shock waves are on target rather than on the kidney. In the older generation lithotriptors (HM3, Dornier) with a large focus (120 mm), the stone remained in the focus, unlike current machines which have much smaller foci. These reduce renal cell damage, but require better and continuous visualization of the target. Some

RML incorporate respiratory gating (through a sensor applied to the chest) which prevents the machine firing if a patient takes a deep breath.

Irradiation dose during radiologically monitored lithotripsy
The dose of irradiation received by the patient has been calculated from film badges. These are not affected by shock waves [1] and can be placed in watertight rubber gloves when testing immersion type (HM3) lithotriptors.

The patient's skin receives 1–30 rem, average 10 rem (100 mSv) per treatment on the affected side, and 0.1–21 rem from the opposite fluoroscopy unit. Exit dose at the lower abdomen averages 13 rem, and female gonadal dose 100 mrem (1.2 mSv) [1]. In comparison, a KUB X-ray gives 1.5 mSv, an intravenous pyelogram 4.6 mSv, a computerized tomography of the abdomen 4.6 mSv, and a radionuclide renal study 0.7 mSv (these are effective doses derived from a weighted sum of equivalent doses – in millisieverts – to a number of tissues, where the weightage depends upon the risk of fatal malignancy for low dose radiation). Skill in moving the gantry reduces radiation dose [2], with entrance dose varying from 2.64 rad when experienced surgeons are doing the procedure, to 3.38 rad for inexperienced ones. Fluoroscopy imaging time may vary from 2–3.5 minutes. Irradiation of personnel during lithotripsy is considered in Chapter 32.

Because patients will be subjected to further ionizing radiation from X-rays during follow-up, and as stone disease is recurrent, lithotriptors which do not utilize ionizing radiation as the sole monitoring modality should be preferred.

Ultrasound monitored lithotriptors (USML)

USML can localize both radiopaque and radiolucent calculi, allowing treatment of urate stones and gallstones. The disadvantage of USML lies in the inability to visualize sections of the ureter. Ureteric stones up to 2 cm below the lower pole of the kidney can be easily visualized as can those below the level of the ischial spine [3]. The extent to which the remaining ureter can be identified is operator dependent [4], but obesity, close proximity to the transverse process and intestinal gas can interfere with localization. For the ureter, we have defined sections in order to assist physicians in identifying which sections can be easily located on ultrasound [3].

The inability to visualize stones in the middle sections of the ureter adds to the cost of therapy as the stones have to be pushed up before therapy.

Whilst localization of ureteric stones becomes more difficult on USM lithotriptors, we have used ESWL for 57% of our ureteric stone patients in 1990, a proportion similar to others using RM lithotriptors [5]. Additionally the push-up rate is not higher when using USM: of the patients treated for ureteric stones, 39% were treated by ESWL *in situ*, only 18% (compared with 21% in Schmidt's series) needing push-up [3]. Schmidt *et al.* [5] compared localization and treatment on radiological and ultrasound monitored lithotriptors and reported similar success rates. Not all stones are easily visualized even on the RML. Cole and Shuttleworth [6] using Dornier HM3, a RML, attributed their failure with RM lithotripsies to inability to localize the stone. Middleton *et al.* [7], in a double-blind study, has

Table 11.1   Comparison between lithotriptors with piezoelectric shock wave generation and electrohydraulic shock wave generation

Author	% with stone size			Lithotriptor	% stone free
	< 2 cm	2–3 cm	> 3 cm		
Kim *et al.*	81.5	13.8	4.7	Piezoelectric	73.4 (95.6 for stones < 1 cm and 52.6 for > 3 cm)
Miller *et al.*	91.0	9.0	–	Piezoelectric	36–55 (55–65 for ureteral particles < 4 mm)
Talati *et al.*	58.3	27.1	14.6	MPL9000 ESWL	60.7 (72.8 at six months)

Reproduced by permission of Williams & Wilkins from Talati J. *et al.* Extracorporeal shock wave lithotripsy for urinary tract stones using MPS 9000 spark gap technology ultrasound monitoring. *J Urology* 1991;146:1482–86 [a]. Please see references 8 and 10 for data from Kim *et al.* and Miller *et al.*

shown the ability of ultrasound to detect 91–96% of stones. Urologists educated in previous decades, during the period of ascendancy of the X-ray, were initially averse to using ultrasound. Current urologists are more at home with ultrasound monitored lithotriptors.

Thus USM when combined with electro-hydraulic shock wave generation is not a real disadvantage. In fact, ultrasound monitoring has the additional advantage over RM, of treating urate stones. The ultrasound probe can also be used for pre-operative evaluation of patients with stone and post-treatment assessment of hydronephrosis and adequacy of fragmentation.

Monitoring and shock wave combinations

It is advantageous to purchase a machine with electro-hydraulic shock wave generation and ultrasound monitoring, and perhaps ideally have both X-rays and ultrasound control as in the MPL-X.

The extracorporeal piezo-electric (EPL) shock waves have the special advantage of producing a very fine powder, and hence *steinstrassen* are an infrequent complication, prophylactic stenting is unnecessary and the ancillary procedure rate is low. Another advantage is that the treatment is almost pain free. However, treatment on EPL requires a larger number of repeat visits. Even with small stone burdens, Kim *et al.* [8] report that the average number of sittings as 1.6 per patient (see Table 11.1). Patients with stones less than 1 cm needed two sittings and those with stones greater than 3 cm needed up to nine sittings. This has to be balanced against the fact that renal damage may be less, as evidenced by no or minimal changes on the CT scan and MRI, and that there is lower urinary enzyme loss after EPL as compared to ESWL; all are attributable to the narrow focus and the fact that ultrasound monitoring targets shock waves onto the stone more consistently.

Successful lithotripsy can however be performed by EPL, as has been shown by a group in The Netherlands (see Chapter 36).

References

1. Bush WH, Jones D, Gibbons RJ. Radiation dose to patient and personnel during ESWL. J Urol 1987;138:716–19.
2. Chen WC, Lee YH, Chen MT *et al.* Factors influencing radiation exposure during ESWL. Scand J Urol 1991;25:223–6.
3. Talati J, Khan LA, Noordzij J *et al.* The scope and place of ultrasound monitored ESWL in a multi-modality setting and the effects of experiential audit evoked changes on the management of ureteral calculi. Br J Urol 1994;73:480–6.
4. DiClemente L, D'Andrea R, DiNardo A *et al.* In situ treatment of ureteral stones with the drum lithotriptor MPL 9000. Domin User Letter, December 1991;7:12–16.
5. Schmidt A, Rasswieler J, Gumpinger R *et al.* Minimally invasive treatment of ureteric calculi using modern techniques. Br J Urol 1990;65:242–9.
6. Cole RS, Shuttleworth KED. Is ESWL suitable treatment of lower ureteric stones? Br J Urol 1988;62:525–30.
7. Middleton WD, Dodds WJ, Lawson TL *et al.* Renal calculi, sensitivity for detection with US. Radiology 1988;167:239–44.
8. Kim SC, Moon YT, Kim KD. Extracorporeal shockwave lithotripsy monotherapy: Experience with piezoelectric second generation lithotriptor in 642 patients. J Urol 1989;142:674.
9. Talati J, Shah T, Memon A *et al.* ESWL for urinary tract stones using MPL 9000 spark gap technology and ultrasound monitoring. J Urol 1991;146:1482–6.
10. Miller HC, Collins LA, Turbow AM *et al.* Initial EDAP LT01 lithotripsy group experience in the United States. J Urol 1989;142:1412.

12. Bioeffects of shock waves: An overview

JAMES E. LINGEMAN

Shock wave lithotripsy (SWL) clearly induces acute injury to the kidney and surrounding tissues in a majority, if not all, SWL patients. All patients who receive more than 200 shocks show gross haematuria as a result of direct damage to the renal parenchyma. Approximately 63–85% of all SWL patients exhibit one or more forms of acute renal injury as determined by MRI and quantitative radionuclide renography. A majority of SWL patients have elevated serum and urinary enzymes, implying significant acute trauma to the kidney and adjacent tissues such as the liver and skeletal muscle. While gastric or duodenal erosion are the most common extrarenal complications of SWL, other complications include myocardial infarction, cerebral vascular accidents, pulmonary contusion, ileus, pancreatitis and brachial plexus palsy.

The two most common renal side-effects seen immediately after SWL are haemorrhage and oedema within or around the kidney. Accumulation of perirenal and subcapsular fluid (blood or urine) occurs in up to 32% of patients. Frequently, the kidney is enlarged and there is a loss of corticomedullary demarcation, both suggestive of acute intrarenal oedema. While the perirenal fluid disappears within a few days, the subcapsular fluid or blood may take six months or more to be reabsorbed. At times, the haemorrhage may be so severe as to reduce renal blood flow, sometimes permanently, and to require blood transfusions. Knapp *et al.* first suggested that patients with existing hypertension were more likely than normotensives to develop perinephric haematomas. Newman and Saltzman confirmed this suggestion. In addition, they noted that patients with coagulopathies and thrombocytopenia had an even higher risk of developing subcapsular haematomas after being treated with SWL. The significance of a subcapsular haematoma to chronic changes in renal function has not been determined.

Histopathological studies performed on biopsy material from SWL-treated kidneys at about one week post-SWL showed marked tubular, vascular, and interstitial changes localized to the plane of the pressure wave. Interstitial oedema and haemorrhage extended from the capsule to the corticomedullary junction. Most renal capsules in these areas were disrupted, while the tubules showed mild degenerative changes and accumulation of haemosiderin granules and cast material. Alterations in the microvasculature included dilatation, endothelial damage and thrombus formation. These observations suggest that all portions of the kidney are

J. Talati et al (eds) The Management of Lithiasis, 95–105
© *1997 Kluwer Academic Publishers. Printed in Great Britain.*

vulnerable to shock waves, but that the microvasculature may be the most susceptible.

Acute changes in renal function have not been fully characterized in SWL patients; only a few studies have attempted to follow renal function post-SWL. Kaude *et al.* found an immediate decrease in effective renal plasma flow, measured by renal scans, in 30% of kidneys treated with SWL. Several investigators noted delayed or no excretion of contrast media by treated kidneys in the absence of ureteral obstruction, and acute renal failure has been reported in a few patients. Others have observed transient, SWL-induced increases in the excretion of tubular enzymes or albumin which suggest, respectively, damage to tubules and glomeruli. All of these studies indicate that renal function is altered in one way or another by SWL, and they disagree with the initial reports by Chaussey who found improved renal function after SWL; however, renal obstruction was present in some of his patients prior to treatment and improved function would be expected once the obstruction was removed. What is not known at this point is whether renal function is altered in every patient treated with SWL, or only in a subset of patients, and whether changes in renal function persist? Moreover, it is not known whether patients with two kidneys tolerate SWL better than those with one kidney. Another interesting observation is that some patients with pre-existing hypertension require higher doses of their blood pressure medication following SWL, suggesting that pre-existing hypertension is a risk factor for adverse effects of SWL.

To date, little information exists on chronic changes in blood pressure after SWL, but new information has been accumulating. Several centres have reported an increase in new onset hypertension following SWL. Lingeman *et al.* reported in 1991 that diastolic pressure was elevated several years post-SWL. The calculated elevation was small (0.78 mmHg), but since it represented an annualized value it had the potential to presage a significant, long-term elevation of blood pressure. The pivotal question to be asked regarding that observation was not whether it represented a physiologically significant elevation of blood pressure, but whether or not it reflected an annual rate of rise of blood pressure that could be expected to occur in subsets of SWL patients. At that time, as well as now, this report represented the largest group of patients from which follow-up information on post-SWL blood pressure has been obtained.

Lingeman *et al.* have recently reported a four-year follow-up on blood pressure in this group of patients. Their findings are both interesting and puzzling. Diastolic pressure remained significantly higher than that in the non-SWL treated controls. The annualized rise in diastolic blood pressure that had been detected at the follow-up date was no longer apparent at the four-year follow up; indeed, blood pressure seemed to have stabilized, although diastolic pressure was significantly lower in the non-SWL treated controls. The investigators concluded that, four-years post-SWL, small but detectable differences in diastolic blood pressure persist between patients who have been treated with SWL and patients who have not. The task at hand for the present would therefore seem to be to determine the functional significance of the elevated blood pressure in some SWL patients.

Additional reports have added to the growing suspicion that, at least for some patients, SWL may pose a risk for the development of hypertension. Indeed, Yokoyama *et al.* reported a statistically significant elevation of diastolic pressure (approaching 5 mmHg) in patients who had received 3000 or more shocks. This report underscores the earlier findings by Lingeman *et al.* and points to the possibility that a subgroup of SWL patients may be at greater risk of developing hypertension.

The study of Yokoyama *et al*, which also included annualized blood pressure data derived from 192 patients, has been cited as contradictory to the findings of Lingeman *et al.* in that Yokoyama *et al.* did not detect a statistically significant elevation of diastolic blood pressure (annualized). It merits mentioning, however, that Yokoyama *et al.* calculated an annualized increase in diastolic blood pressure of 0.78 mmHg, which is identical to the value that was calculated by Lingeman *et al.* Whereas the increase seen by Lingeman *et al.* was statistically significant, that seen by Yokoyama *et al.* was not. However, since the study of Yokoyama *et al.* was more than four times smaller than that of Lingeman *et al.*, it is quite likely that the difference in statistical interpretation reflects this large difference in sample size (765 vs. 192 patients).

In view of the foregoing indication that SWL may be associated with gradual long-term elevations of blood pressure, renal damage caused by SWL could be the causative factor. Williams *et al.* observed a significant decrease in effective renal plasma flow at 17–21 months post-SWL in patients with two kidneys, and Brito *et al.* have noted that patients with a solitary kidney showed elevated serum creatinine levels five years post-SWL. Williams and Thompson have reported a permanent reduction in renal blood flow coupled with hypertension in patients treated with SWL.

All the above data have been collected in adult patients. However, 1–3% of all urolithiasis cases occur in the paediatric population. The successful use of SWL in adults has led to its use in the treatment of renal stones in paediatric patients. However, only a few report on the effects of SWL in children have been published. It has been suggested that fewer shock waves should be delivered in children, and that the positioning of the paediatric patient is more important than it is for adults. Firm conclusions cannot yet be drawn about the safety of SWL in children.

Bioeffects of shock waves

FARHAT ABBAS

In recent years, the potential of shock waves to induce biological damage has commanded much attention. Clinical and experimental studies have defined structural and functional changes in the kidneys and adjacent organs, and questioned their effects on renal growth in children. New onset hypertension in patients exposed to shock waves has been an issue of debate. A mutagenic effect on embryos and female ovaries has been speculated, as, simultaneously, application of focused shock waves for therapy of solid human neoplasms has emerged. Radiation exposure to the patients in X-ray imaged machines is an additional risk unrelated to shock waves, which however is absent in ultrasound-imaged machines.

Therapeutically, shock wave lithotripsy (SWL) has undoubtedly revolutionized stone disease management; but how safe is SWL? From existing data we can attempt to derive recommendations for minimizing biological damage. The important issues to comprehend are the nature and underlying mechanism of injury, tissue susceptibility, factors promoting tissue damage and the long-term sequelae. In spite of growing concern, extracorporeal SWL (ESWL) appears to be well tolerated with a mortality of 0.02% (in 62 000 patients – AUA Lithotripsy Committee, 1987) with most deaths not a direct result of SWL.

Renal structural changes

Transient haematuria, observed in almost all patients, occurs from localized parenchymal trauma, and not from the shrapnel effect from stone fragments.

Grantham *et al.* [1] noted that renal enlargement is seen in IV urograms in 26% of patients immediately after SWL, but most cases in his series had obstructing ureteral stones. Others note a 9% increase in size of treated kidneys on computed tomography (CT) [2]. Evaluation with MRI has shown post-ESWL renal enlargement in 69–84% [3–5]. This is thought to indicate parenchymal and perinephric fluid collection. Other acute changes include intrarenal and subcapsular haematomas, loss of corticomedullary demarcation and low intensity perinephric fat changes. These studies were done on the Dornier HM3 lithotriptor which is a powerful machine with relatively large shock wave focal size. No morphological alteration was detected on MRI in 20 cases following extracorporeal piezo-electric lithotripsy (EPL) [6]. In a comparative study, Miller *et al.* [7] found evidence of acute injury on MRI in only 6.7% of patients after EPL (on the Wolf-Piezolith) as compared to 50% after electro-hydraulic (EH) SWL (on the Dornier HM3). This

J. Talati et al. (eds) The Management of Lithiasis, 98–105
© *1996 Kluwer Academic Publishers. Printed in Great Britain.*

difference was attributed to the mode of shock wave generation and the small focus in EPL. Morris *et al.* [8] confirmed larger areas of acute change with EH and electromagnetic (EM) lithotriptors compared to EPL, in rabbits, but there was no difference in functional derangement or extent of pathologic damage at four weeks.

Perinephric haematomas have been reported in 0.66% of 3208 patients treated on HM3 [9]. In subsets of hypertensives the incidence of haematomas was 2.5%; in poorly controlled hypertensives the incidence of developing haematomas was 3.8%. There was no correlation with the number or energy of shock waves [9]. Other investigators have also identified uncontrolled hypertension, and also diabetes mellitus, aspirin and non-steroidal analgesic use as risk factors for subcapsular haematoma formation [10, 11]. Bleeding diathesis, unless fully corrected, is an absolute contraindication to SWL.

Biological damage may follow septic complications and urinary tract obstruction, which are discussed in other chapters.

Factors influencing biological damage by shock waves have been studied in various animal models. The morphological alterations appear to be dose-dependent [12–14]. In the initial studies by Chaussey, no acute or chronic histological changes were detected in dogs subjected to 500 shock waves [15]. Later studies on the same animal model by Thibault *et al.* [16], Jaeger *et al.* [17], and Neisius *et al.* [18] (who used clinical doses of shock waves) showed parenchymal and subcapsular haematomas, venous thrombi and tubular damage. The number of intraparenchymal haematomas seen on MRI increases with the number of shock waves [19, 20] and applied energy (voltage) [21]. Splicing out required large doses into multiple small dose treatments reduces damage [14, 22].

Data addressing long-term structural changes in humans following SWL are limited. In clinical studies complete resolution of acute renal and perirenal changes is seen at three months on MRI [5], and no adverse effects can be seen at three years on plain X-ray (KUB) and ultrasound [23]. Animal studies suggest that acute damage may progress to focal areas of fibrosis involving up to 1% renal volume, usually without concomitant functional deterioration. In a minipig model, large scars have been seen at the injury site on MRI evaluation at six months [24]. In dogs, diffuse interstitial fibrosis, calcification, nephron loss, dilated veins and cortical scars extending into the medulla, are seen at four weeks after 1800–8000 shocks [25].

Alterations in renal function

Various physiological parameters have been studied to detect functional derangement following shock wave application. Glomerular filtration rate (GFR) remains unaffected [26], or shows a transient suppression which returns to baseline in most cases [27]. Significant reduction in GFR was seen after 2792 shock waves in patients with solitary kidneys [28], but there was minimal change with 1600 [27] and 2253 [26] shocks. In a dog model, 1500 shock waves produced no change in GFR [29], but marked reduction in GFR, which however returned to normal in 24 hours, was demonstrated with 3000 shocks [30]. A dose-dependent suppression in GFR which normalized at six months was noted in a minipig model [24]. In animal studies GFR returns to normal in the long term [31, 32]; but in patients with chronic renal failure or solitary kidneys, Chandhoke *et al.* [33] noted depressed GFR at 41.5 months post-SWL.

An immediate decrease in effective renal plasma flow (ERPF) following lithotripsy has been noted in 33% patients treated on HM3 [3], but there is no significant change following EPL [34]. ERPF, unlike GFR, is unaffected in patients with solitary kidneys [28]. Suppression in ERPF is dose-dependent in some animals [24, 35], but Evans *et al.* [36] and Miller *et al.* [31] found no immediate or long-term suppression in ERPF in a minipig model respectively. Chaussey [15] showed normal function on iodohippurate renal scan in patients at four years, whilst Williams and Thomas [37] found a significant decrease in ERPF at 17–21 months after SWL. Simultaneous bilateral treatment could result in permanent functional deterioration as evidenced by a clinical [38] and experimental animal study [35]. Tubular function appears to be only transiently reduced in clinical studies [6, 26, 27] and rapidly reverts to normal. Blood chemistry is not altered [32] and only mild cellular changes are observed [39].

Enzyme studies

Renal and adjacent tissue injury following SWL has been assessed by monitoring specific urinary and serum enzymes as markers of biological damage. Elevation in urinary N-acetyl-glucosaminidase (NAG) and alkaline phosphatase (ALP) has been shown to be a sensitive and specific marker of proximal tubular damage [26, 28, 40, 41]. Enzymuria however, is transient and in most studies reverts to normal in two to three weeks. Also, the level of elevation appears to correlate with the number of shock waves administered. Enzyme studies also suggest that the degree of tissue damage could be dependent on the shock wave focal size and the type of machine [13, 42, 43]. Damage to muscle, liver and spleen could follow exposure to large doses of shock waves as demonstrated by elevated urinary excretion of lactate de-hydrogenase (LDH), glutamic oxaloacetic transaminase (GOT), glutamic pyruvic transaminase (GPT) and gamma glutamyl transferase (GGT) [42, 43, 44]. Again the changes are transient and rapidly return to normal. As expected, no long-term de-rangement in enzyme levels has been demonstrated following lithotripsy.

Hypertension following SWL

Development of hypertension as a long-term sequela to SWL remains a controversial issue. Retrospective studies have shown an incidence of 0.65–8.2% of new-onset hypertension in patients having undergone SWL [45–49]. Worsening of pre-existing hypertension is reported. The hypothesis that SWL produces small vessel changes in the kidney resulting in hypertension could not be substantiated by other workers who failed to demonstrate any significant long-term elevation in blood pressure [50–52]. Similarly the incidence of hypertension in patients having had shock wave treatment should be matched with the expected yearly incidence in the general population which Lingeman *et al.* [50] calculated to be 2–3.5% in white men aged 25–54 years. Although at present there is significant concern, the issue remains unresolved and controlled prospective studies are required to provide more definitive answers.

Extra-renal side-effects

Most patients tolerate SWL well without any serious side-effects. Shock waves are however known to damage chick embryo [53], and pregnancy is hence an absolute contraindication. Lung parenchyma is damaged if exposed during treatment and should be shielded by styrofoam, especially in children and adults with chest deformities. Most of the reported complications have occurred in a small number of patients and include gastric or duodenal erosions [54], colonic injury [55], pancreatitis [56, 57], pneumonitis [56] and nerve palsies. Shock waves can induce extrasystole and special recommendations should be adhered to while subjecting patients with a pacemaker to lithotripsy [58].

McCullough *et al.* [59] demonstrated no adverse effects of SWL on rat ovaries. It is difficult to extrapolate this information for clinical use on young women undergoing lithotripsy for pelvic ureteral calculi. Newman *et al.* [25] showed no spinal cord damage in a dog model using 2000–6000 shock waves, but epiphyseal growth plate abnormalities have been noted in experimental immature rats [60], though no bone growth abnormalities are described in humans.

At present SWL appears to produce no long-term damage to adjacent organs.

Renal growth

Do shock waves induce any growth restriction in paediatric kidneys? In infant rabbits, focal cortical and capsular scarring did not lead to long-term growth restriction or functional deterioration [61, 62]. Paediatric sheep kidneys exposed to 2000 shocks at 21 kV exhibited only marginally reduced weight compared to the contralateral control kidneys, with no difference in GFR or ERPF at one year [63]. One study in rhesus monkeys has shown a dose-dependent reduction in ERPF, especially after bilateral ESWL, but growth has not been studied [35]. In view of limited data, especially in humans, more studies are needed to establish the safety of shock wave treatment in the paediatric age group.

Minimizing biological damage

Given the present day understanding of mechanisms and factors responsible for biological damage, we can attempt to formulate certain recommendations to ensure minimal biological damage.

–   The renal morphological and functional abnormalities appear to be dose-
    dependent. Two recent studies suggest 1000 [64] and 2000 [65] shock waves at
    18 kV on the Dornier HM3 lithotriptor as the maximum safe limit per session.

Food and Drug Administration (FDA) guidelines restrict the patient to 2000 shocks/kidney/day on the electro-hydraulic lithotriptor.

– The lowest possible level of energy power (kilovoltage) should be used for stone fragmentation since it may be an important determinant of tissue damage [21, 24].

– Rapid firing (100 shocks versus 1 shock per second) [66] and administering shock waves in pairs [67] could augment damage.

– Dividing a large shock wave dose into multiple small dose treatments (bi-weekly) produces less acute and chronic damage [14, 22].

– A minimum of 2–5 days is recommended as a safe interval between treatments [68].

– Stone size, stone composition and location determine the number of shock waves required for fragmentation. Combining SWL with other modalities or alternate modes of treatment should be considered where a large dose of shock wave is anticipated. Unfortunately the safe upper limit is not known.

– The extent of damage could be related to the shock wave focal size and the type of shock wave generator. Less damage is anticipated with machines utilizing a small focal size [8].

– Accurate stone focusing and avoidance of 'blast path' lithotripsy is likely to require a lesser number of shock waves and hence less damage.

– Fegan *et al.* [69] have suggested pretreatment use of mannitol or verapamil to protect kidneys from relative hypoxic injury due to capillary disruption and tissue oedema following SWL.

– Obstruction distal to stone should be corrected or bypassed with a stent, and pre-existing hypertension, urinary tract infection and diabetes mellitus should be properly controlled prior to SWL to prevent avoidable complications causing renal damage.

– Uncontrolled bleeding diathesis and pregnancy are absolute contraindications to SWL.

– Platelet inhibiting medicines such as aspirin and non-steroidal antiinflammatory agents should be withheld 2–3 weeks prior to therapy to minimize the chances of sub-capsular haematoma formation.

– Whenever possible, simultaneous bilateral treatments for renal stones should be avoided. Very careful treatment with regular monitoring is advised in patients with a solitary kidney and those with chronic renal failure.

– Infection and urinary tract obstruction following SWL should be promptly and aggressively treated.

– Children undergoing SWL should have their lungs shielded with styrofoam padding. The lowest possible energy and number of shock waves should be used for treatment.

References

1. Grantham JR, Millner MR, Kande JV *et al.* Renal stone disease treated with extracorporeal shock wave lithotripsy: Short term observation in 100 patients. Radiology 1986;158:203–6.

2. Rubin JI, Arger PH, Pollack HM *et al.* Kidney changes after extracorporeal shock wave lithotripsy: CT evaluation. Radiology 1987;162:21–4.

3. Kaude JV, Williams CM, Millner MR *et al.* Renal morphology and function immediately after ESWL. Am J Roentgenol 1985;145:305–13.

4. Baungartner BR, Dikey KW, Ambrose SS *et al.* Kidney changes after extracorporeal shock wave lithotripsy: Appearance on MR imaging. Radiology 1987;163:531.

5. Dyer RB, Karstaedt N, McCullough DL *et al.* Magnetic resonance imaging evaluation of immediate and intermediate changes in kidneys treated with extracorporeal shock wave lithotripsy. J Lithotripsy Stone Dis 1990;2:302.

6 Vahlensieck Jr, W, Kurz HJ, Steinhauer H *et al.* Side effects of extracorporeal piezoelectric shock wave lithotripsy (EPL). Urol Res 1990;18:53–6.

7. Miller GL, Wilson WT, Hussman DS *et al.* Deleterious effects of four models of renal stone removal: How does lithotripsy fare? J Urol 1990;143:361A.

8. Morris JS, Husman DA, Wilson WT *et al.* A comparison of renal damage induced by varying modes of shock waves generation. J Urol 1991;145:864–7.

9. Knapp PM, Kulb TB, Lingeman JE *et al.* Extracorporeal shock wave lithotripsy induced perirenal haematomas. J Urol 1988;139:700–3.

10. Saltzman B. Clinically apparent subcapsular haematomas following shock wave lithotripsy. Identification of potential etiologies. J Urol 1990;143:272A.

11. Rius H, Saltzman B. Aspirin induced bilateral renal hemorrhage after extracorporeal shock wave lithotripsy: Implications and conclusions. J Urol 1990;143:791.

12. Recker F, Rubben H, Bex A *et al.* Morphological changes following ESWL in rat kidney. Urol Res 1989;17:229.

13. Robert DM, Eric AS, Sally JC *et al.* Pressure threshold for shockwave induced renal haemorrhage. J Urol 1990;143:230A.

14. Morris JS, Hussman DA, Wilson WT *et al.* Temporal effects of shock wave lithotripsy. J Urol 1991;145:881–3.

15. Chaussey C. *In vitro* and *in vivo* studies on biological systems. In: Chaussey C, editor. Extracorporeal shock wave lithotripsy: Technical concept. Experimental research and clinical application. Basel: S. Karger, 1986;21–68.

16. Thibault P, Doty J, Cotard JP *et al.* Lithotripsy by ultrashort pulsation: Experimental study in renal lithiasis in the dog. Ann Urol (Paris) 1986;20;20.

17. Jaeger P, Redha S, Alund G *et al.* Do shock waves damage the kidney? Morphologic and functional changes of the kidney following exposure to shock waves. Schweiz Med Wochenschr 1989;119:944–9.

18. Neisius D, Seitz G, Gebhardt T *et al.* Dose-dependant influence on canine renal morphology after application of extracorporeal shock waves with Wolf Piezolith. J Endourol 1989;3:337–45.

19. Brendel W. Effect of shock waves on canine kidney. In: Gravenstein JS, Peter K, editors. Extracorporeal shock waves lithotripsy for renal stone disease: Technical and clinical aspects. Stoneham: Butterworths, 1986:141.

20. Delius M, Enders G, Xuan Z *et al.* Biological effects of shock waves: Kidney damage by shock waves in dogs – dose dependance. Ultrasound Med Biol 1988;14:117–22.

21. Muschter R, Schmeller NJ, Schen W *et al.* ESWL and renal damage: An experimental study using the modified Dornier lithotriptor HM 3. Proceedings of the Fifth World Congress on Endourology and ESWL, Cairo, Egypt, 1987:233.

22. Ryan PC, Jones BJ, Kay EW *et al.* Acute and chronic bioeffects of single and multiple doses of Piezoelectric shockwaves (EDAP LT. 01). J Urol 1991;145:399–404.

23. Wolfson B, David R, Fuchs A *et al.* Long-term observations on function and morphology of kidneys receiving multiple treatments with ESWL. J Urol 1990;143:298A.

24. Evan AP, Willis LR, Connors B *et al.* ESWL induces dose dependant changes in renal structure and function in the young mini-pig. J Urol 1990;143:232A.

25. Newman R, Hackett R, Senior DF *et al.* Pathologic effects of ESWL on canine renal tissue. Urology 1987;29:194 200.

26. Karlsen SJ, Berg KJ. Acute changes in kidney function following extracorporeal shock wave lithotripsy for renal stones. Br J Urol 1991;67:241 45.

27. Gilbert BR, Riehle RA, Vaughan JR. Extracorporeal shock wave lithotripsy and its effect on renal function. J Urol 1988;139:482–5.
28. Karlsen SJ, Berg KJ. Acute changes in renal function following ESWL in patients with a solitary functioning kidney. J Urol 1991;145:253–6.
29. Karlsen SJ, Smevik B, Stenstorm J *et al.* Acute physiological changes in canine kidneys following exposure to extracorporeal shock waves. J Urol 1990;143:1280–3.
30. Jaeger P, Constantinides C. Canine kidneys: Changes in blood and urine chemistry after exposure to extracorporeal shockwaves. In: Lingeman JE, Newman DM, editors. Shock wave lithotripsy II. Urinary and biliary lithotripsy. New York: Plenum Press, 1989:7–10.
31. Miller GL, Wilson WT, Hussman DS *et al.* Deleterious effects of four models of renal stone removal: How does lithotripsy fare? J Urol 1990;143:361A.
32. Begun FP, Kuoll CE, Gottlieb M *et al.* Chronic effects of focused electrohydraulic shock waves on renal function and hypertension. J Urol 1991;145:635–9.
33. Chandhoke PS, Albala DM, Clayman RV. Long term comparison of renal function in patients with solitary kidneys and/or moderate renal insufficiency undergoing extracorporeal shock wave lithotripsy or percutaneous nephrolithotomy. J Urol 1992;147:1226–30.
34. Daniel MP, Burns JR. Renal function immediately after piezoelectric extracorporeal lithotripsy (abstract). J Urol 1990;143:298A.
35. Thomas R, Neal DE, Cerniglia FR *et al.* Pediatric extracorporeal shock waves lithotripsy – an animal model. J Urol 1992;147:256A.
36. Evan AP, Willis LR, Connors B *et al.* Shock wave lithotripsy-induced renal injury. Am J Kid Dis 1991;XVII:445–50.
37. Williams CM, Thomas WC. Permanently decreased renal blood flow and hypertension after lithotripsy. N Engl J Med 1989;321:1269–70.
38. Thomas R, Frentz GD. Effect of simultaneous bilateral extracorporeal shock wave lithotripsy on renal function (abstract). J Urol 1992;147:218A.
39. Silverio FD, Gallucci M, Gambardella P *et al.* Blood cellular and biochemical changes after extracoporeal shockwave lithotripsy. Urol Res 1990;18:49–51.
40. Sakamoto W, Kishimoto T, Nakatani T *et al.* Examination of aggravating factors of urinary excretion of N-acetyl-beta-D-glucosaminidase after extracorporeal shock wave lithotripsy. Nephron 1991;58:205–9.
41. Trinchieri A, Zanetti G, Tombolini P *et al.* Urinary NAG excretion after anaesthesia-free extracorporeal lithotripsy of renal stones: A marker of early tubular damage. Urol Res 1990;18:259–62.
42. Kishimoto T, Senju M, Sugimoto T *et al.* Effects of high energy shock wave exposure on renal function during ESWL for kidney stones. Eur Urol 1990;18:290–8.
43. Karlin GS, Schulsinger D, Urivetsky M *et al.* Presence of persisting parenchymal damage after extracorporeal shock wave lithotripsy as judged by excretion of renal tubular enzymes. J Urol 1990;144:13–14.
44. Kishimoto T, Yamamoto K, Sugimoto T *et al.* Side effects of extracorporeal shock wave exposure in patients treated by extracorporeal shock wave lithotripsy for upper urinary tract stone. Eur Urol 1986;12:308–13.
45. Williams CM, Kaude JV, Newman RC *et al.* Extracorporeal shock wave lithotripsy: Long term complications. Am J Roentgenol 1988;150:311–15.
46. Yokoyama M, Shoji F, Yanagizawa R *et al.* Blood pressure changes following extracoporeal shock waves lithotripsy for urolithiasis. J Urol 1992;147:553–8.
47. Zwergel TBH, Neisius D, Zergel UE *et al.* Hypertension after extracorporeal shock wave lithotripsy: Incidence following treatment with Dornier HM-3 lithotriptor or Wolf Piezolith 2300 lithotriptor. In: Lingeman JE, Newman, DM, editors. Shock wave lithotripsy: Urinary and biliary. New York: Plenum Press, 1989.
48. David RD, Wolfson B, Khan M *et al.* Effects of multiple ESWL-procedures. J Urol 1992;147:323A.
49. Lingeman JE, Woods JR, Toth PD. Four year follow up of blood pressure changes following various forms of treatment for nephrolithiasis. J Urol 1992;147:219A.

50. Lingeman JE, Woods JR, Toth PD. Blood pressure changes following extracorporeal shock wave lithotripsy and other forms of treatment for nephrolithiasis. J Am Med Assoc 1990;263:1789–94.
51. Sandlow JI, Winfield HN, Loening SA. Blood pressure changes related to ESWL. J Urol 1989;141:242A.
52. Puppo P, Germinale F, Ricciotti G *et al.* Hypertension after extracorporeal shock wave lithotripsy: A false alarm. J Endourol 1989;3:401.
53. Moran ME, Sandock D, Drach GW. Effects of high energy shock waves on chick embryo development. J Urol 1990;143:167A.
54. AL-Karawi MA, Mohammad AR, El-Etaibi KE *et al.* ESWL induced erosions in upper gastrointestinal tract. Prospective study in 40 patients. Urology 1987;30:224–7.
55. Cass AS. Colonic injury with ESWL for an upper ureteral calculus. In: Newman DM, Lingeman JE, editors. Shock wave lithotripsy. New York: Plenum Publishing, 1988.
56. Drach GW, Dretler SP, Fair WR *et al.* Report of the United States Cooperative study of extracorporeal shock wave lithotripsy. J Urol 1986;135:1127.
57. Lingeman JE, Newman DM, Mertz JHO *et al.* Extracorporeal shock wave lithotripsy: The Methodist Hospital of Indiana experience. J Urol 1986;135:1134.
58. Cooper D, Wilkoff B, Masterson M *et al.* Effects of extracorporeal shock wave lithotripsy on cardiac pacemakers and its safety in patients with implanted cardiac pacemakers. PACE 1988;11:1607–16.
59. McCullough DL, Yeaman LD, Bo W *et al.* Effects of shock waves on the rat ovary. J Urol 1989;141:666.
60. Yeaman LD, Jerone CP, McCullough DL. Effect of shock waves on structure and growth of the immature rat epiphysis. J Urol 1989;141:670.
61. Jones BJ, Connolly JA, Nowlan P *et al.* Paediatric extracorporeal shock waves lithotripsy (abstract). J Urol 1992;147:256A.
62. Kurzweil SJ, Smith JE, Van Arsdalen K *et al.* Effects of extracorporeal shockwaves on skeletal and renal growth in the infant rabbit. J Urol 1988;139:32A.
63. Fusia TJ, Bova S, Langley MJ *et al.* The effect of extracorporeal shockwave lithotripsy on the developing sheep kidney and its function. J Urol 1990;143:231A
64. Thomas R, Roberts J, Sloane B *et al.* Effect of extracorporeal shockwave lithotripsy on renal function. J Endourol 1988;2:141–4.
65. Haupt G, Haupt A, Donovan JM *et al.* Short term changes of laboratory values after extracorporeal shockwave lithotripsy: A comparative study. J Urol 1989;142:259–62.
66. Delius M, Jordan M, Eisenhoefer, H *et al.* Biological effects of shock waves: Kidney haemorrhage by shock waves in dogs – administration rate dependence. Ultrasound Med Biol 1988;14:689–94.
67. Delius M, Mueller W, Goetz A *et al.* Biological effects of shockwaves: Kidney haemmorhage in dogs at a fast shock wave administration rate of fifteen Hertz. J Lithotripsy Stone Dis 1990;2:103–10.
68. Smith LH, Drach G, Hall P *et al.* National high blood pressure education program (NHBPEP). Review paper on complications of shock wave lithotripsy for urinary calculi. Am J Med 1991;91:35–641.
69. Fegan JE, Alexander M, Husmann DA *et al.* Preservation of renal function following extracorporeal shock wave lithotripsy (abstract). J Urol 1992;147:255A.

13. Laser fragmentation of urinary calculi

GRAHAM WATSON and TARIQ K. SHAH

Laser fragmentation techniques use intense light energy to produce a mechanical effect – fragmentation of calculi.

Mechanism of stone destruction

Destruction occurs by photodisintegration, which depends upon the light absorption behaviour (and hence the chemical composition of the stone) as related to the wavelength of the laser, and pulse energy. Light absorption produces charge carriers such as free electrons. Ions and free electrons allow plasma ignition. When the initial electrons absorb energy from the laser, they release further electrons through impact ionization. This creates a plasma, which further heats up under laser energy and expands, and causes a shock wave front at its boundary which fragments the stone, assisted by cavitation and microjets. Once the plasma is ignited by non-linear absorption, stone absorption behaviour and laser wave length cease to be important.

Calcium oxalate dihydrate, monohydrate and calcium carbonate stones and mixed stones reach their plasma thresholds when the laser power density at the stone exceeds 0.8 MW/mm², for a wave length of 755 nm.

Tissue effects of lasers

The effects are thermal, and at higher energy levels tissue ablation can occur. Haemoglobin does not absorb 755 nm. Compared to 500 nm, tissue damage with 755 nm is less. Furthermore the low absorption rate of tissue for 755 nm wave lengths, results in a high threshold for plasma formation. Hence if a plasma is formed due to direct irradiation of the ureteric wall, most of the energy has already been expended in producing the plasma and not much is left for a direct irradiation effect.

As laser light can be transmitted through a very fine fibre, small endoscopes can be used to great advantage when treating ureteric stones by fragmentation.

Early history

The first attempts to fragment calculi were made [1, 2] using continuous wave Nd YAG lasers at 70 W. These lasers proved ineffective and hazardous. Pensel *et al.*

J. Talati et al. (eds) The Management of Lithiasis, 107–112
© 1997 Kluwer Academic Publishers. Printed in Great Britain.

[2] used single giant Q switched pulses (0.00000001 s) of Nd YAG laser energy to fragment certain calculi by focusing the beam onto the stone surface in air. These pulses were greater than 1 joule/pulse and could not be transmitted through quartz fibres. The action was either to fragment the calculi into several large daughter fragments or to have no visible effect at all. Fair [3] showed that an optico-mechanical coupler could be used to produce a shock wave. In this technique again a Q switched Nd YAG laser was directed at a thin layer of aluminium confined between glass and brass. This research confirmed that a measurable shock wave could be produced by a laser pulse. The technique was limited however because the stone could not be broken just by holding the device adjacent to the stone. An Nd YAG laser with a longer pulse duration (100 microseconds; 0.00001 s) using trains of pulses could be transmitted through quartz fibres to fragment certain dark calculi, uric acid calculi and gallstones under water with the fibre in contact with the stone [4]. Uric acid and gallstones could be fragmented well. Pale calculi could only be fragmented if the calculi were stained black.

Because of the obvious importance of stones colour, a Beckman spectrophotometer with integrating sphere was used to study the transmission and remittance of light from 250 to 2500 nm by Watson *et al.* [4]. Back scattered and forward scattered light was collected using the integrating sphere. Any light not leaving the stone was therefore absorbed. Urinary calculi had a common pattern: absorption was powerful in the ultraviolet range with gradually reducing absorption through the visible range from blue to red, reaching a minimum at 1 micron. With increasing wavelength through the infrared, stones absorb according to their chemical composition. Phosphate absorbs at 1.4 microns and water at 2.3 and 10 microns. Knowledge of these data started the development of the first clinical system – the pulsed dye laser [5].

The problems that had to be overcome were to find: a pulse duration that could be transmitted through a fibre; a fibre that would withstand the optical and mechanical phenomenon at the site of stone fragmentation; and a wavelength absorbed sufficiently well by the stone, yet poorly by the surrounding tissue of the ureter. The potential for thermal damage to the tissue had also to be low. The parameters chosen were a pulse duration of 1 microsecond, green light (504 nm) a 200 or 320 micron fibre, and a pulse repetition rate of 5–20 Hz. Though these were designed to be optimal parameters, it was recognized that there were many possible laser systems for stone fragmentation and these will be mentioned below.

The mechanism of stone fragmentation

Stone fragmentation occurs through production of a shock wave. A plasma is a recognized mechanism for the production of a shock wave.

In the initial experiments on stone fragmentation using microsecond laser pulses it was considered that the peak power densities were too low for plasma production.

Plasma formation is characterized by the production of light of multiple wavelengths and a noise. The proof of plasma formation was provided by Teng *et al.* [6], at the Massachusetts General Hospital Wellman Laboratories, who demonstrated both the formation of light of wavelengths other than the initial laser wavelength and a shock wave deformation.

The range of lasers capable of fragmenting calculi

The following range is described in order that each hospital or individual can select the laser that will be most cost-effective for their use. A multipurpose laser will be of less use in a pure urology set-up.

Excimer lasers

These lasers have a very suitable action on the stone with an ablation action on the stone surface creating predominantly vapour and a fine silt. The problems with Excimer lasers are that the standard 10 nanosecond pulses are difficult to transmit through quartz fibres and that the wavelength of the Excimer lasers (which are in the ultraviolet range), is powerfully absorbed by the surrounding tissue. The problem of fibro-transmission is partially solved by increasing the pulse to 100 nanoseconds. However the powerful absorption of the wavelength by tissue results in a laser that can be used to incise tissue. There is less thermal action however than with the longer pulsed lasers, as for example the holmium laser.

Pulsed dye lasers

These operate efficiently at a pulse duration of 1 microsecond which is ideal for stone fragmentation. These lasers can emit at wavelengths from the ultraviolet to the red according to the dye chosen; 504 nm has been selected because of the maximum differential absorption between stone and ureter occurring at this wavelength. In another laser system 590 nm has been chosen because it is probably the most efficient dye rather than because of its being a preferred wavelength.

Alexandrite lasers

The alexandrite laser is a solid state laser of composition Cr: BeAl (2:04) emitting at 720 nm. It is a solid state Q switched laser coupled to a 200 μm quartz fibre. The energy delivery varies from 30–80 mJ. The pulse lasts 625 ns at 30 mJ and 325 ns at 80 mJ. It delivers 1.5–7.8 MW/mm^2 at the stone surface. The pulse duration is typically 10 nanoseconds but this can be stretched to 100 nanoseconds to facilitate fibre transmission. At 10 nanoseconds the relatively poor absorption of 720 nm is not significant because of the short pulse duration and therefore high peak power. The disadvantage is that the fibre erodes rapidly during fragmentation of a stone. Tiny pieces of quartz within the ureteric lumen are of no significance since these will pass. However in an experimental animal model pieces of fibre were found embedded within the ureteric lumen. The longer pulsed alexandrite lasers have a spiky profile. Fibre transmission is significantly improved. Pale calculi are fragmented relatively inefficiently because of the unfavourable absorption at this wavelength.

Titanium sapphire lasers

These are semiconductor lasers and therefore have the potential to be significantly smaller than other lasers. They emit at approximately 850 nm. One author (Watson) has tested the titanium sapphire laser at pulse durations of 3 microseconds and 13 microseconds but with a spiked pulse profile in the former case and a spiked initial profile followed by a smooth tail in the case of the longer pulse duration. The shorter pulse duration was the more efficient, requiring pulse duration of 100 to 200 ms to fragment calculi. The action on pale calculi was relatively inefficient. There was also a prominent impulse on the stone. Perhaps the most awkward of all was the finding that the laser had a variable effect from pulse to pulse as the stone surface altered. There was not the smooth transition on rising above threshold through controlled breakage of small fragments to a more strong mode with cleavage of major fragments and increased propulsion of the stone. However the possibility of developing a semiconductor laser is attractive because of the potential of reducing the size and cost.

Continuous wave neodymium YAG lasers

As with any other continuous wave laser these should never be used to fragment urinary calculi. Pulsing the Nd YAG laser will allow fragmentation but this does not include using a continuous wave Nd YAG laser for short exposure times. The 100 microsecond laser has already been described as having the capability of fragmenting uric acid calculi and gallstones, but not pale calculi. The 10 ns Nd YAG laser has been used at pulse energies of 30 mJ via 100 micron core fibres to fragment calculi. The high peak power allows fragmentation in spite of poor absorption. At these low pulse energies the fibre transmission is feasible. However the distal end of the fibre is at risk of destruction should it touch the stone. Therefore two solutions were developed. One was to shape a lens on the distal end of the fibre [7] and the other was to place a metal cap on the end of the fibre which formed a shock wave in the manner of Fair [3]. These attachments increase the cost of the fibre.

Holmium lasers

The holmium laser emits at 2.0 to 2.1 microns (depending on the precise formulation of the holmium rod). This wavelength band is absorbed well by water. All stones will absorb this wavelength well because of the water both within the stone and on the stone surface. The pulse duration is typically 200 microseconds. This in turn means that pulses of 500 ms to 1.0s will be required for official fragmentation. Fibre transmission requires the use of a low water content fibre but is otherwise straightforward. A typical regimen is to use 1 J pulses at 5 Hz via a 320 micron fibre. Recent *in vitro* studies performed in this unit have shown that the holmium laser at 1 K in a 300 microsecond pulse duration is equivalent to 70 mJ in a 1 microsecond pulse duration using a pulsed dye laser. Tissue absorbs this wavelength powerfully. This regimen has a significant action on normal ureter should the laser fibre touch it during delivery of a burst of laser pulses. This is in contrast to the situation with the pulsed dye laser where tissue damage is trivial.

The holmium laser has the advantage of being a multipurpose laser; the fragments are tiny and there is very little momentum imparted to the stone. The disadvantage however is that it tends to drill into the stone and it does cause significant tissue damage if incident on tissue.

Laser, extracorporeal shock wave lithotripsy or lithoclast?

The miniaturized ureteroscope revolutionized ureteroscopy, by making it easier and safer. Whereas from 1987 to 1989, the laser was the only modality which could be used through a miniaturized ureteroscope, the development of electro-hydraulic and miniaturized ultrasound fragmentation probes and the lithoclast allow all these modalities to be used with the same ureteroscopic advantages [8, 9]. The electro-hydraulic probe is currently available in 1.9 and 3 F probes. The generator is significantly cheaper than a laser. If a unit only uses a modality sporadically, this is the cheapest choice. However the cost of the probes makes the lithoclast a cheaper modality once 50 probes have been consumed (and this may be after fewer than 50 treatments). If multipurpose lasers are considered, the holmium laser may be indicated. The laser fibres can be reused frequently, making the disposable costs minimal. The pulsed dye laser and alexandrite laser are significantly more expensive. They can only be justified by a unit with significant ureteric stone practice. The high initial cost of the laser is justified once a unit performs a number of stone fragmentations per year. This number is in the region of 50 cases in the USA and 200 cases in the UK.

This relationship between numbers and the laser is unfortunate because the unit performing ureteroscopic stone therapy only sporadically has the greatest need of the safest modality. The lithoclast would probably therefore be more appropriate for the sporadic user than the electro-hydraulic probe. Many units are treating more and more calculi with extracorporeal shock wave lithotripsy. This is clearly the least invasive modality. Provided that the stone can be imaged, less expertise is required. However endoscopic management of ureteric calculi remains important. If a stone is causing significant obstruction that obstruction can be relieved more certainly and more rapidly by endoscopy. The development of smaller ureteroscopes is now making it increasingly possible to treat patients without recourse to general anaesthesia. The patient can be treated with no more discomfort than shock wave lithotripsy. We therefore predict that laser fragmentation will become more widely used as these local anaesthetic techniques become adopted, as non-laser modalities are less suited to use with small flexible ureteroscopes and cause more discomfort under these conditions.

References

1. Tanahashi Y, Orikasa S, Ciba R *et al.* Disintegration of urinary calculi by laser beam: Drilling experiment in extracted urinary stones. Tohoka J Exp 1979;128:189–96.
2. Pensel J, Frank F, Rothenburger K *et al.* Destruction of urinary calculi by neodymium YAG laser irradiation. In: Kaplan S, editor. Laser surgery IV. Proceedings of Fourth International Symposium on Laser Surgery, Jerusalem. New York: Academic Press, 1981; 10:4–6.
3. Fair HD. *In vitro* destruction of urinary calculi by laser induced stress waves. Med Instrumentation 1978;12:100–5.
4. Watson GM, Wickham JEA, Mills TK *et al.* Laser fragmentation of renal calculi. Br J Urol 1983;55:613–16.
5. Watson GM, Dretler S, Parrish JA. The pulsed dye laser for fragmenting urinary calculi. J Urol 1987;138:195–8.
6. Teng P, Rishioka WS, Anderson RR *et al.* Optical studies of pulsed laser fragmentation of biliary calculi. Appl Phy B 1987;42:73–8.
7. Hofmann R, Hartung R, Schmidt-Kloiber H. First clinical experience with a Q-switched neodymium YAG laser for urinary calculi. J Urol 1989;141:275–9.
8. Yorreuther R. Minimally invasive ureteroscopy using adjustable electrohydraulic lithotripsy. J Endourol 1992;6:47–50.
9. Hofbauer J, Hobarth K, Karberger K. Lithoclast: New and inexpensive mode of intracorporeal lithotripsy. J Endourol 1992;6:429–32.

14. ESWL today: Spectrum of stone disease treated on the extracorporeal lithotriptor

JAMSHEER TALATI

In this chapter, we review the results of treatment of 350 patients treated on the lithotriptor in 1991, in our unit by three faculty members. The sex distribution was 79% male, 21% female, mean age was 37 ± 14 years (range 3–86 years), average weight was 65 ± 16.7 kg (range 10–109 kg) and body mass index averaged 32.81. Three urologists took care of these patients supported by a dedicated full time lithotripsy staff. The ASA (American Society of Anesthesiologists) grade recorded in 233 patients was ASA 1 in 60%, ASA 2 in 30%, and ASA 3 in 10%. Thus 40% were less than completely fit individuals.

The projected area in two dimensions (stone surface area) for patients with one stone was 248.5 ± 375.6 mm^2 (range 6–2925 mm^2). Sixty-nine per cent had a stone in the kidney, 23% in the ureter and 8% in the bladder; 65.4% had a single stone, 10% had two stones, 2.6% had three stones, 0.57% had four stones, and 2.86% more than four stones. Forty-five per cent had an obstructed system which was completely obstructed in 33% (of all patients).

The treating consultant expected treatment to be complete within two sittings in 69%, within four treatments in an additional 20%, and within six treatments in an additional 8% patients; but 49% completed therapy in one sitting, and a cumulative total of 72% in two sittings. Eleven per cent required three, 6% had four, 5% had five, 1% had six and 1% had more than treatments.

Twenty-four per cent of patients were treated by extracorporeal shock wave lithotripsy (ESWL) after insertion of a double J stent (DJS) of which 65% were inserted because of the stone size; 5.6% were inserted beside a ureteric stone; 3.4% were inserted for a pelviureteric junction (PUJ) stone; 13.5% were inserted after a stone was pushed up; and the remainder were inserted for other causes. The DJS was retained for mean of 50.3 days ± 65.3 days.

Six (1.7%) had a percutaneous nephrolithotomy (PCNL); 2.6% required a PCNL pre-ESWL; and 2.9% had surgery prior to ESWL. No patient required post-ESWL PCNL. Nine (2.5%) required push-up of residual fragments.

Results

A total of 671 treatments were required for 350 patients; 56% were given in the supine, 35% in the lateral, and 10% in the prone position. An average of 2.1 treat-

J. Talati et al. (eds) The Management of Lithiasis, 113–114
© *1997 Kluwer Academic Publishers. Printed in Great Britain.*

ments ($\pm$ 1.5) was used. Voltage (and hence power) was adjusted on the consultant's assessment of stone bulk and fragility, and patient size; 25% were treated by a maximum voltage of 14 kV; 14% required a voltage up to 17 kV; 39% had a maximum voltage of 18–19 kV; 21.8% required voltage up to 20–21 kV; and 50% patients were treated by a mode voltage of 14 kV. The average time taken for treatment was 50 $\pm$ 35 minutes. An average of 2051 shock waves were used per treatment.

Eighty-five per cent were treated as outpatients. Fifty per cent were admitted because they had to undergo a surgical procedure; 1.9% were admitted because of preoperative hypertension, 3.7% because of diabetes, and 5.6% and 1.9% required admission post-ESWL because of renal colic and pyrexia respectively.

Within 30 days 42.3% were stone-free; an additional 18.9%, 7.1% and 3.5% stone-free were within 90, 180 and beyond 180 days respectively. Urinary tract infection was seen in 13 patients (3.7%).

X-rays of patients with residual calculi were analysed in 60 patients. Nine per cent of the calculi were in the ureter, the remainder in the kidney.

15. Management of renal stones by operation

JAMSHEER TALATI

In a patient with renal calculus, surgery may be required solely for removal of the calculus; or additionally for correction of associated anatomical abnormalities, removal of a lower calyx which was acting as a sump, or removal of kidneys which are contributing little to overall renal function and causing ill health, sepsis, or hypertension.

The role of partial nephrectomy is very limited today and a recent review from Britain, over three decades [1] has shown a dramatic decrease from an average of 13.2% of all nephrectomies per year to 2.7%. Very few patients we see would specifically benefit from partial nephrectomy.

Anatrophic nephrolithotomy is performed very infrequently today, in view of the availability of percutaneous nephrolithotomy (PCNL) and extracorporeal shock wave lithotripsy (ESWL), though a comparison of PCNL and anatrophic nephrolithotomy has shown a higher stone-free rate with the latter [2].

Pyelolithotomy and nephrolithotomy are well-known options. Laparoscopic nephrectomy has come of age, and retroperitoneal laparoscopic pyelolithotomy is now becoming an option [3]. Both these procedures require a high degree of technical skill and are more appropriate for previously unoperated kidneys.

Renal damage after open surgery

Conventionally we accept that ESWL and PCNL damage the kidney, but conveniently forget that nephrolithotomy, an adjunct to pyelotomy, can also do so. Nephrolithotomy produces a greater decrease in DMSA uptake than does pyelolithotomy [4].

Nephrectomy rate: An indicator of poor health care cover?

In a hospital for industrial workers in Karachi, from 1969–75, 13% of all stone operations in the male, and 33% in females were nephrectomies [5]. In this period there were no ureteroscopes at this hospital, and no lithotriptors. The case mix included patients with late diagnosis, superadded infection and renal destruction. In the social security hospitals, only the workers were given health cover. Even when

I. Talati et al. (eds) The Management of Lithiasis, 113–117
© 1997 Kluwer Academic Publishers. Printed in Great Britain.

this was extended to the families, the women were usually left behind at home in the villages, and had no health service to fall back on.

A review of open operations in 1978 by Farrakh Khan from Punjab, reports nephrectomies in 7% of 178 patients, pyelolithotomies/nephrolithotomies in 70% and ureterolithotomies in 23%.

A review of 47 nephrectomies in a four-year period (1990–93) at the Aga Khan University Medical Center (AKUMC), showed that 45% were for destruction of the kidney by stone, and an additional 7% for xanthogranulomatous pyelonephritis often accompanied by stone. By comparison, 26% were performed for tumours. At AKUMC, nephrectomy for stone as a proportion of all open surgery for stone has declined from 4.65% (6/129 patients) in 1987 to 2.5% (7/281) in 1990; and relative to hospital admissions has declined from 0.039% of 17 756 admissions to 0.028% of 21 529 admissions.

Nephrectomy for stone-related causes epitomizes the failure of the nation to cope effectively with stone disease. Most stone-related nephrectomies are done for pyelonephritis, xanthogranulomatous pyelonephritis, pyonephrosis or gross hydronephrosis, many of which are unsuitable for laparoscopic approach.

Justification for nephrectomy

In the 1960s, surgeons had little concern about removing a kidney, reassuring patients that the other kidney was adequate. It was felt that as all of the 1.5 litres of urine would have to be evacuated through one collecting system, the flow rate of urine would be faster and hence would discourage stone nuclei aggregation and hence stone formation in the remaining kidney.

This is unfortunately not true for Pakistan. The remaining kidney may be subject to the same metabolic forces that caused the first stone, and is likely to form another. Passage of the stone into the ureter may cause anuria in a patient who has had a kidney removed. Such a person often does not seek aid until he is in dire straits: in severe pulmonary oedema, and hyperkalaemia.

In the rat fed ethylene glycol, unilateral nephrectomy increases the incidence of lithiasis in the remaining kidney [6].

In Pakistan, a kidney conserving approach is recommended. Even when renal function is impaired and the renal cortex is thinned out into a shell, we would still contemplate removing, say, the urethral calculus rather than the kidney if there is no gross infection. A large hydronephrotic kidney, by virtue of the large total square area, contains many glomeruli. Renal function tested by DTPA in the presence of obstruction will not give a true picture of the ability of the kidney to recover. Measurement of single kidney urine output, its specific gravity and sodium conserving ability, a week after percutaneous nephrostomy, will give a more accurate representation of renal function watched over a week. Inability to concentrate urine or conserve sodium indicates poor renal function. A repeat DTPA at this stage will also give a better assessment of returning renal function. If little urine is produced, there is great sodium loss, poor concentrating ability, and a small percentage contribution to total renal function on a DTPA done some days after the nephrostomy, nephrectomy is justified. We have conserved kidneys with gross hydronephrosis when there has been no associated urinary tract infection, because these large kidneys still retain a large number of glomeruli and can eliminate water and potassium if a stone blocks off the opposite kidney.

Patients with xanthogranulomatous pyelonephritis, shrivelled shrunken kidneys, or pyonephrotic renal destruction will require nephrectomy.

References

1. Kubba AK, Hollins GW, Deane RF. Nephrectomy, changing indications 1960–1990. Br J Urol 1994;74:274–7.
2. Assimos D, Boyce WH, Harrison LH *et al.* Role of open surgery since ESWL. J Urol 1989;142:263–7.
3. Gaur DD, Agarwal DK, Purohit KC *et al.* Retroperitoneal laparoscopic pyelolithotomy. J Urol 1994;151:927–9.
4. Katayama Y. Influence of renal stone surgery on renal function – evaluation of renal function with 99m Tc DMSA renal scintigraphy. Nippon Hinyokika Gakkai Zaashi 1991;82:1588–93.
5. Haziq ul Yakin. Urolithiasis in industrial workers. JPMA 1975;25:274–8.
6. Liu YH, Hwang WC, Chang LS *et al.* Uninephrectomy enhances urolithiasis in ethylene glycol treated rats. Kid Int 1992;42:292–9.

16. ESWL for kidney stones and options for calyceal calculi

JAMSHEER TALATI

The vast majority of renal stones are today amenable to extracorporeal shock wave lithotripsy (ESWL) monotherapy, but best results will be obtained by selective therapy. Which patient should be treated on the lithotriptor?

Suitability for ESWL

Stone characteristics, the status of the outflow tract, and the condition of the patient, should be considered when choosing the most suitable therapy for renal stone. The ideal patient for ESWL has a body mass index (weight in kilograms/square of the height in metres) of 20–28, is younger than 60 years, and has a single stone (measuring 1 cm^3) in the renal pelvis [1].

Suitability for ESWL: The patient

ESWL produces minimal changes in normal haemodynamics and very ill patients who are unfit for surgery can be treated by ESWL after bringing them to an optimal condition. Three major contraindications remain: pregnancy, pacemakers and bleeding disorders. Patients with the latter two conditions can be made fit for ESWL, as can other high-risk patients (see Section III).

Suitability for ESWL: The kidney outflow tract and stone site

An unimpeded outflow tract is essential for clearance of stones. Distorted (horse-shoe and sigmoid) kidneys, pelvic and transplanted kidneys, and solitary kidneys require special management.

Patients with pelviureteric junction (PUJ) stenosis or strictures of the ureter should have these conditions corrected before ESWL. In horseshoe kidneys (encountered in 0.25% patients) [2], stones lying in the medial, interconnecting bar of tissue are difficult to target and may require a prone position. Stones beyond the reach of target focus (F2), have been crushed, presumably because of the energy available beyond the F2 focus [3]. ESWL is suitable for small stones, but a large stone burden, proximity to the vertebra, and poor drainage, set the stage for poor results [4].

J. Talati et al. (eds) The Management of Lithiasis, 119–123
© *1997 Kluwer Academic Publishers. Printed in Great Britain.*

Solitary kidneys should not be subjected to too many shocks at one time, and need special attention to prevent obstruction during therapy. Even staghorn calculi have been treated without stents [5], but many authors [6, 7] caution that complications arise in 50% in spite of stenting, when the stone burden is large. Stenting is therefore preferable. ESWL is suitable for friable stones, in solitary kidneys, but some other form of treatment should be considered for solitary kidneys with large stones or stones appearing dense white on X-ray. Properly selected and post-stenting ESWL should not cause deterioration of renal function beyond that noted in percutaneous nephrolithotomy (PCNL) (22–29%) [8], and should achieve a stone-free rate in about 86% of patients [9]. Large series (52 solitary kidneys) and long follow-up, have demonstrated hypertension in only one patient after 12–56 months' follow-up, an 8% recurrence rate, and 5% regrowth of residuals [10].

Stones impacted at PUJ, fragment well *in situ* and do not require to be pushed back into the pelvis. If the entire stone length is visible on the ultrasound, we commence treatment from the lower end. If only the upper interface between stone and the dilated ureter is identified, then we have satisfactory results by treating in the head-down position. Fragmentation is started from the upper end of the stone. The head-down tilt allows fragments to fall away from the stone into the kidney. Removing them from the main stone increases the effectiveness of shock wave delivery, and allows the operator to see the part of the stone still unaffected by treatment. However, passage of fragments back into the kidney delays clearance. Once the stone bulk has fragmented to some extent, as is evident by the change in the ultrasound reflex from a crescent to oval, furosemide 10 mg, may be administered to produce diuresis, loosen up the fragments, and clear particles down the ureter. Larger doses produce such intense diuresis that the patient may require to void during lithotripsy.

Stones in renal transplants and pelvic kidneys can be treated in a prone position [11]. Stones occur in up to 20% of polycystic kidneys and can be treated without major complications, though they may occasionally require cyst puncture [12]. Stones in medullary sponge kidneys can also be effectively treated by ESWL [13]. A 100% stone-free rate [14] has been reported, though more often the stones are multiple and it is unwise to spread shock waves all over the kidney to eliminate small stones in this condition.

The calyceal stone
The calyceal stone was considered innocuous in the 1970s, and there was no mechanism whereby it could be removed with minimal problems to the patient. Approach through an intrarenal pelvis was difficult and it was felt that it was not justified to remove such a calculus by a nephrotomy; the stone was therefore left alone. Calyceal stones should be treated, as these stones tend to grow, and can cause ureteral obstruction when expelled from the calyx. Airline companies and armies require their removal before employment in active service.

Untreated, only 11% remain symptom-free beyond 10 years; 68% get infected, and 45% increase in size in an average 7.5 years of observation per stone [15]. Delay in surgery leads to complications. In Hubner and Porpaezy's series of 32 patients operated on, eight had developed staghorns, eight had acute obstruction with incipient sepsis, three had chronic urinary tract infection, and one had loss of renal function [15]. As 16% pass spontaneously [15], a period of observation for three months is appropriate [16].

In some patients the stone is associated with pain. Very often, the pain is out of proportion to the small stone impacted in a non-dilated inferior calyx. With the advent of PCNL and ESWL it is very easy to treat these stones. Should all be treated? Are these patients really harbouring asymptomatic stones with somatization of a stress problem? Lee *et al.* [17] noted that complete pain relief occurs in 79% and significant relief of pain in an additional 21%, 3–15 months after ESWL. Pain-free status is achieved even when the stone is not cleared – 85% of the stone-free group and 29% patients with residuals were pain free [17]. Stone-free and pain-free status may be achieved in only 32% [16]. Others report stone-free rates of 39% [17] to 50% [16]. For patients with psychiatric problems the stone should not be treated before their adequate management. Asymptomatic small stones will have to be treated in airline pilots, who will not be allowed to fly until stone free. Asymptomatic calyceal stones behind a narrow calyceal neck are unlikely to move out. The stone causing pain or infection will need treatment.

Treatment modality
Calyceal stones should be treated by ESWL [18]. The lower calyx is not an impediment to fragmentation, but the calyx tends to collect the gravel. Normal calyces empty by peristalsis, but in many patients with long-standing calyceal stones, the calyceal wall has lost its expulsive power. Tapotement, or application of a vibrator-massager, in the head-down position in the follow-up period may be helpful. Citrate therapy may prevent recongealing of fragments. If the powder recongeals, a PCNL evacuation or irrigation through a PCNL may be required. Patients with an abnormal IVP have a lower clearance [17]. A cobra catheter inserted into the lower calyx could be used for irrigation during lithotripsy, to promote egress of the stone fragments [19]. Because of these problems, percutaneous removal should be contemplated as the first choice if the stone is greater than 10 mm, in a dilated lower calyx [20], whilst stones in a middle calyx, and smaller than 1 cm are best treated by ESWL (see Chapter 41).

Stones in a calyceal diverticulum
If the calyceal diverticular opening is wide, ESWL is successful in obtaining a stone-free rate in 58%, and relief from pain in 86% [21]. Those rendered pain free remained free of pain but infection persisted in those who had pre-ESWL infection. If the calyceal neck is narrow, laser division of the neck at flexible ureteroscopy has been effective. If the stone is asymptomatic and small, an alternative is to leave it alone. A pilot will be grounded until such a stone is removed, and occupation may determine whether an asymptomatic stone is treated.

When an intravenous pyelogram shows a stone at the site of a calyx which fails to visualize, a pyocalyx should be suspected, especially if the patient has a fever. Such patients are at risk for sepsis during ESWL [22]. A preferable form of treatment is removal by PCNL followed by infundibulectomy.

Suitability for ESWL: The stone

Most problems associated with lithotripsy arise from large stone bulk, multiplicity and awkward stone site. Partial and complete staghorns require special attention, and are dealt with separately in Chapter 18. Stones less than 90 mm² fragment with ease [7] with any type of shock wave. The shape of the stone, and surface irregularities determine the total amount of energy transmitted to the stone. This factor determines outcome when treating irregular faced calculi such as staghorns [23] but mixed or phosphate stones fail to respond to extracorporeal piezo-electric lithotripsy therapy [7]. On any lithotriptor, as the stone size increases to greater than 10 mm, stone-free rates with ESWL decrease from 90.6 to 77.8%, the number of shock waves needed rises, and the number of secondary treatments increases.

Assessment of stone size
The longest diameter gives some idea of the size of the stone but does not give a good approximation of stone volume. Surface area measurements from two longest diameters is better, but stones can be very complex in shape, and many stones may be present. Planimetric evaluation of the perimeter and hence surface area is cumbersome for routine use. Stone volume requires a third dimension which cannot be easily obtained by conventional radiographs. Ultrasound is helpful only in spherical stones as the dense acoustic shadow cast by the stone precludes measurement. The CT scan gives a better idea of the stone volume but this can hardly be recommended routinely. The most practical and best approximation (to an accurate volume determined by immersion of the stone in water) comes from Ackerman *et al.* [1] who have devised the formula:
Stone volume = surface area$^{1.27}$.

Simultaneous bilateral lithotripsy

Bilateral stones should be treated simultaneously with caution. Melser *et al.* [24] treated bilateral stones with an average stone burden of 22 mm, simultaneously in 75 patients; 65% had no complications. Due to the risk of creatinine increase, bilateral ureteral obstruction must be carefully evaluated. Bilateral simultaneous treatment is acceptable if there is a small stone which fragments completely into fine powder on the first treatment on one side.

In unilateral ESWL, the effective renal plasma flow (ERPF) was disturbed if the shock wave burden (number of shocks × voltage) was greater then 45 000. However 50% of patients undergoing bilateral ESWL showed a decrease of ERPF irrespective of the shock wave burden. In a reported series of 361 patients who received simultaneous lithotripsy, 95% in the same session, none developed acute renal failure and follow-up three months later showed no increase in serum creatinine [25]. The stone-free rate was 47% (61% for renal pelvis to 33% for lower calyceal stone) [25].

Comment

In our unit, 76% of stones were treated by ESWL from January to June 1995, and 93% of renal calculi were treated by ESWL. The question 'which patient should be treated on the lithotriptor?' appears redundant, but nevertheless demands attention, because refinements in therapy are needed to treat some categories of these patients.

References

1. Ackerman DK, Fuhriman R, Pflinger D *et al.* Prognosis after extracorporeal shockwave lithotripsy of radio-opaque renal calculi: a multivariate analysis. Eur Urol 1994;25:105–9.
2. Ohyama A, Asar Y, Amano Y *et al.* ESWL for urolithiasis in horseshoe kidneys. Hinyokika kiyo 1991;37:1627–31.
3. Whelan JP, Finlayson B, Welch J *et al.* The blast path: Theoretical basis, experimental data and clinical application. J Urol 1988;140:401–4.
4. Esuvaranathan K, Tan EC, Tung KH *et al.* Stone in horse-shoe kidney, results of treatment by ESWL and endourology. J Urol 1991;146:1213–15.
5. Numa H, Yoshida K, Yoneshina H *et al.* Clinical application of ESWL to 5 solitary kidney patients with upper urinary tract stone. Hiayokika Kiyo 1991;37:845–9.
6. Ishii T, Imanishi M, Kohri K *et al.* Clinical study of ESWL for stones in solitary kidneys. Nippon Hinyokika Gakkai Zaashi 1991;82:1466–72.
7. Cohen ES, Schmidt JD. ESWL for stones in a solitary kidney. Urology 1990;36:52–4.
8. Cass AS. Renal function after ESWL to solitary kidneys. J Endourol 1994;8:15–19.
9. Sarica K, Kohle R, Kunit G *et al.* Experience with ESWL in patients with a solitary kidney. Urol Int 1992;48:200–2.
10. Zanetti GR, Montanari E, Guarneri A *et al.* Long-term followup after extracorporeal shock wave lithotripsy treatment of kidney stones in solitary kidneys. J Urol 1992;148:1011–14.
11. Jones DJ, McNicholas TA, Carter SS *et al.* Lithotripsy and endourological therapy for renal calculi in renal transplants. J Urol 1989;141:402A.
12. Martinez-Sarmiento M *et al.* ESWL in polycystic kidneys. Actas Urol Esp 1994;18:35–8.
13. Nakada SY, Erturk E, Monaghan J *et al.* Role of extracorporeal shock-wave lithotripsy in treatment of urolithiasis in patients with medullary sponge kidney. Urology 1993;41:331–3.
14. Bhatia V, Biyana CS. Calculus disease in duplex system role of extracorporeal shockwave lithotripsy. Urol Int 1993;50:164–9.
15. Hubner W, Porpaezy P. Treatment of calyceal calculi. Br J Urol 1990;66:9–11.
16. Hendrix AJ, Bierkins AF, Debruyne FM. Extracorporeal shockwave lithotripsy for small asymptomatic calculi: is it effective? Urol Int 1991;47:12–15.
17. Lee MH, Lee YH, Chen MT *et al.* Management of painful calyceal stones by ESWL. Eur Urol 1990;18:211–14.
18. Kriegnair M, Schuller J, Schmeller N *et al.* Diverticular calculi of the kidney calyces – ESWL, PCNL or OS. Urology (A) 1990;29:204–8.
19. Nicely ER, Maggio MI, Kuhn EJ. The use of cystoscopically placed cobra catheter for directed irrigation of lower pole calyceal stones during extracorporeal shock wave lithotripsy. J Urol 1992;148:1036–98.
20. Lingeman SE, Siegel YI, Steele B *et al.* Management of lower pole nephrolithiasis, a critical analysis. J Urol 1994;151:663–7.
21. Streem SB, Yost A. Treatment of calyceal diverticular calculi with ESWL, patient selection and extended follow up. J Urol 1992;148:1043–6.
22. Meretyk S, Bigg S, Clayman RV *et al.* Caveat emptor; Calyceal stones and the missing calyx. J Urol 1992;147:1091–5.
23. Pittomvils G, Vandeursen H, Hellemans J *et al.* Stone geometry and structure and dependence on ESWL. J Endourol 1993;7:357–62.
24. Melser MA, Littleton RM, Cerny JC. Simultaneous bilateral ESWL. J Urol 1989;141:405A.
25. Cass AS. Bilateral lithotripsy for renal stones. J Urol 1990;143:299A

17. Percutaneous nephrolithotomy for renal stones

TARIQ SHAH and SARWAT HUSSAIN

Percutaneous nephrolithotomy (PCNL) entails endoscopic removal of renal stones by extraction or disintegration via a nephrocutaneous track. Extracorporeal shock wave lithotripsy (ESWL) has reduced the indications for PCNL. However, when ESWL is not availble, PCNL assumes a primary role in the management of renal and upper ureteric calculi.

All patients for PCNL should be fit, even if the procedure is to be done under local anaesthesia, as complications from PCNL may necessitate open surgery and hence general anaesthesia. Bleeding disorders must be corrected before PCNL.

Combination PCNL–ESWL therapy

When ESWL is availble, PCNL is chiefly used to debulk larger stones and remove stubborn residue from inferior calyces. Combination therapy (PCNL–ESWL) may be used for any stone greater than 4 cm in size. ESWL may precede or follow PCNL, or be sandwiched between two PCNL sessions. When employing the combination treatment, it is wiser to remove the stones from the pelvis and the dependent portion of the kidney through a lower polar puncture. The upper and middle polar calyceal stones are then left to be dealt with by ESWL, thus averting the need for multiple punctures. For combined therapy, a 24–26 Fr nephrostomy tube is left *in situ* so that the fragments evacuate rapidly rather than pass slowly down the ureter.

PCNL as monotherapy

PCNL can be employed as a primary procedure for complete removal of the stone in preference to open surgery. Pelvic and inferior calyceal stones can be removed through one puncture. For complicated stones multiple punctures and more than one sitting may be required. If there are residual stones after the first sitting a large bore nephrostomy tube is left in to stabilize the tract which is then used for future clearances. With patience, perseverance and good planning very large and complicated stones have been cleared.

Percutaneous antegrade access can be used for pyelolysis or dilatation of secondary pelvi ureteric junction obstruction, calyceal neck stenosis or upper ureteric

J. Talati et al. (eds) The Management of Lithiasis, 125–132
© *1997 Kluwer Academic Publishers. Printed in Great Britain.*

strictures at the same time as treating the stone. This obviates the need for retrograde dilatation of the pelvi-ureteric junction and DJ stent insertion, which does not always work. Stones in calyces with narrowed infundibular necks or in calyceal diverticulum require a direct puncture on the particular calyx and removal of the stone.

Logistics technique and armamentarium

PCNL is now done as a one-stage procedure with puncture, dilatation and extraction of stone all being done in one session. Alternatively, the puncture could be performed in the radiology department, and the extraction in the operating room. Operating suites equipped with facilities for radiological screening work are ideal for a 'one window' operation but an image intensifier has to be used as a substitute.

Teamwork is the key to success. During the early learning period the procedure tends to be prolonged and complications during the operation are seen much more often. At this time, a radiologist with experience in interventional radiology and three-dimensional fluoroscopic imaging is more helpful than a general radiologist.

The procedure requires the cystoscopic placement of a ureteric balloon catheter, establishment of a track to the pelvi-calyceal system and endoscopic fragmentation and extraction. The ureteric ballon catheter allows opacification and distension of the pelvi-calyceal system and prevents stone fragment egress into the ureter.

Cystoscopy and placement of the balloon catheter

Cystoscopy can be done on the screening table, in the radiology department, with the patient supine (legs spread wide apart), a cushion under the sacrum for obliteration of the pelvic angle. A ureteric occluding balloon catheter is threaded and advanced over a guide wire and placed just under the pelvi-ureteric junction, and inflated with 0.5–2 ml urografin diluted to half its strength with sterile water. The cystoscope is then removed and a size 14–16 Fr Foley catheter is passed into the bladder alongside the ureteric catheter, and the two catheters are then fixed to each other with adhesive tape. Contrast medium is injected via an extension tube from which air has been removed. This is intermittently checked on fluoroscopy.

Radiological puncture and tract dilatation

The patient is turned over into a prone oblique position (Figure 17.1) with the affected side up, the upper arm supported on an arm rest, a pillow between the legs, and wedged sponges under the loin to lift it up and flatten the upper loin. Indelible ink is used to mark the twelfth rib, paraspinal muscle border and the iliac crest.

The operation site is prepared and draped for sterile puncture. A water proof drape on either side with funnelled ends draining into the collection buckets should be fashioned (purpose-built PCNL drapes are good but costly). The C-arm image intensifier unit can be very neatly draped using the sterile leggings for the lithotomy

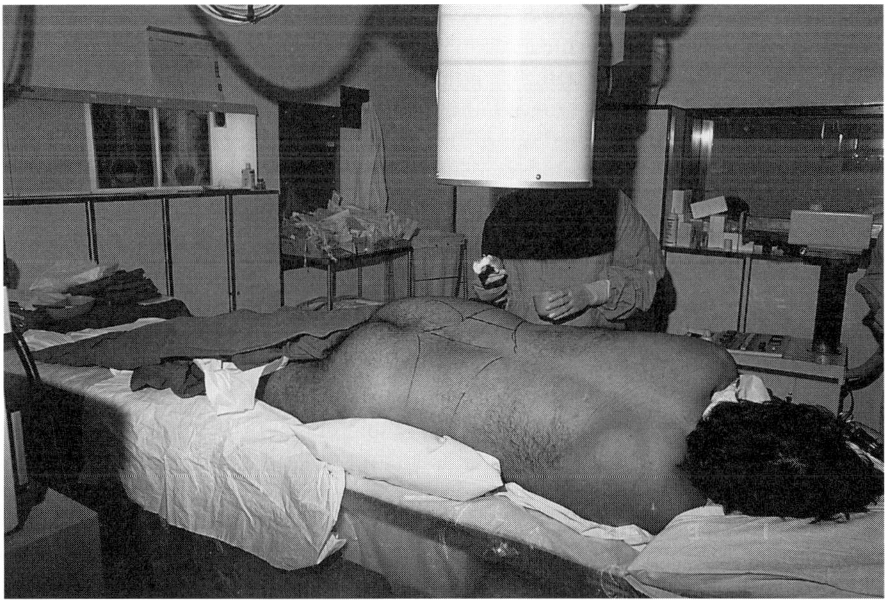

Figure 17.1 Patient in prone oblique position

work. If a fixed ceiling mounted unit is being used, the controls should be covered by a sterile sheet.

Once fully draped, the image intensifier unit is brought into position to image the puncture site. A radiopaque object, such as long artery forceps or spinal needles, is placed over the puncture site to align with the calyx selected for puncture (as seen after injection of radiocontrast) in the most direct approach at an oblique angle, damage the parenchyma minimally and obtain a straight and direct tract for subsequent nephroscopy. This direction in the two planes is noted and the point of puncture is incised with a No. 11 blade.

The 18-gauge long dwell needle is advanced through this incision in the appropriate direction. If biplanar fluoroscopy or C-arm facilities are not available, and the puncture is being done under the ceiling mounted X-ray beam, the advance and position of the needle is checked and corrected by parallax method by rocking the patient on the table while screening. To avoid an angulated tract the puncture should be done during mid-inspiration. As the needle enters the kidney, it can be seen to swing with the movement of the kidney during respiration.

The stylet is now withdrawn out of the needle. If the renal collecting system has been entered, a free flow of dye urine should be seen. If free flow does not occur, a 5 ml syringe is attached to the cannula and a gentle suction is done while the needle is slightly advanced or gradually withdrawn until urine starts flowing freely.

On confirming the needle to be in the selected calyx at the desired angle, the soft guide wire is introduced through the cannula into the calyx. The needle is then advanced slightly over the guide wire into the calyx to acquire a stable position. The guide wire is ideally threaded through the calyceal neck into the pelvis, or even into the ureter, if possible, to provide a secure position for subsequent dilatation.

Once the needle is stabilized, the guide wire is withdrawn and replaced by a Lunderquist guide wire; this will avoid the kinking that may occur in a soft guide wire, which may also get pulled out of the collecting system when the dilators are introduced over it.

A metal fascial dilator is threaded over the Lunderquist into the calyx, and possibly through the calyceal neck into the pelvis, which will not only stretch the thoraco-lumbar fascia but also allow the reintroduction of the soft guide wire through it alongside the Lunderquist, to act as a second, safety guide wire. The needle is then removed and the safety guide wire coiled and anchored on one side, out of the operative field. This wire becomes useful if during dilatation the Lunderquist is inadvertently pulled out of the system.

The olive tip central metal guide for telescopic dilators is now introduced and positioned securely. The telescopic dilators are threaded one over the other with a gentle screwing and pushing action up to the olive tip of the central guide where they are locked.

Occasionally a tough thoraco-lumbar fascia is encountered which cannot be easily stretched; in such a situation the fascia is incised with a blade on a long handle (or with one of the purpose-built lumbotomes) by two cuts made at right angles to each other to give a cruciate incision. The depth of this incision is determined from the plain X-ray. The central guide is kept firm and steady with a slight pull, against the push of the dilators, with the position being regularly checked on the monitor.

The dilatation is normally done up to 24 Fr, following which the 26 Fr or 30 Fr Amplatz sheath is to be used, further dilatation should be carried on with the telescopic dilators to 26 or 28 Fr respectively, and the sheath introduced over the largest dilator. Having secured the position of the Amplatz sheath, the whole assembly of the dilators along with the Lunderquist is removed *en bloc.*

Multiple or 'Y' tracts

Variations in making the track are required for complex or multiple stone. This is seldom necessary if PCNL is to be combined with ESWL. A 'Y' (in fact a V) tract may be needed when calculi are located in parallel or adjacent calyces and cannot be approached through a single tract. Once the first calyx has been cleared, the Amplatz sheath is pulled to lie just outside the kidney; it is then angled to face the second calyx. The second puncture is made by the needle passed through the repositioned Amplatz into the calyx. Guide wire and Lunderquist are positioned and dilatation is carried out as described previously, up to the second stone; finally the Amplatz is passed over the last dilator and the calyx cleared of stone. Stones which cannot be reached through the Y tract because of their location require new punctures and separate tracts.

Upper polar or middle polar stones in a high lying kidney may necessitate a supra-twelfth rib puncture. The technique is essentially the same as in lower pole tracts. However to avoid the pleura the tracts should be formed as lateral as possible.

Unusual situations may require minor variations in the puncture technique. For stones located in isolated calyces or in a calyceal diverticulum, direct puncture over the stone or into the diverticulum is done. Since there is little space for anchoring the guide wire, care should be taken during dilatation not to lose the tract.

Nephroscopy

Once satisfied about the position of the stone and the Amplatz sheath, the image intensifier is moved out of the field of action but within easy reach, to be brought in if required during endoscopy. Endoscopy begins with profuse irrigation of the kidney to wash away all blood and clots which can also be removed by grasping in biopsy forceps. Suction may be needed if the clots do not wash away easily. If the sheath has moved out of the kidney, pale fatty tissue is encountered. Fluoroscopy with retrograde injection of the contrast will help identify whether the sheath is lying in the perinephric fat or has been pushed too far out of the pelvis. By gently manipulating the sheath under vision, the sheath can usually be repositioned into the system. Following the safety guide wire, if it can be seen, is very helpful in re-locating the sheath into the collecting system. However if the sheath is lying too far out, repositioning is done by dilatation of the tract up to the collecting system over the guide wire which is reintroduced through the sheath. The pelvi-calyceal system can be identified by the free flow of the irrigation fluid in space which is often clearly seen lined by the smooth urothelium.

Once a clear view is obtained, the position should be identified by locating the uretero-pelvic junction and the infundibular necks. The stone usually comes into view at this time (Figure 17.2 – see p iv) If the stone has been displaced, this should be confirmed on fluoroscopy and the nephroscope can then be manoeuvred to the right place.

Stone extraction and fragmentation
Stones up to 1.2 cm in their largest axis can be removed intact by grasping forceps through a 30 Fr Amplatz sheath. Sheaths of 24, 26, and 28 Fr would allow stone sizes of 0.6, 0.8, and 1 cm respectively to be pulled out comfortably. Most stones can be removed with the alligator forceps. Triradiate forceps are used for larger, ir-regular and awkwardly placed calculi. Very occasionally a Dormia type basket is required for retrieving stones from the ureters or from inside a calyx which cannot be removed by the forceps.

Calculi which are too large to be extracted intact are fragmented *in situ* by ultra-sonic or electro-hydraulic means. If the stone is too hard to be broken up by these lithotriptors, a Maumeyer stone punch can be used for fragmentation of such calculi, with caution – the instrument requires a large space for manipulation and should not be used if space in the pelvis is limited. If soft the grabbing forceps can be used for crushing and removing piecemeal.

The ultrasonic system generates ultrasound at a frequency of 23–27 kHz, from the piezoceramic elements in their transducers. This is transmitted to the stone by a metal probe that vibrates and drills into the stone. The probe is hollow and is connected to a foot-operated vacuum roller pump which sucks away the debris as the stone disintegrates. Continuous irrigation is required to provide a good view. If the probe comes in contact with the pelvic wall it does not produce anything more than a bruise unless forcibly pushed through the wall. Later modifications of ultrasound probes transmit ultrasound shock waves to the stone.

Lithotripsy is commenced from one edge of the stone and gradually worked to reduce the stone size. If large fragments of the stone break off, these should be disintegrated first before the main stone. Forceps may be used to remove fragments to expedite the process.

The advantage of the ultrasound lithotriptor is its safety and efficiency in removing the debris at the same time as the stone is being disintegrated. Hard stones may be difficult to fragment with ultrasound, and electro-hydraulic (EHL) disintegration may be required. Ultrasound disintegration is a slow process and some large stones can take quite a few hours before complete clearance is achieved.

EHL works by producing a shock wave generated by passing an ultra-short high voltage through the spark gap between two electrodes placed underwater. As the electric current is passed between the two electrodes the fluid around it is vaporized and a bubble is formed that propagates at the speed of sound. The kinetic energy of the bubble dissipates as sound waves at the surface of the stone to produce shearing force; this overcomes the structural adhesive force of the stone, which fragments with repeated application of the shock wave.

The EHL electrode is long, thin and flexible and can be easily passed through the working port of the nephroscope. It is connected by a lead to the externally placed capacitor discharge power unit which is controlled by a foot pedal. The advantage of the EHL system is its capacity to break very hard calculi into smaller fragments which can be retrieved by the forceps. The process is also fairly quick compared to the ultrasonic system. Its major disadvantage is in the trauma it can produce if the probe slips off the stone on to the wall of the collecting system which can be very easily perforated. A good precaution is to put the unit on only when the probe is in good contact with the stone and there is good vision all around; also the power should be switched off before withdrawing the probe from the nephroscope. A spark discharge too near the nephroscope can fracture the lens; each time the shock wave is generated there should be a minimum gap of 2–3 mm between the probe end and the urothelium and nephroscope lens. Another disadvantage of the EHL system is that the electrodes can be very rapidly destroyed by the repeated application of the shock waves and have to be replaced; this increases the cost of the treatment.

Special kidneys and special stones

PCNL can be done in children. The tract is short and small and great care should be exercised during dilatation. It is usually difficult to opacify the pelvi-calyceal system retrogradely, and usually a combination of ultrasound and intravenous pyelography is required.

In horseshoe kidneys the calyces are more posterior and medial than normal and therefore the puncture needs to be more medial than usual. Often the paraspinal muscles have to be dilated to form a satisfactory tract. Because of the obviously long distance of the stone from the skin, a longer Amplatz sheath may be required.

Stones in the upper third of the ureter may be approached through the upper pole in patients in whom retrograde ureteroscopy has failed. Now that there is greater success with ESWL, this approach is seldom necessary.

Results

PCNL, like ureteroscopy, has poorer results during the learning curve. Seventy patients (52 males) aged 14–63 years (mean 42 years), were treated between June 1987 and June 1989 in the early part of our experience at the Aga Khan University Medical Center. Sixteen per cent had recurrent urinary tract infection. Stone size ranged from 0.7 cm to complete staghorns, 37% having multiple calculi. Access was gained through the lower pole posterior calyx in 94%, and middle calyx in 4%. Malrotated kidney and bleeding and obscuration of the tract by contrast resulted in failure in two patients.

Planned debulking or complete removal were achieved in 66 of the 68 patients (97%). In two patients the procedure was abandoned because of haemorrhage, necessitating open pyelolithotomy in one and a calyceal neck stricture in another. Seventeen per cent of stones were small enough to be removed in one piece, 44% required mechanical fragmentation, 54% had ultrasonic litholriesis, and 15% had additional electro hydraulic lithotripsy.

Twenty-one per cent develop post-PCNL infection requiring antibiotics. Care needs to be taken that the cap of the surgeon does not mar the sterile field. In 3% of patients, the procedure was abandoned because of bleeding, and an additional 3% needed transfusion and balloon tamponade with an 8–10 Fr Foley catheter for delayed haemorrhage. Fragments can pass down the ureter, especially if the ureteric occlusion catheter is not properly inflated. Most fragments will pass spontaneously but ureteroscopy was required in one of the four patients who had ureteral fragments. Stones or stone pieces may be lost in the nephrostomy tract (in the soft tissues) if an Amplatz sheath is not in place. A nephroscope should be passed immediately down the tract. Usually it is not possible to retrieve the calculus. We have lost one fragment in the tract prior to routine use of the Amplatz sheath.

After removal of the nephrostomy tube, urinary leakage may continue from the nephrostomy tract for 3–6 days. This spontaneously ceases, and persistent leak indicates calcular fragment in the ureter or other causes of ureteric obstruction.

Colonic perforation occurred in one patient. Fortunately this is a very rare complication, and results from a lateral position of the colon with a pocket of peritoneum behind the kidney, in very thin individuals, old men or young females. The descending colon more often than the ascending colon falls into this recess, exposing the patient to the risk of colonic injury during any percutaneous renal fossa intervention. If suspected, a CT scan would delineate the anatomical boundaries of the peritoneal surfaces. The fistula was discovered on removal of the nephrostomy tube, failed to close spontaneously, and required formal operative closure which was successful.

Advantages of PCNL

Though PCNL is not a totally non-invasive procedure, it produces much less tissue trauma and patient morbidity than open surgery. There is a significant reduction in hospital stay and in the loss of working days for the patient. Typically the patient is discharged home on the second or third post-PCNL day, and can resume work in a week. When used in conjunction with ESWL, PCNL reduces the number of treatments and expedites stone clearance.

In our series, the average length of stay was 5.6 days. This included the early learning phase, when caution delayed hospital discharge. Significant delay was noted in four patients; in three there were complications, and in the fourth, repeated instrument failure after successful puncture was responsible.

Conclusions

Recent advances have provided various options to the urologists and radiologists treating urinary stone disease. At one end of the spectrum is open surgery, at the other is ESWL with its substantial advantages. Somewhere in between lies the minimally invasive procedure of PCNL with its own set of indications and usefulness. The indications for each technique are not absolute. They depend upon a variety of factors, including availability of technology, affordability and expertise. Each presenting stone may initiate a different treatment plan. Patient factors that affect a management decision are body habitus, urinary anatomy, and medical history. Stone factors that affect decisions are the size, site within the collecting system, and fragility. Availability of the equipment and the expertise and motivation of the radiologist's and the urologist's teams are also important.

18. Management of staghorn calculi

JAMSHEER TALATI

Partial and complete staghorns constitute 15% of all the calculi treated in our unit, and 12.5% of the stones treated in the West [1]. Partial staghorns extend from the pelvis into one calyx. Complete staghorns branch into two (C4 type) or three or more (C5 type) calyces.

Treatment options

Staghorn calculi can be treated by extracorporeal shock wave lithotripsy (ESWL), percutaneous nephrolithotomy (PCNL), operation, or a combination of any of these modalities. A few, composed of urate, can be dissolved by oral alkali therapy or percutaneous irrigation. What is the best treatment?

Unselected treatment of all staghorns by ESWL can yield unsatisfactory results. Large stones require an average of four treatments, with patients requiring up to seven treatments (mean 2.1) on even the HM3 [2]. Unselected ESWL yields low clearance rates (52–55%) [3–5] and a high incidence of ureteral obstruction (up to 43%), fever (35%), colic (31%) and peri-renal haematoma (3.7%); there is a greater need for a DJS (in 15%), percutaneous nephrostomy (PCN) (in 25%), and PCNL for removal of fragments (in 2.7%). Auxiliary procedures may be required in 41% and clearance is slow (68% either stone-free or with particles less than 4 mm at three months; 75% stone free at one year) [2]. C4 calculi clear more readily on ESWL. Larger stones can be treated by ESWL monotherapy, with good results, especially when furosemide is used during therapy, gentler shocks are used to produce an erosive rather than explosive effect, and therapy is spaced to allow clearance of debris. Clearance of urate and struvite stones can be assisted by citrate [6]. Percutaneous irrigation with citrate, magnesium and EDTA containing solutions, used pre-ESWL for stones with high radiodensity and post-ESWL for residual fragments, improves results.

Surgery is an infrequently used option today, but is effective in clearing large bulky bilateral stones simultaneously through midline laparotomy incisions. Preoperative use of Doppler ultrasound during surgery and hypothermia assists stone clearance. Anatrophic nephrolithotomy may be needed.

Now that ESWL is available as a backup, PCNL monotherapy should be reserved for the staghorn extending into inferior calyces which are not dilated and communicate freely with the pelvis and which can be cleared by a maximum of two

J. Talati et al. (eds) The Management of Lithiasis, 133–136
© *1997 Kluwer Academic Publishers. Printed in Great Britain.*

punctures [7]. PCNL gives good clearance for stones smaller than 500 mm². It is inappropriate to use transpleural tracts for the upper stones so readily amenable to ESWL. Using PCNL monotherapy, excellent results have been obtained in expert hands, but treatment of complex stones by PCNL alone should only be undertaken in units doing large numbers of PCNL. With the advent of ESWL, training for PCNL becomes limited, expertise grows more slowly, and it is preferable to use combination methods where indicated.

PCNL or ureteroscopic [8] debulking prior to ESWL is expensive, but reduces the number of ESWL treatments and increases stone-free state.

Thomas *et al.*'s [9] figures demonstrate the usefulness of the combined ESWL–PCNL approach: 76 patients with mono-ESWL required 2.8 treatments, PCN in 29% and left residuals in 48%; 66 patients with mono-PCNL needed 2 or more tracts in 71%, blood transfusion in 21%, and left residuals in 18%. In the 22 patients with one track-PCNL/ESWL, 9% were transfused and 13% had residuals.

The cost of combination therapy is however high. Staghorn ESWL monotherapy in Karachi costs Rs 25 000–45 000 (US$ 850–1500), PCNL–ESWL costs well over Rs 50 000 (over US$ 1600), whereas surgery costs Rs 15 000–20 000 (US$ 500).

Critical decisions on use of ESWL, ESWL–PCNL or surgery

The stone bulk, its distribution between calyces and pelvis, the degree of dilatation of calyces, and the composition of the stone, determine treatment outcomes and therefore choice of therapy.

Clearance rates with ESWL monotherapy are low for oxalate stones (57% stone free at 3 months) [5], and largely carbonate-containing stones (14.3%) [10], whilst urate and struvite stones have an 83% and 86% stone-free rate respectively [5], with 100% clearance of struvite stones in non-dilated systems. In Japan, an affluent nation, most staghorns are either struvite/carbonate (easy to fragment) or apatite [11]. Few are cystine, whewellite or brushite (difficult to fragment). In Pakistan, many are composed of difficult to fragment whewellite.

Silverio *et al.* [12] have suggested that therapy be modified according to stone composition and pelvi-calyceal structure, and we have combined their suggestions and those of Alken [7] and others in a comprehensive table (see Table 18.1). The American Urological Association Nephrolithiasis panel has made useful recommendations and suggestions for the treatment of staghorn calculi [13].

Asymptomatic staghorn calculi

Asymptomatic stones should be treated, as progressive destruction of the renal cortex and infection may occur. Struvite stones retain organisms within them [14], and untreated they will destroy the kidney and cause death in a significant propor-

Table 18.1   Rational therapy choices in staghorn calculi

Modifying factors	Preferred option
Previously operated kidney	Operation fraught with more risk; prefer alternative
Partial non-bulky staghorn, calyx not dilated	Treat with ESWL monotherapy with DJ stent
Partial staghorn non-bulky but overflowing into a dilated lower calyx	PCNL
Complete staghorn, of urate or struvite	Repeated ESWL, low voltage shocks, 2000–4000 shocks per treatment
Complete staghorn, dense white stone without coraliform appearance on X-ray (suspected calcium oxalate monohydrate)	PCNL combined with ESWL Avoid ESWL monotherapy Surgery a valid option
Large staghorn, major bulk pelvic, extensions into a grossly thinned out kidney	Operation best choice
Staghorns in which 70% clearance possible with single puncture PCNL	PCNL with ESWL
Staghorns following previous open clearance by PCNL expected to be < 70%	Review possibility of open surgery
Peripheral bulky stone, high density, non-dilated calyces	Open surgery with ESWL; preferable to ESWL monotherapy
Pyonephrosis	Nephrectomy
Hydronephrosis, infected hydronephrosis	PCNL or operation, ESWL to be avoided
Poor functioning kidney with normal contralateral kidney in an elderly[a] patient	Nephrectomy
Ureteral stenosis, ureteral displacement and kinking from previous surgery	Open surgery
Children	Avoid psychological trauma of multiple treatments

[a] Elderly should be defined in the context of the average lifespan of the local population.

tion of patients [15]. There is a small risk of carcinoma of the renal pelvis. A recent survey of 1032 patients with staghorns showed that four had renal pelvic tumours, of which only two were positive on cytology [16].

All large calculi should be treated, except those in patients with a short remaining life span, little and non-progressive renal cortical destruction on serial IVP or ultrasound, and absence of urinary infection.

Conclusion

In Europe, 23% of staghorns are removed by surgery, 31% by PCNL, 31% by ESWL, and 15% by a combination [7]. Eisenberger and Schmidt [17] from Germany (1987) treated staghorn calculi by ESWL in 2.5%, PCNL in 13%, combination in 80% and surgery in 4.5%. These percentages will vary according to the local stone population. In Pakistan, expertise with PCNL is available in few centres. Furthermore, the predominance of hard whewellite stones often makes open surgery or surgery with ESWL for residual fragments the best option.

References

1. Gallibondo F, Mendoza-Valdes A, Feria G *et al.* ESWL of staghorn (monotherapy) and ureteral calculi using a second generation lithotriptor (lithostar) on an outpatient basis. J Urol 1989;141:406A.
2. Wirth MP, Theiss M, Frohmuller HG. Primary extracorporeal shock wave lithotripsy of staghorn renal calculi. Urol Int 1992;48:71–5.
3. Gleeson MJ, Griffith DP. ESWL monotherapy for large renal calculi. Br J Urol 1989;64:329–32.
4. Gleeson M, Lerner SP, Griffith DP. Treatment of staghorn calculi with ESWL and PCNL. Urology 1991;38:145–51.
5. Fuchs GJ, Chaussy CG. ESWL for staghorn stones: Reassessment of our treatment strategy. World J Urol 1987;5:237–44.
6. Cicerello E, Merlo F, Gambaro G *et al.* Effect of alkaline citrate therapy on clearance of residual renal stone fragments after extracorporeal shock wave lithotripsy in sterile calcium and infection nephrolithiasis patients. J Urol 1994;151:5–9.
7. Alken P, Scharfe T, Hammer C *et al.* Percutaneous treatment of staghorn calculi. In: Jonas U, Dabjoiwala NF, Debruyne FMJ, editors. Endourology. Berlin, Heidelberg: Springer-Verlag, 1988;121–32.
8. Dretler SP. Ureteroscopic fragmentation followed by ESWL, a treatment alternative for selected large or staghorn calculi. J Urol 1994;151:842–6.
9. Thomas R, Figueroa TE, Macaluso J. Combination treatment in the management of staghorn renal calculi. J Urol 1989;141:286A.
10. Hatano Y, Segawa A. The treatment of staghorn calculi. Hinyokika Kiyo 1993;39:1087–91.
11. Takeuchi H, Yoshida O. Treatment of staghorn calculi on the basis of composition and structure. Hinyokika Kiyo 1993;39:1071–6.
12. Silverio FD, Galluci M, Alpi G. Staghorn calculi of the kidney, classification and therapy. Br J Urol 1990;65:449–52.
13. Segura JW, Preminger GM, Assimos DG *et al.* Nephrolithiasis clinical guidelines panel summary report on the management of staghorn. The American Urology Association Nephrolithiasis Clinical Guidelines Panel. J Urol 1994;151:1648–51.
14. Nemoy W, Stamey TA. Surgical, bacteriological and biochemical management of infected stones. J Am Med Assoc 1971;215:470.
15. Koga S, Arakaki V, Matsnoka M *et al.* Staghorn calculi, longterm results of management. Br J Urol 1991;68:122.
16. Nakatsu H, Masai M, Okano T *et al.* Urinary cytology in patients with urolithiasis. Nippon Hinyokika Gakkai Zasshi 1991;82:1281–5.
17. Eisenberger F, Schmidt A. Staghorn stones surgery or PCN and ESWL. In: Guiliani L, Pufpo P, editors. Controversies on the management of urinary stones. Basel: Karger, 1988:145.

19. Management of ureteric stones

JAMSHEER TALATI

Patients with ureteric stones present in many ways. Ureteric colic is dramatic, painful and distressing to even the observing relative. Anuria is disastrous. Many physicians in the third world do not realize the significance of obstructive anuria and treat it by forcing fluid or furosemide. Both colic and anuria are emergencies that require attention. Ureteric stones can also lie undiscovered, whilst insidiously destroying the kidney, a not too uncommon event.

Ureteric colic is a common emergency in Pakistan. It accounted for 2.6% of 3480 patients who sought help at the emergency room (ER), in a two-month period at the Aga Khan University Medical Center (AKUMC). An ER visit for colic occurs predominantly in the young with an average age of 31 years (range 17–70) for males, and 25 years for females (14–81) years.

Management of the patient with ureteric colic

Ureteric colic demands immediate relief, and intravenous hyoscine achieves this instantaneously. We have noted rapid dilatation of the ureter on administration of hyoscine during ureteroscopy. Continuous administration of hyoscine is not advisable, as it may interfere with propulsion of the stone by peristalsis of the ureter, but it is useful for acute colic. Some patients may require stronger analgesics or narcotics such as pethidine. Non steroidal antiinflammatory drugs reduce pain. They reduce the production of PGE_2 in the renal medulla, reducing afferent arteriolar dilatation and glomerular filtration. Those against the use of this drug warn that reduction of PGE_2 removes the protective mechanism that ensures adequate perfusion in the face of increasing luminal pressures from obstruction. Recent reports suggest that they cause lowering of ureteric motility.

Our current policy requires that patients seen in ER with colic should have an emergency limited intravenous pyelogram (IVP). If there is complete obstruction further films are taken, and if a nephrogram persists for more than 6 hours, a percutaneous nephrostomy is done. Patients with stones in the ureter of a solitary kidney, or a stone unlikely to pass because of size are admitted. Compliance with the protocol is low. Some patients refuse even a KUB X-ray as they have come to our hospital because they cannot reach their usual physician for this emergency, stating that they will have investigations as ordered by him/her. Only 50 (54%) of 92 patients

J. Talati et al. (eds) The Management of Lithiasis, 137–150
© *1997 Kluwer Academic Publishers. Printed in Great Britain.*

attending ER in a two-month period had a KUB done, and 22 (24%) had a limited IVP. Of these, only 12 demonstrated a stone. Only 3 of the 92 required admission for unremitting colic (data collected by Dr Navaid Alam). Chia [1] has also noted that 50% of IVP were negative in emergency patients and that if both microscopy of urine and KUB were negative, the IVP was normal in 90%. The colic may have been caused by the passage of gravel, the stone may have passed or the emergency physician may have made an error in diagnosis. A policy avoiding IVP under such circumstances will be cost-effective.

In acute colic, it is preferable not to force diuresis either by fluid loading or diuretic. The stone will best move down by peristalsis. Forced diuresis and continued hyoscine will produce a dilated, peristaltic ureter. Percutaneous nephrostomy restores ureteric peristalsis and speeds stone expulsion. Recently, acute obstruction has been urgently treated with extracorporeal shock wave lithotripsy (ESWL) [2].

Treatment of anuria

Anuria kills through fluid overload (and pulmonary oedema) and hyperkalaemia. Percutaneous nephrostomy aborts the emergency, allows fluid to drain and electrolytes to normalize. Subsequent therapy can then be undertaken safely and with less mishap. Calculus associated anuria is a major problem and constituted 4% of admissions to a nephrourology department in Pakistan [3].

The extent of the problem

In the pre-ESWL era (1986–87), at AKUMC, 43% of surgery for stone was for ureteric calculi. In 1995 (January to June), six years into ESWL, 30.6% of stones treated by all interventional modalities are ureteric stones. Many more patients with ureteric stones contact us as outpatients and are not included in these statistics.

In specialized centres, in the West, 26–40% of stones were ureteric [4], and up to 26% of stones treated on the lithotriptor were ureteric [5]. At AKUMC, 20–28% of stones treated on the lithotriptor were ureteric (1988–94).

In poorer populations in Pakistan, ureteric stone is less frequent, or less frequently reported. Ureteric stones accounted for 10.5% [6] to 20% [7] of stones in all age groups, and 4.1% [8] to 8.4% [9] in the paediatric age group. At AKUMC, only 5% of the 132 patients with ureteric stones subjected to ESWL from 1990–91, were under 20 years of age, with 27%, 36%, and 20% in their third, fourth and fifth decades.

Ureteric stones in Pakistan are often neglected once acute colic has subsided. They are generally larger ($11.9 \pm 5.0 \times 7.4 \pm 4.3$ mm) (1991) than in the West. Of 132 stones (1990–91), 22% were over 15 mm long, 33% were 10–15 mm long, 16% were wider than 10 mm, and 60% had a D1 $\times$ D2 area of more than 50 mm^2, 31% being more than 100 mm^2.

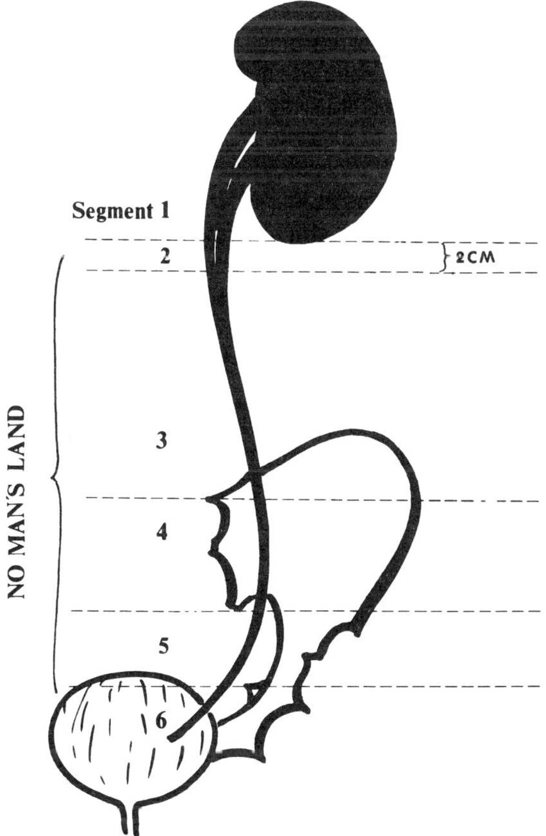

Figure 19.1 Ureteric stone: convenient segments for ESWL

Definitions of ureteric sections, stone-free status and impacted calculi

Comparison of results from different series is difficult as the terms upper, middle and lower ureter are used to indicate different sections of the ureter. We have proposed a classification into six sections [10] which has practical applications in decisions regarding therapy: section 1 extends from the uretero-pelvic junction to the level of the lower border of the kidney; section 2, for the next two centimetres; section 3, up to the upper border of the sacro-iliac joint; section 4, over the region of the joint; section 5, below the joint, up to the ischial spine; and section 6, from the ischial spine to the bladder (Figure 19.1).

Ultrasound monitored lithotriptors can easily identify ureteric stones up to the lower border of the kidney as the kidney provides a good landmark. Stones in a dilated ureter can often be identified with certainty up to 2 cm below that level. Hence the need to identify this segment of ureter. Level 4 is supported posteriorly by a bony structure and hence will require prone position during treatment even on radiologically controlled extracorporeal lithotriptors. Stones below the ischial spine will be easily localized by ultrasound using the acoustic window of a bladder filled with saline.

There is a problem with differentiating level 5 from 6, as the stone in the ureter will variously appear high or low depending on the position of the X-ray tube relative to the umbilicus. The X-ray should therefore be standardized.

A patient should be declared stone free only when there is no visible stone fragment on a KUB X-ray, or on ultrasound [11]. This is especially important in the case of the ureter, where a contrasting form of therapy (ureterolithotomy) provides 100% clearance.

An impacted calculus is one in which initial attempts at passing a guide wire or ureteric catheter past the stone failed [12], or the stone cannot be pushed back into the pelvi-calyceal system [13].

Options for interventional management of ureteric calculi

Three major options are available for interventional management of ureteral calculi – ureterolithotomy (UL), endoscopic fragmentation and extraction, and ESWL. The effectiveness of each procedure develops with experience, but is aided by a few guidelines, listed below, for each of these three procedures.

Ureterolithotomy

In third world countries, 14.5%–17% of ureteric stones may still require UL [14]. Throughout the world it is by far the commonest method of removing ureteric calculi [15], especially as large ureteric stones are common, and ESWL and ureteroscopy (URS) are available in very few centres even in 1995. In the early days of lithotripsy, we attracted many patients with large stones, and 29% of ureteric stones were operated either primarily or after failed URS [10]. Today (January to June 1995) only 2% are treated by ureterolithotomy. In the West, in units which use open surgery for only 2% of stones, 20% of the open operations are UL [16].

The complication rate for ureterolithotomy has been reported to be as high as 18% [17]. Some techniques to reduce complications are:

- An X-ray on the morning of operation detects sudden unsuspected movement of the stone. In the case of radiolucent stones, a limited IVP on the morning of surgery, or a retrograde pyelogram on the operating room table instilling radio-contrast so gently that it does not to dislodge the stone, is useful.
- The choice of incision based on the surface marking of the stone, and proper positioning of the patient, are crucial to a quick and successful UL. The stone position is plotted in relation to the disc space between L3 and 4 vertebrae (the umbilicus on surface marking) or the anterior superior iliac spine, or crest of the iliac bone, all landmarks easily felt or seen.

- Stones over the bony pelvis are best treated in the supine position with a sand bag under the ipsi-lateral gluteal region. Stones at the level of the umbilicus or above are best treated in a lateral kidney position so that if the stone slips into the kidney, it can be extracted.
- An incision planned two-thirds above and one-third below the surface marking of the stone, facilitates early taping of the ureter above the stone.
- Muscle splitting incisions yield strong wounds. If ureteric stones are at two different sites (e.g. over the sacrum and deep in the pelvis), use one incision for the skin and the external oblique, and a separate incision in the deeper muscles. These will be small and the grid-iron nature of the incision can be preserved.
- Occlusion of the ureter above the stone by a tape or silicone tubing, before handling the section of the ureter bearing the stone, prevents upward migration. With the tape secure, the ureter can be angulated to occlude it. Alternatively a second loop of tape can be thrown around the ureter. Upward migration complicates the operation unnecessarily, especially when the patient is in a supine position and the incision is for a lower ureteric stone in section 3 or 4.
- An incision on the posterolateral aspect of the ureter prevents leakage as the ureteric incision lies against the psoas. This is facilitated by rotating the ureter on its axis. Urine is obtained from the proximal dilated ureter via syringe and needle and sent for culture. An incision is then made (between stay sutures) long enough to allow the maximum transverse diameter of the stone to be delivered. Wounds heal from side to side, and no attempt should be made to forcibly and blindly extract an impacted stone through a small incision. Such a manoeuvre is fraught with the risk of leaving behind gravel imbedded in the ureteric mucosa, or in the distal ureters. Under such conditions it is better to make an incision as long as the long diameter of the stone, and use a Watson–Cheyne dissector to free the stone from the oedematous ureteric mucosa. All particles of stone should be picked out by fine non-toothed forceps such as Waugh's. In unimpacted stones, a transverse incision in the ureter is preferred, as it heals more readily and is associated with a lower incidence of postoperative urinary leakage.
- Ensuring that the lower ureter is patent by passing a ureteric catheter down the ureter also minimizes the risk of leak. Small fragments of calculi present in the upper ureter or the kidney may be swept into the lower ureter as the tape is released. This can be prevented by keeping the ureteric catheter in the lower ureter until the tape release.
- Fine closely applied sutures (chromic catgut 4/0 or vicryl 4/0) diminish urinary leak.
- Levering the stone out of the ureter by a Watson–Cheyne dissector, rather than handling it with a forceps of any kind, prevents crumbling.
- A tube drain allows any leaked urine to be carried away and prevents a disastrous sclerosing urinoma (collection of urine around the ureter). A suction drain is more appropriate for pelvic ureteric incisions, where urine leak will fall into a sump difficult to empty by a tube drain. Otherwise an ordinary red rubber tube will be adequate and preferable as suction drains at times perpetrate leakage.

The drain should be so placed that it does not lie across the ureter, and does not lie in direct contact with the suture line in the ureter. The drainage should decrease to less than 20 ml per day before drain removal is contemplated. The patient may be discharged when ambulant, and return later for removal of sutures and tubes; these should not be removed in a hurry.

- If UL is to follow URS, a DJ stent or open-ended catheter that is passed up to the level of the stone at cystoscopy could be pulled up into the kidney at the time of open surgery. Its correct positioning should be confirmed by X-ray before reversing anaesthesia. If the stent is found coiled in the dilated upper ureter, cystocopy is necessary for readjustment; the stent can be pulled out partially so that its tip emerges at the urethral meatus, a guide wire inserted through it into the kidney and the stent repositioned correctly. A pull through stent with attached nylon thread is preferable, as the patient does not then need a second admission.

- The operation is done extraperitoneally. If the peritoneum is opened accidentally, it is sutured at the start of the operation, to avoid urinary contamination of the peritoneal cavity.

- The stone should be retained to show it to the patient's relatives the same day, as soon as the operation is over, and the patient the next day. The stone should not be delivered to the relatives; it will be taken home for proud display, and it will not be possible to retrieve it for analysis. Showing the stone to the patient in the recovery room may not be beneficial, as the patient is often so much under the influence of narcotics that he cannot remember having seen it.

- It is important to show the stone before sending it for analysis. Many a patient tells us in his history that he had an operation, and the doctor told him that a stone was removed, but never showed it to him; implying sceptically that it was not found at operation.

Advantages of ureterolithotomy

In an unsophisticated environment, UL is the most effective method of removing ureteric stones expeditiously at low cost. Even in a multimodality setting with ultrasound lithotriptors, ureterolithotomy remains the most cost-effective procedure for large calcium oxalate monohydrate stones in the mid-ureter with a dilated ureter and gross hydronephrosis.

UL, without a preliminary attempted ureteroscopy, utilizes less operating time compared to URS – 20 minutes for section 3 and 4 stones in a non-teaching environment. The number of staff involved in a ureterolithotomy is minimal. A UL can be done with an anaesthetist, single runner nurse, and single scrub nurse, and no other personnel in the theatre. A first assistant is helpful but not mandatory. A radiographer is not required in the operating room. An additional advantage is that the stone is always available for analysis, something that is becoming rare when the stone is treated by ESWL, in spite of encouraging and coercing patients to collect stone debris.

Ureterolithotomy requires only the conventional instruments available in any hospital. Capital costs of a lithotriptor, ureteroscope and C-arm increase the cost of procedures other than UL.

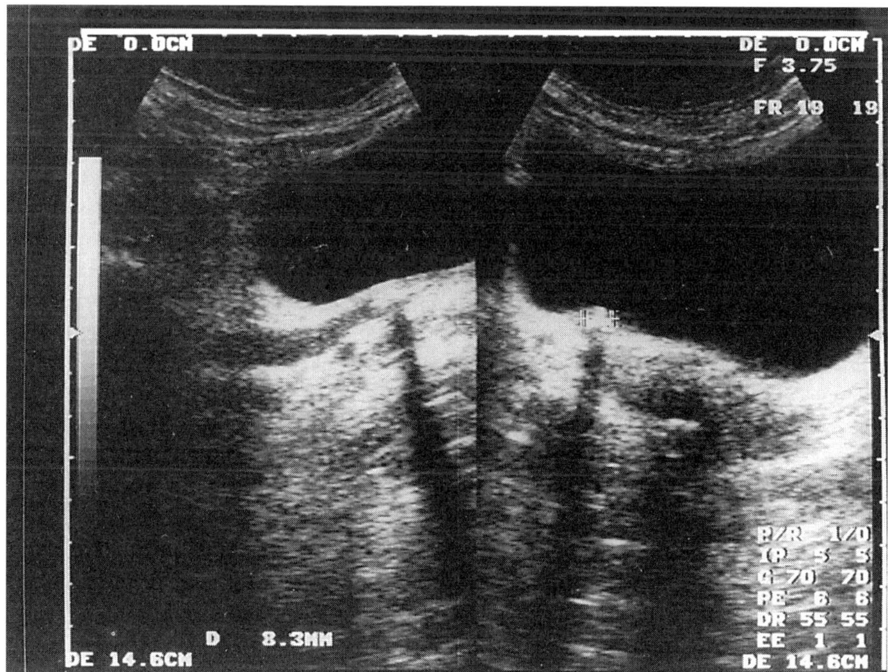

Figure 19.2 Stone in lower ureter visualised through a bladder distended with saline. The stone casts an acoustic shadow. The dilated ureter can be seen below the bladder in the left half of the ultrasound image

Ureteroscopy equipment is fragile. In a setting with multiple users there are likely to be one or two breakages per year, especially when residents are in training or laser is being used. Disposable ureteroscopes at $ 1000 each cannot be purchased for a third world setting. Ureterolithotomy requires only one visit to hospital for treatment unless a DJ stent has been utilized. Though the patient needs admission, the hospital stay is short (mode four days) and the total costs to the patient are of the order of US$ 500 for UL compared to US$ 500–750 required for ESWL (but the charges for ESWL are heavily subsidized). Incisional hernias should be uncommon if muscle splitting incisions are used and carefully reapproximated.

Ureteroscopy

URS is an efficient way of managing *steinstrasse* after ESWL and small lower ureteric stones. In the third world and emerging countries, large stones, gross hydronephrosis, and high costs make it less suitable.

Ureteroscopy requires a high capital outlay and maintenance budget, for ureteroscopes and ancillaries such as laser, electro-hydraulic (EHL) and ultrasound intracorporeal lithotriptors, and C-arm. Ureteroscopy has to be done in an operating room setting, and requires a dedicated team which include a radiographer, scrub person and anaesthetist, whose skill has to keep pace with the surgeon. Success rates of 89–93% have been quoted [14, 18]. Success and complication rates will vary according to protocols for treatment, size of stones, sites of ureter tackled, and equipment available. Difficulties will be encountered in the obese, with impacted stones, non-dilatable ureters and patients with strictures below the stone. Success is dependent on the quality of endoscopes and fragmenting modality. Ureteroscopic skills are learnt slowly [19] and there is a variable complication rate with distressing complications from the interference with the sanctity of the ureteric orifice and perforation and stricturing of the ureter. Inexperience adds hazards. Learning curves are shorter with the current small instruments. Lithoclast and lasers perforate the ureter less frequently than EHL. Judicious use of buscopan or nifedipine after induction of anaesthesia, and judicious use of dilatation of the ureteric orifice when using larger instruments, increase success rates.

Some series have reported ureteric perforation in up to 17% [20]. The majority will occur in the proximal ureter [18]. Minor perforations heal without sequelae on stenting. Infected urine, sepsis, a large leak or enlarging or persistent collection require aspiration. Forced introduction of the scope may cause it to bend, which causes the visual field to alter from a disc to a 'half moon' appearance. Gentle handling, and a readiness to abandon the procedure if half-mooning of the visual field occurs, reduces chances of injury.

URS requires intermittent radiological imaging with entry site doses for the patient ranging from 0.6–15 rad, with exposure times of 2–4.3 minutes. Lead aprons reduced general exposure to surgeons but the fingers and neck may receive 97 rem per case [21].

Like ESWL, ureteroscopy (URS) can be done as a day admission. This reduces the real costs in comparison to ESWL. Patients are usually stone free at the end of the procedure; and only one additional visit to the operating room is required for removal of a stent. This visit can be eliminated by using stents with a pull-through suture, or using an open-ended catheter as a temporary splint.

Success and safety

In the absence of small instruments and lithoclast, a two-stage policy of stenting the ureter at the initial procedure in difficult cases adds costs but increases safety. Consigning large stones to operation gives better results. The temptation to persevere with endoscopic management because the patient has been referred by another urologist who has attempted endoscopy and failed, and who has referred the case for non-operative removal, must be resisted. Arguing on the basis that a UL could just as easily have been done by the referring doctor, often in another town many miles away, a UL at the tertiary centre does not seem an attractive option and can push decisions to non-operative management, sometimes to the detriment of the patient. Every surgeon needs to remember that UL has a definite place in the management of ureteric stones, and that after adequate attempts at URS, the procedure should be abandoned without reflection on his/her expertise rather as an accolade to his/her judgement. Stubborn persistence may result in higher complication rates and more serious complications.

All patients for URS should therefore be advised of the possible need for UL, and this fact should be entered in their consent form. Conversion to UL can then occur under the same anaesthetic after reasonable attempts at URS extraction.

What constitutes reasonable attempts? If endoscopists do not diligently struggle in the initial years of their experience, their skills at URS will be very limited. It is only by persevering that success is achieved. But this perseverance must be tempered by judgement. There is no place for the use of sheer force. Direct UL has a very low morbidity, whereas unsuccessful URS followed by UL has a 25% complication rate, utilizes more operation room time and anaesthesia time, and prolongs hospital stay [9]. The lithoclast and laser have revolutionized ureteric stone endoscopy. Smaller instruments and video camera monitored teaching have made the procedure easy to learn. Ureteroscopy will assume greater importance in the management of lower ureteral calculi in well-equipped clinics.

Each physician should determine his/her percentage of success for different types and sizes of stones; this enables prediction of URS success on a particular patient and suggestion of appropriate first-line therapy.

ESWL for ureteric stones

Barring restrictions from inability to localize stones in certain sections of the ureter, ESWL is the first-line treatment for ureteric stones. At times, ESWL cannot be used because the stone is out of reach of the second focus, F2. Most stones (except those very close to the transverse processes of the lumbar vertebrae and those that are radiolucent) will be visualized on radiologically monitored lithotriptors. Many will not be visible on ultrasound lithotriptors and will therefore need push-up, some by ureteric catheter, others at ureteroscopy.

As with renal calculi, ESWL of ureteric stones therefore demands that the unit be competent in ureteroscopy. When choosing ESWL as therapy for ureteric stones, much will depend upon the type of machine available and the level of development of ureteroscopic skills in the unit.

Because UL and URS have a potential for producing a stone-free patient on day one, the aim of ESWL should be to have the patient stone free in the shortest possible time, without the need for any pre-ESWL or post-ESWL procedures or anaesthesia. Treatment should therefore minimize need for push-ups or stenting and should not leave behind recalcitrant fragments which fail to clear. It should be completed in a minimal number of sittings and should be safe.

Stones in the ureter require 20 kV, but will seldom require more than 2000 shocks if less than 10 mm long. The need for more powerful shocks has been demonstrated by Parr *et al.* [22] on synthetic stones. The amount of stone that disintegrated when the stone lay free (243 ± 18 mg) was much more than when it was held confined (62 ± 18 mg) or impacted (22 ± 8 mg). Too many shocks, however, produce oedema and hinder particle elimination [23]. Treatment should be stopped as soon as an end-point is reached.

Experience improves results. Though the mean size of stones treated at AKUMC increased in 1991 compared to 1990, 85% compared with 55% were treated in one session only, and 7.5% required a third treatment. Forty per cent required only 1001–2000 shocks but 4% needed more than 4000 shocks. Six per cent required ureteroscopy for extraction of fragments after ESWL.

Stone clearance

Ureteric stones sometimes take a long time to clear. A KUB X-ray, the morning after ESWL, may show little change in the calculus, other than subtle change in the ratio of length to breadth. After 2–3 days, a repeat X-ray may show complete disappearance of the stone. This is because the fragmented stone is held closely by the ureter in spasm. Specific changes in the ultrasound reflex obtained from the stone on the in-line scanner are of help in some cases. In the lower ureter, ultrasound (US) of the unfragmented stone gives a sharp convex linear reflex. This becomes broad and egg-shaped as the stone fragmentation allows US waves to penetrate the stone. Still later a serpentine wave of urine can be seen passing through the stone, indicating that sufficient fragmentation has occurred.

Cumulative clearance rates could be of the order of 17% on day 7, 64% by day 30, 83% by day 90 and 87% by day 180 (AKUMC statistics, 1990–91) at the start of the experience. Today, we use a smaller number of shock waves and clearance is seen within the first few weeks, often within seven days.

Push-up before ESWL or in situ *treatment?*

Our experience has shown that ESWL *in situ* is very successful. Stones which cannot be visualized on either the US or radiologically monitored lithotriptor will require push-up. Difficulties in localization of stone on the fluoroscope screen when using radiologically monitored machines result from obesity, a stone too close to the spine, or skeletal abnormality. On the US monitored lithotriptor, stones in sections 3, 4 and 5 will require push-up. Overall, the number requiring push-up on US monitored machines will be a only little higher than on radiologically monitored lithotriptors. It could be argued that if a ureteroscope is to be used to push up a stone, why can it not be used to extract the stone. The reason for not doing so is that multiple passes will be required to clear the fragments, of necessity through the narrower distal ureter, thus increasing the risk of trauma.

Stones in sections 1, 2 and 6 are easily visualized on ultrasound monitored lithotriptors. Stones in other sections will either need push-up for ESWL [10, 24] or some other modality of therapy. Experience and dedication can increase the number of stones that can be localized on either US or radiologically monitored lithotriptors. Using the MPL 9000, and US monitored lithotriptor, we treated 83% of 69 section 1, 2 and 6 stones *in situ*, compared to 68% of 63 in 1990. DiClemente *et al.* [25] treat all stones at all levels *in situ*. Their expertise is unique. Treatment of 100% of section 1, 2 and 6 stones *in situ* should be aimed for.

Treatment *in situ* eliminates the need for anaesthesia, admission and instrumentation and its attendant risks. Push-up into systems that are dilated will delay clearance.

Stenting for ureteric stones

Stenting does not improve results [26–28] but may be required for flushing with contrast to localize urate stones on radiologically monitored lithotripsy.

Facilitating endoscopic manoeuvres complimentary to ESWL
Consent for the above manoeuvres should include all options: push-up, ureteroscopy, UL and general spinal or epidural anaesthesia.

To avoid anaesthesia, the use of flexible instruments is suggested to help push up stones. However, these instruments do not have a beak to assist push-up.

All push-up procedures are done with full preparation for ureteroscopy, in an operating suite where any additional equipment will be available and open operation can be done without risk of sepsis. An image intensifier is used. The tabletop needs to be radiolucent. After induction of anaesthesia a prophylactic antibiotic is given because of the risk that high pressures generated in the pelvis may provoke bacteraemia and endotoxaemia. The patient is positioned as for cystoscopy. Hyoscine given IV or nifedepine given sublingually is of value in dilating the ureter and countering the effects of muscle relaxants which can cause ureteric spasm. Nifedipine is a smooth muscle relaxant which dilates the ureter and is beneficial in ureteroscopies. It has not been found effective in treating ureteric colic, as the ureter continues to become increasingly distended due to the fact that nifedipine does not reduce glomerular filtration rate [30].

A cystoscope is passed under vision and the ipsilateral ureteric orifice is cannulated with an open-ended 6F ureteric catheter. The following steps are taken in sequence, only proceeding to the next step if necessary.

1. An open-ended catheter is passed under vision to the site of the stone which is then gently and repeatedly nudged by the catheter to displace it back into the pelvis.
2. Saline is injected under pressure. Perez-Castro [31] recommends the use of carbon dioxide, instead of saline.
3. A guide wire is passed through the 6F catheter and the catheter withdrawn. A balloon catheter is introduced up to the stone and wedged between the stone and the ureteric wall. The balloon is inflated and deflated a number of times, advancing the catheter a little each time, to create a space parallel to the stone.
4. The balloon catheter is deflated and withdrawn a short distance and saline injected under force. If this and balloon catheter nudging fails, a guide wire is inserted through the catheter and the catheter and cystoscope are withdrawn completely. A ureteroscope is introduced to the stone guided by the wire. Rotation of the beak of the scope can often disimpact the stone, under vision. Currently we dilate the ureteric orifice when using the larger scopes, but not the entire lower ureter, relying on hydrostatic pressure from a syringe to dilate the ureter. Eshgi *et al.* [32] have demonstrated that hydraulically dilated ureters are less traumatized than ureters dilated mechanically with bougies or balloons. There is also less chance of pushing epitheliums outwards into the subepithelial layers to produce Brunn's nests.
5. If all this fails, disimpaction of the calculus can be undertaken by electro-hydraulic lithotripsy or US lithotriesis.
6. If laser is available then all steps should be skipped; If the calculus is declared impassable (impacted) it should be dislodged by laser [15].

7.   Lignocaine 1% instilled into the ureter counters the effects of muscle relaxants which increase the contractility of the ureter [33]. The use of deep halothane anaesthesia without muscle relaxants has been recommended.

8.   As an alternative to push-back, Perez-Castro [31] inserts a catheter up to the stone and irrigates with saline during ESWL to flush away particles.

9.   Others have used a stone brush to remove debris so that shock waves could reach the stone core effectively [13].

10.   If push-back fails in the absence of sophisticated methods, a simple open ended ureteric catheter with multiple holes should be introduced past the stone, or a DJ stent passed for later (two-stage) ureteroscopy.

Position during ESWL

We now prefer the lateral position for section 1 and 2 stones. Stones pushed back into the kidney are treated in the supine position, and stones in the lower ureter (level 6) in the prone position. Treatment for section 6 stones is assisted by controlled filling of the bladder with saline from an IV fluid bottle, via a three-way catheter. Distension of the bladder allows the visualization of the stone through the acoustic window of the full bladder. Once localized with surety, the bladder should be emptied partially to maximize patient comfort. This is not necessary for radiologically monitored ESWL. Feria *et al.* [5] suggest a prone position when the ureteric stone cannot be localized or brought into focus on the radiologically monitored machine.

Open surgery, ureteroscopy or ESWL?

ESWL is the preferred treatment for most stones in the ureter. However, ureteric stone bulk is greater in the third world, and Table 19.1 shows how stone size determines the treatment decision.

In our initial enthusiasm to minimize UL, we incorrectly treated many large stones by URS only to have to convert them to UL. A retrospective review showed that 83% of the stones that were treated by UL after URS were greater than $50 \, mm^2$, compared with only 42% of those treated successfully by URS. However 22% of stones treated successfully by ESWL were greater than 15 mm long axis, and 68% were greater than $50 \, mm^2$ with 31% greater than $100 \, mm^2$.

Stone site is the next most important determinant of choice of therapy. In our 1990–91 experience (132 stones), 43% of stones were in section 1, 18% in section 2, 30.3% in section 6, and the rest in sections 3–5. In 1990, 78% of stones at section 6 were treated by ESWL; today we treat all except those behind a structure by ESWL. Sixty-two per cent of stones at sections 1 and 2 were treated by ESWL; today we would attempt ESWL as first-line therapy for all.

Table 19.1   Size of stones treated on different modalities

ESWL	$74.5 \pm 50.3 \, mm^3$
URS	$81.8 \pm 82.9 \, mm^3$
UL[a]	$122.9 \pm 93.4 \, mm^3$

[a]   UL includes all patients treated by UL, including those treated after failed URS.
(Reproduced by permission from the *British Journal of Urology*).

A large stone, greater than 10×5 mm at section 3 or 4 is best tackled by ureterolithotomy. PUJ and section 1 and 2 stones are best treated by ESWL. Section 5 stones are best treated by URS. It is not advisable to push back a stone into a dilated system, as clearance from a lower calyx will be difficult. An attempt should be made to localize and focus on stones in sections 3, 4 and 5. It may be possible to treat them on radiologically monitored lithotriptors. If not then push-up/ureteroscopy should be planned.

Personal experience will sway decisions. Those with great expertise in URS such as Perez-Castro will use it as the first modality. Most recommend ESWL as first-line therapy. Fuchs *et al.* [34] have however shown in a randomized trial, treating ten stones by ESWL and ten by URS, that URS was successful in 100% whilst only six of the ten ESWL patients were stone free without ancillary procedures even after two treatments. The greater success with the lower compared to upper ureter stones and the fact that costs are 50% of ESWL led Sloane *et al.* [35] to recommend URS as the procedure of clearance for lower ureters. For section 6 stones, there is no doubt that ESWL is the most successful with 100% stone-free rates obtainable in a week.

Cases which are difficult for URS are mid-ureteric and proximal ureteric stones; stones in obese patients; non-dilatable ureters; and stones above a stricture. All these difficulties will be compounded by inexperience with the method, and hampered by the lack of availability of small ureteroscopes, laser and lithoclast.

An alternative to UL must be considered for such stones. The main disadvantages of ESWL are the number of visits of the patient to the hospital for treatment and follow-up; the long time that it takes to clear a stone; and the unavailability of stone material for analysis. These are more than offset by the elimination of the need for anaesthesia (except for push-back and DJS insertion) and the possibility of day-care therapy without admission. Follow-up is very important in ureteric stones. Our general follow-up rate was 80% in 1991 and was only achieved by diligent audits. Letters to patients (if phone calls fail to achieve results) are constantly required.

References

1. Chia SJ. A review of ureteric colic – the outcome and value of initial investigations. 2nd Asian Congress of Urology. Bangkok: Asian Urological Association, 1994.
2. Cass A. In situ ESWL for obstructing ureteral stones with acute renal colic. J Urol 1992;148:1786–7.
3. Hussain U, Ali B, Lal M. Calculus renal failure. Review of 360 cases. First International Symposium, Sindh Institute of Urology and Transplantation, 1995:167.
4. Gschwend J, Weber HM, Miller K *et al.* Experience with ultrasound guided ESWL. Urologie A 1991;30:207–10.
5. Feria G, Madonza A, Gabelando F. In situ treatment of ureteral calculi using an electromagnetic generator. J Urol 1990;143:248A.
6. Rizvi SAH. Calculous disease. A survey of 400 patients. J Pak Med Assoc October, 1975;25:268–74.
7. See Table 3.4, p. 27 this book
8. Rizvi SAH. Pediatric nephrolithiasis in Pakistan. J Pak Med Assoc 1982;32:177–82.

9. Khan MN, Islam S, Afzal S *et al.* Urolithiasis in children, a comparison of Western and Pakistani data. Pak J Surg 1991;7:757–60.

10. Talati J, Khan LA, Noordzij JW *et al.* The scope and place of ultrasound monitored ESWL in a multimodality setting and the effects of experiential, audit evoked changes on the management of ureteral calculi. Br J Urol 1994;73:480–6.

11. Talati J, Shah T, Memon A *et al.* ESWL for urinary tract stones using MPL 9000 spark gap technology and ultrasound monitoring. J Urol 1991;146:1482–6.

12. Morganteller A, Bridge SS, Dretler SP. Management of the impacted ureteral calculus. J Urol 1990;143:263–6.

13. Niezarello J, Rubenstein MA, Norris DM. ESWL and the ureter stone brush. J Urol 1990;143:261–2.

14. Guo YL, Guo FL, Zhang JL *et al.* Vicissitudes in the management of ureteral stones. Chinese Med J 1990;103:131–3.

15. Dretler SP. Alternatives for the management of ureteral calculi. Pak J Surg 1989;5:50–61.

16. Boyle E, Segura JW, Patterson DE *et al.* The role of open surgery in stone disease. J Urol 1989;141:243A.

17. Furlow WL, Bucchiere JJ. The surgical fate of ureteral calculi; review of the Mayo clinic experience. J Urol 1976;116:559–61.

18. Stoller ML, Wolff JS, Hoffman R *et al.* Ureteroscopy and outcome assessment. J Urol 1991;145:298A.

19. Adolfsson J, Lindstrom AC, Carbin BE *et al.* Ureteroscopic manipulation of stones in the upper ureter, a four year experience. Scan J Urol Nephrol 1990;24:113–15.

20. Kramolowsky EV. Ureteral perforation during URS treatment and management. J Urol 1987;138:36.

21. Bagley D, Gardman A. Radiation exposure during ureteroscopy. J Urol 1989;141:175A (abstract 24).

22. Parr NJ, Pye SD, Ritchie AW *et al.* Mechanisms responsible for diminished fragmentation of ureteral calculi: An experimental and clinical study. J Urol 1992;148:1079–83.

23. Parr NJ, Ritchie AW, Moussa SA *et al.* The impact of extracorporeal piezoelectric lithotripsy on the management of ureteral calculi – relationship between number of shocks delivered and success. J Urol 1991;145:270A.

24. Schmidt P, Rassweiler J, Gumpinger R *et al.* Minimally invasive treatment of ureteral calculi using modern techniques. Br J Urol 1990;65:242–4.

25. DiClemente L, D'Andrea R, DiNardo A *et al.* In situ treatment of ureteral stones with the drum lithotriptor MPL 9000 Dornier. User Letter 1991;7:16–22.

26. Psihramis K, Jewett MA, Bombardier C *et al.* Lithostar extracorporeal shock wave lithotripsy, the Toronto experience. J Urol 1992;147:1006–9.

27. Albala DM, Meretyk S, Clayman RV. ESWL for ureteral calculi; to stent or not to stent. J Urol 1991;145:299A (abstract 345).

28. Fetner CD, Preminger GM, Kettlehut MC *et al.* Morbidity of ureteral stenting during ESWL. J Urol 1989;141:270A (abstract 402).

29. Tubaro A, Miano L, l'Aquila *et al.* Lithiasis of the pelvic ureter, ESWL in prone and sitting position on a sonolith 3000 lithotriptor. J Urol 1990;143:249A.

30. Ghonheim GM, Dilworth JP, Roberts JA. Nifedipine sublingual for acute ureteral obstruction. J Urol 1989;141:414A.

31. Perez-Castro EE. Ureteral stones, how to manage them, In: Giuliani L, Puppo P, editors. Controversies in management of stone disease. Basel, Munchen, Paris: Karger, 1988:88–9.

32. Esghi M, McLamed D, Chaudhary M. ESWL in the treatment of distal ureteral stones in the supine position without stenting or anesthesia. J Urol 1989;141:208A.

33. Ryan PC, Jones BJ, Hargaden KM. Pharmacological dilatation of the human ureter for ureteroscopy, an experimental study. J Urol 1990;143:363A.

34. Fuchs G, Steryl A, David R. ESWL vs URS in stones below the pelvic brim. J Urol 1989;141:411A.

35. Sloane B, Thomas R, Macaluso J. Management of ureteral stone – should there be a controversy? J Urol 1989;141:272A.

20. Clinical results of laser fragmentation of ureteric stones

GRAHAM WATSON and TARIQ SHAH

For those wishing to read the chapters on laser in continuity, the following sequence is suggested: read Chapter 13 first, then this chapter, and finally the Appendix on non-visual laser lithotripsy.

A total of 2200 ureteric calculi have been treated in our unit using the pulsed dye laser; 30 have been treated with the holmium laser. In the initial phase the pulsed dye laser was compared with 5F electro-hydraulic (EHL) probes in fragmenting calculi embedded in the lower third of the ureter of the pig [1]. Laser fragmentation produced no tissue damage in contrast to the electro-hydraulic discharges. However these differences were less significant than the injury produced by the uretero-scopes in the lower third of the ureter. The calibre of the ureteroscope was the most significant parameter affecting the ureter, and the pulsed dye laser was successful in clinical practice partly because of the simultaneous development of a miniaturized ureteroscope (Candela Corporation). This was the 7.25F tip miniscope with a dual channel [2] that made ureteroscopy possible without dilatation.

We have recently reviewed our clinical experience with the pulsed dye laser [3]. The first 100 patients were instrumented with an 11.3F rod lens ureteroscope. Successful access to the stone on the first attempt was only achieved in 73%. There were seven perforations of the ureter. Twelve patients required temporary nephros-tomy drainage following treatment in the lower third of the ureter. The second 100 patients were instrumented using a range of ureteroscopes from 8.5 to 11.5F. Access to stone was successful on first attempt in 94% of cases. In this group there were three ureteric perforations, a nephrostomy was required in six cases, and two patients subsequently developed a stricture in the lower third. By contrast, in the first 200 patients treated by miniscope or occasionally a flexible ureteroscope, access to the stone was successful in 99% of cases; there were no perforations of the ureter, no nephrostomies and no strictures. Clinical experience therefore mirrored the experience on the pig ureter model.

The next period when using the pulsed dye laser was one in which our trainees were also performing ureteroscopy, initially supervised and later unsupervised. In a larger series of 2000 patients treated by all grades of urologist at our unit the success rate on first attempt was 97%. The failures were treated successfully by performing a second attempt retrogradely in 42 cases and antegradely in 17 cases. There were no cases treated by open ureterolithotomy. Two patients had a ureteric

J. Talati et al. (eds) The Management of Lithiasis, 151–153
© *1997 Kluwer Academic Publishers. Printed in Great Britain.*

perforation and one patient required nephrostomy. No patient developed a ureteric stricture.

Thus the miniaturization of ureteroscopes which has developed alongside laser fragmentation of calculi has been of profound significance.

Not only is the ureteroscope important but so also are other accessories. We have now made it our routine to attempt a complete stone clearance at the time of ureteroscopy. In a survey of our experience with 224 patients [3] in the lower third of the ureter 36%, 54% and 80% of patients respectively were clear at the end of the procedure, and after one and three months. When a basket was used subsequent to laser, 61%, 81% and 91% were clear of stones.

Recently we have performed 34 laser fragmentations with a holmium laser. We have used 1.4 per pulse at 5 Hz using a 300 microsecond pulse duration and a 320 or 400 micron fibre. Provided that care is made to avoid any direct lasering of the ureter, treatment is safe. The holmium laser has the advantage [4] of being a multi-purpose laser; the fragments are tiny and there is very little momentum imparted to the stone. The disadvantage is that the holmium laser tends to drill into the stone and it does cause significant tissue damage if incident on tissue.

EHL, laser or ESWL?

Whereas from 1987 to 1989 only the laser could be used with a miniaturized ureteroscope, the development of other miniaturized fragmentation devices – EHL probes, ultrasound probes and the lithoclast – now means that all these modalities can be used [5, 6]. The EHL probe is currently available in 1.9F and 3F probes. The generator is significantly cheaper than a laser. If a unit only uses a modality sporadically then this is the cheapest choice. However the cost of the probes makes the lithoclast a cheaper modality once 50 probes have been consumed (and this may be after fewer than 50 treatments). If alternative uses are considered, the holmium laser may be indicated. The laser fibres can be reused frequently, making the disposable costs minimal. The pulsed dye laser and alexandrite laser are significantly more expensive. They can only be justified by a unit with significant ureteric stone practice. The high initial cost of the laser is justified once a unit performs a number of stone fragmentations per year. This number is in the region of 50 cases in the USA and 200 cases in the UK. This relationship between numbers and the laser is unfortunate because the unit performing ureteroscopic stone therapy only sporadically has the greatest need of the safest modality. The lithoclast would probably therefore be more appropriate for the sporadic user than the EHL probe.

Many units are treating more and more calculi with extracorporeal shock wave lithotripsy (ESWL), clearly the least invasive modality. Provided that one can image the stone it requires less expertise. However endoscopic management of ureteric calculi remains important. If a stone is causing significant obstruction, that obstruction can be more certainly and more rapidly relieved by endoscopy. The development of smaller ureteroscopes is now making it increasingly possible to treat patients without recourse to general anaesthesia. The patient can be treated with no more discomfort than shock wave lithotripsy. We therefore predict that laser fragmentation will become more widely used as these local anaesthetic techniques become adopted, as non-laser modalities are less suited to use with small flexible ureteroscopes and cause more discomfort under these conditions.

References

1. Watson GM, Murray S, Dretler S *et al*. An assessment of the pulsed dye laser in the pig ureter. J Urol 1987;138:199–203.
2. Watson GM, Wickham JEA. The development of a laser and a miniaturized ureteroscope for ureteric stone management. World J Urol 1989;7:147–50.
3. Watson GM, Landers B, Nauth-Miser R *et al*. The importance of ureteroscopes and accessories associated with laser lithotripsy. World J Urol 1993;11:19–25.
4. Watson GM, Smith N. A comparison of the pulsed dye and holmium lasers for stone fragmentation, *in vitro* and clinical experience. In: Katzir, Anderson, editors. Laser surgery: Advanced characterization, therapeutics and systems. IV Proceedings of SPIE, 1993.
5. Vorreuther R. Minimally invasive ureteroscopy using adjustable electrohydraulic lithotripsy. J Endourol 1992;6:47–50.
6. Hofbauer J, Hobarth K, Marberger M. Lithoclast: New and inexpensive mode of intracorporeal lithotripsy. J Endourol 1992;6:429–32.

21. Management of vesical and urethral stones

ZIAUL AMIN HOTIANA and JAMSHEER TALATI

Bladder calculi

In children, bladder stones cause irritation of the trigone, and cause the patient to constantly hold or pull on the penis. The most expedient way to remove such calculi is by cystolithotomy. We have used extracorporeal lithotripsy for small stones in children older than two years, with good success. We protect the testis by wrapping the scrotum in aluminium foil, which reflects the sound waves. We do not treat female children, because of the inability to protect gonads. Patients are treated prone, as described for adults (see below).

In the adult, stones may be discovered during investigation of lower urinary tract symptoms suggestive of prostatism. Many are associated with obstructive benign prostatic hyperplasia, and may represent calculi descended from the ureter or kidney, or formed *de novo* in the partially stagnant pool of urine in the post-prostatic pouch. A characteristic symptom not seen very often is the history of sudden jerky shift in the body posture during micturition to restart the urinary stream which was interrupted as the stone rolled over the internal meatus.

Three methods can be used for treating bladder stones in the adult – cystolithotomy, endoscopic extraction (at times after fragmenting the stone) or extracorporeal shock wave lithotripsy (ESWL). In adults, bladder outflow obstruction must be treated concurrently. Cystolithotomy is the best alternative for very hard and very large stones (such as those illustrated in Figure 21.1), and is the most sensible method of extracting the stone if a transvesical prostatectomy is to be done. Cystolithotomy can follow a trans-urethral resection of the prostate (TURP) under the same anaesthetic, if the stone is large.

Cystolithotomy is a simple low-skill procedure which can be performed by anyone with basic general surgical training. No special instruments are required. Perhaps this modality of treatment is still ideal for very large or multiple stones and is the commonest and sometimes the only method used in district hospitals all over Pakistan. Meticulous two-layer closure of the bladder after cystolithotomy in children has allowed catheter-free postoperative care.

Prior to TUR, smaller stones can be easily crushed by mechanical means – either a Mauermyer punch or strong forceps with crushing jaws. Very small stones can be washed out by Ellick's evacuator, or held in the jaws of a biopsy forceps and removed *in toto*. Large stones could be treated endoscopically, but now that we

J. Talati et al. (eds) The Management of Lithiasis, 155–158
© *1997 Kluwer Academic Publishers. Printed in Great Britain.*

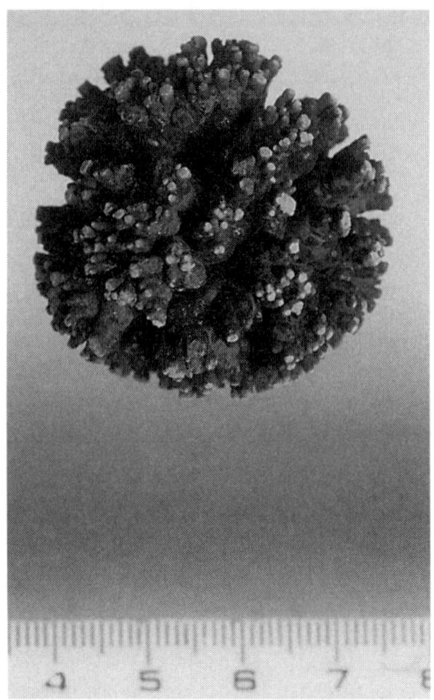

Figure 21.1 Large jackstone vesical calculus. Such a calculus is hard to break by ESWL or intracorporeal lithotripsy

know that these stones can be treated successfully by ESWL, it is inappropriate to introduce these large instruments through the urethra, risk stricture, and prolong the anaesthesia time and operating room utilization.

ESWL is conveniently used prior to TURP [1]. Large stones will require repeat treatments, which can be scheduled two to three days before TURP. Combined treatment by ESWL and TURP has been earlier reported by Bosco and Niels [2]. They used epidural anaesthesia for ESWL (using Dornier HM3 lithotriptor) and performed TURP later under the same anaesthesia. We have used ESWL for bladder stone effectively and safely [1] since December 1989. Hospitalization and anaesthesia are not required in adults and large stones are effectively fragmented. In our experience, the number of sessions and shock waves depends as much on the size of the stone as on the experience of the operator. As more experience is gained, fragmentation can be achieved more effectively, and a greater proportion will be treated by ESWL.

Patients are treated in the prone position, utilizing the acoustic window provided by a bladder filled with saline via a three-way Foley catheter. This can be retained up to the day of the TUR. Mild vesical mucosal congestion and petechial haemorrhages have been noted at the time of TUR. Fragment egress occurs better without a catheter but the catheter should not be dispensed with until coexisting bladder outflow obstruction is treated. Electrohydraulic (EHL) and ultrasound fragmentation have an important place in the management of vesical calculi in hospitals where ESWL is not available. EHL probes can jump off the stone onto the mucosa, and cause perforation. EHL is expensive and more than one probe may be needed for a single stone; the probe is however fine where the instrument for ultrasound is of larger calibre, and increases the risks of urethral injury and stricture. The ultrasound probe has to be pressed against the stone and can cause erosion of the bladder mucosa, resulting in transmigration of fluid into the retroperitoneal or even peritoneal space. Sequential drilling of the stone to produce a series of pits, the walls of which are subsequently drilled, prevents the formation of pieces of stone too large to evacuate through the instrument without further crushing.

ESWL and surgery are being increasingly used by us. In the early phase of our experience with ESWL, in 1989, 75% stones were treated by endoscopic means, 20% by cystolithotomy and only 5% by ESWL. In the first quarter of 1991, 54% were treated by ESWL, and 23% each by surgery and endoscopy. In the first half of 1995, ESWL treated 36%, cystolithotomy 9%, and litholapaxy 55%. Cost-wise, ESWL is more expensive.

Treatment of bladder stones has come a long way from the bloody operations designed by Susruta in India, and practised in the time of Samuel Pepys, who survived such an onslaught at the age of 25 years. It is essential to have patient-friendly devices for removal of bladder stones so that patients do not harbour their stone and allow them to grow to gigantic sizes, which causes problems such as vesico-intestinal fistula as reported by Abbas and Memon [3].

Urethral calculi

The majority (88%) of urethral calculi are seen in adult males with women and children each contributing 5.6% [4]. Sixty per cent [4] to 89% [5] present with acute urine retention, others with a sudden slowing of the stream.

In Pakistan, 57% arrest in the prostatic urethra, 15% in the bulbous urethra, 20% in the perineal urethra and 10% in the navicular fossa [4]. In another series, the majority were in the anterior urethra [5]. In females the stone impacts at the external meatus. In males, stricture, meatal stenosis and benign prostatic enlargement are often the cause of the arrest [4]. Other urinary tract calculi may be present in up to 32% [5]. Rarely, urethral calculi may form *in situ* (see Figure 21.2).

Distressing retention brings the patient to the emergency room, where a calculus may be felt in the anterior urethra (some can be felt between the two testes) or on rectal examination when in the posterior urethra. At times, the calculus cannot be felt, and an X-ray is required. The latter must include the entire urethra, and the stone must be specifically searched for, in the area between the symphysis pubes.

Treatment

In the emergency room, anterior urethral calculi can be milked out after copious instillation of lignocaine jelly into the urethra which is occluded proximal to the stone by compression between the thumb and fingers of the operator. Occasionally a meatotomy (of the external meatus) is required.

Stones in the posterior urethra can be pushed back into the bladder by a blunt nosed Nelaton or a Foley catheter. Irrigation with forced instillation of saline assists the push-ups. A Foley catheter is retained until the next operating day when the

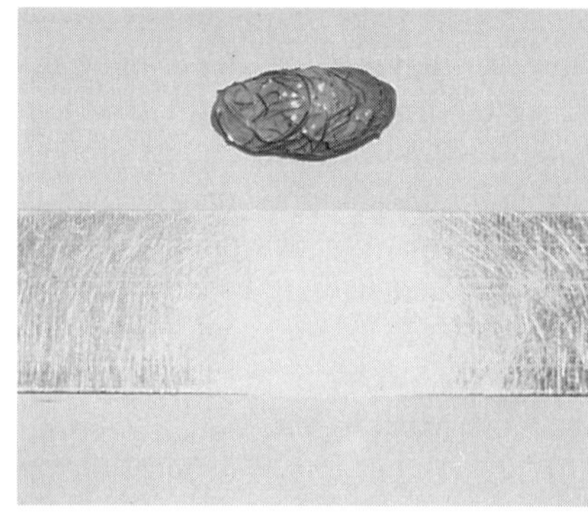

(a)

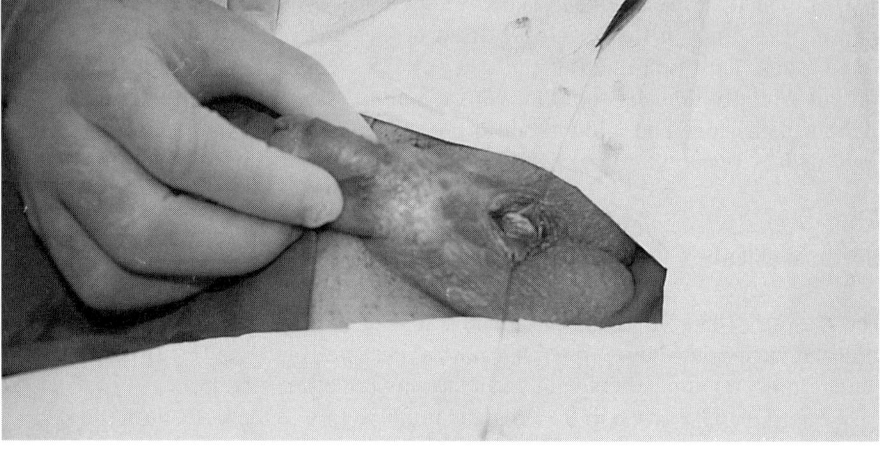

(b)

Figure 21.2 This calculus formed on hair growing from the skin used for a hypospadius repair

stone is crushed in the bladder and evacuated or treated by ESWL. Formal treatment of the stone includes treatment of any associated condition such as a stricture. We have treated one urethral calculus in the anterior urethra with ESWL.

References

1. Hotiana MZ, Khan LA, Talati J. Extracorporeal lithotripsy for bladder stones. Br J Urol 1993;71:692–4.
2. Bosco PJ, Niels PT. ESWL in combination with transurethral surgery for management of large bladder calculi and moderate outlet obstruction. J Urol 1991;145:34–6.
3. Abbas F, Memon A. Colovesical fistula, an unusual complication of prostatomegaly. J Urol 1994;152:479–81.
4. Sheikh M. Urethral calculi. 2nd Asian Congress of Urology, Bangkok, 1994. Asian Urological Association.
5. Amin HA. Urethral calculi. Br J Urol 1973;45:192–9.

Section III
Enhancement of Efficacy and Safety of Treatment

22. Patients at risk for excessive post-ESWL bleeding

MOHAMMED KHURSHEED and JAMSHEER TALATI

Though mild haematuria is an invariable accompaniment of lithotripsy, detectable perinephric haematomas occur in only 0.66% of all patients, 2.5% of hypertensives and 3.8% of poorly controlled hypertensives treated on the Dornier HM3 [1]. Diabetes mellitus, aspirin and nonsteroidal analgesic use are additional risk factors for haematoma formation [2, 3]. Because of the potential for haematomas and haematuria, patients should be screened for haemostatic deficits prior to lithotripsy. Bleeding diathesis is an absolute contraindication to lithotripsy until fully corrected.

Haemostasis is normally achieved by interactions between the vessel wall, coagulation factors and platelets. Defects or deficiency of any of these three elements will give rise to haemostatic deficits.

The commonest inherited (congenital) defects are factor VIII and IX deficiencies, which may be mild or severe. In Pakistan, consanguineous marriages are very common and hence inherited defects – factor VIII, IX and XIII deficiencies and platelet function defects – are more frequent than in the West. The commonest platelet function defects have been Bernard–Soulier and Glanzmann thrombasthenia. Acquired haemostatic problems include coagulation factor deficits secondary to other disease processes such as hepatic dysfunction, and platelet function defects secondary to intake of drugs such as aspirin and non-steroidal antiinflammatory drugs.

Haemostatic screening for deficits

A good history (a haemostatic enquiry) is invaluable. The enquiry determines whether the patient has a tendency to spontaneous bleeding, bleeding out of proportion to common haemostatic stresses such as delivery and dental extraction, or bleeding out of proportion to trauma applied; whether this is an inherited or acquired condition; whether there are any other disease processes that may affect coagulation; and whether there is a history of drug intake and a family history of bleeding. Physical examination should be geared to confirming the history.

It may be possible to localize the defect to the platelets or plasma coagulation system. Platelet deficits result in bleeding from superficial sites, which comes on immediately after trauma, and is controllable by pressure. Bleeding from

J. Talati et al. (eds) The Management of Lithiasis, 161–164
© *1997 Kluwer Academic Publishers. Printed in Great Britain.*

coagulation defects occurs hours or days after surgery, and occurs in subcutaneous tissues, joints and other deep tissues.

Laboratory screening tests include bleeding time and platelet count, whole blood coagulation time, prothrombin time and activated partial thromboplastin time and factor XIII screening tests.

Management of patients with bleeding or coagulation defects

Management of haemostatic disorders is based on the accurate diagnosis and identification of the cause of the haemostatic deficits. Deficiencies of the coagulation factors, platelets, and platelet function, can be managed by adequate replacement of the missing or defective component. The source of the coagulation factors would either be whole blood, fresh frozen plasma, cryoprecipitate, or factor concentrates, and the amount and the time period over which they are given is dependent on the severity of the coagulation factor deficiency. As a general rule, treatment should also include post-therapy infusions. Platelets are given on a similar basis, the source being either fresh blood, platelet rich plasma or platelet concentrates.

Management of acquired defects, which include deficiencies of coagulation factors or platelet deficits, includes replacement of these prior to therapy. Patients with inhibitors may require plasmapheresis prior to treatment.

Aspirin should be withheld for at least seven days, preferably 14 days prior to extracorporeal shock wave lithotripsy (ESWL), as it causes irreversible acetylation of prostagland in synthetase and hence stops production of thromboxane by the platelet. As platelets have no nuclei, Prostaglandin synthetase cannot be produced and thromboxane production capacity will not return to normal until fresh platelets are produced from the bone marrow.

Patients on long-term anticoagulants such as warfarin, can be managed by switching to heparin 48 hours prior to therapy. Heparin is discontinued six hours prior to surgery or ESWL, and recommenced afterwards; it is continued until the risk of bleeding from the procedure is minimal. The patient can then revert to warfarin.

The choice of procedure for treatment of the stone should be one that will result in rapid stone clearance with minimal repetition. Operations should avoid cutting renal substance, and should approach the kidney through a relatively avascular abdominal wall incision such as a midline abdominal incision, or a posterior lumbotomy.

Treatment of haemophiliacs requires careful continuous observation. Bleeding with extensive retroperitoneal haematomas, and haemorrhagic shock [4] can occur in spite of apparently adequate antihaemophilic replacement therapy because of a factor VIII inhibitor, and may require plasmapheresis and embolization [5].

The amount of replacement therapy can be gauged from the following reports. Yokohama and Nasu [6] describe a 44-year-old patient with haemophilia B who was first infused with 1000 units of factor IX which returned the prothrombin time and the partial thromboplastin time to normal. Another 1000 units were infused

30 minutes before ESWL, and subsequently every 12 hours for two days, then every day for eight days. Over the following seven days, 500 units were infused per day. Gross haematuria disappeared on the third day. The patient had received 2363 shocks at 17 kV on the MPL 9000 lithotriptor for a 14 × 22 mm stone [6]. Ultrasound and CT did not detect any perirenal haematoma. Partney *et al.* [7] report on the treatment of a patient with haemophilia, utilizing 7000 units of human anti-haemophilic factor (AHF) preoperatively. The AHF activity was maintained by continuous infusion of 300 units AHF per hour.

A 38-year-old male had a right mid-ureteric 10 × 17 mm calculus and a triangular 20 × 20 × 20 mm left renal calculus with small calcular debris in the lower calyx on the same side. He suffered from alcohol induced liver failure, and with a prolonged prothrombin time (70 vs. control of 17s) and augmented thromboplastin time (100 vs. 35s). Correction by fresh frozen plasma preoperatively was suggested. The operative was to clear both renal tracts on the same day, utilizing ureterolithotomy for the right and pyelotomy for the left. ESWL was considered inappropriate as multiple sessions would be needed. Preoperatively massive infusions of fresh frozen plasma were required. In view of the gross abnormality, it was felt that incisions on both sides would result in an excessive consumption of clotting factors. If there had been no inferior calyceal particles, the left side would have been approached through a lumbotomy incision which would have minimized muscle cutting, and reduced coagulation factor consumption. However, through a lumbotomy, renal handling is limited, a stone and cannot be manoeuvred from the inferior calyx with ease. Operation was therefore restricted to the right side, which was the only obstructed side, and operation on the left was deferred until there was improvement of his hepatic status.

Conclusion

Patients with haemostatic disorders require careful preoperative evaluation and correction of haemostatic deficits prior to therapy. Treatment modes which reduce the need for repetitive replacement of missing factors should be preferred. Thus operation may be preferred to multiple ESWL sessions, and access to the kidney should be through incisions which avoid extensive muscle cutting incisions.

References

1. Knapp PM, Kulb TB, Lingeman JE *et al.* ESWL induced peri renal hematomas, J Urol 1988;139:70–3.
2. Saltzman B. Clinically apparent subcapsular hematomas following shock wave lithotripsy. Identification of potential etiologies. J Urol 1990;143:272A.
3. Rulz H, Saltzman D. Aspirin induced bilateral renal hemorrhage after extracorporeal shock wave lithotripsy: Implications and conclusions. J Urol 1990;143:791.
4. Lauper M, Lammle B, Furlan M, Zehntner C, Zingg E. Hemorrhagic shock nine days after extracorporeal shock wave lithotripsy in a patient with hemophilia B (letter). Thromb Haemost 1988;60:532.

5. Nabeshima S, Hamada H, Nishio S *et al.* ESWL in a patient with hemophilia A: A case report. Nippon Hinyokika Gakkai Zaashi 1994;85:354–7.
6. Yokohama T, Nasu Y. ESWL in a patient with hemophilia B. Nippon Hinyokika Gakkai Zashi 1993;84:566–9.
7. Partney K, Hollingsworth RL, Jordan WR *et al.* Hemophilia and ESWL, a case report. J Urol 1987;138:393–4.

23. Patients with pacemakers

NAGEEB BASIR

Patients with pacemakers may require extracorporeal shock wave lithotripsy (ESWL). The strong shock waves and electromagnetic fields can possibly affect pacemakers and implantable cardioinverters and defibrillators [1].

ESWL shocks are triggered in the refractory period in less than 10 ms after the onset of the R-wave. As a result, shocks cannot be delivered faster than the heart rate but it is unwise to de-link the ECG monitoring, because of the risk of ventricular arrythmias, tachycardia and fibrillation. Direct stimulation of the heart by electrical fields is unlikely [2]. Electrical fields created by side currents in the coupling fluid, in HM3, have a pulse duration less than 1 ms and a density of $5 \times 10^{-4}\,\mathrm{mA/cm^2}$, far less than that required for direct contact pacing [2].

Single or multiple, atrial or ventricular ectopic beats may occur during treatment, even with piezo-electric lithotriptors, in up to 45% of patients [3] both during right and left side treatments. Multifocal ventricular premature beats, ventricular bigeminy and cardiac arrest can occur. It is well-known that a precordial thump can convert a ventricular tachycardia to sinus rhythm or conversely further rhythm degeneration [4]. It is uncertain whether the stimulus to the heart during ESWL is mechanical, electrical or through sympathetic hyperactivity in the anxious patient or because of anoxia produced by respiratory depression induced by sedoanalgesia. A rise in catecholamines has been suspected but has never been demonstrated [5]. Patients with severe underlying heart disease and a history of complex arrhythmia should be monitored by ECG during treatment even by piezo-electric lithotripsy. Sedated patients and those with underlying heart problems should have their oxygen saturation measured continuously and should receive additional oxygen.

Patients with pacemakers require special care. A knowledge of pacemakers is essential for those intending to treat these patients. Lithium batteries used for pacing show decreased pacing efficiency as voltage declines at end-of-life (7–12 years for single chamber and 4–8 years for dual chamber). Most permanent pacemakers are programmable (by radiofrequency), to optimize pacing rate, voltage and sensitivity and a number of other more sophisticated variables. An international five-letter code describes various modes of pacing [6].

The VVI mode is still the commonest method of pacing though it is not the method of choice. In this the chamber paced is the ventricle; the chamber sensed is the ventricle; and the sensing circuit in the pacemaker inhibits (turns off) the pacemaker to prolong battery life if the patient's heart rate is more than the

J. Talati et al. (eds) The Management of Lithiasis, 165–167
© *1997 Kluwer Academic Publishers. Printed in Great Britain.*

minimum programmed rate. Spontaneous ventricular beats are sensed and suppress the pulse generator. A slow pace is set (about 50/min), if it is prophylactic for occasional sinus pauses causing syncopal attacks. A faster setting is used in complete heart block. Today the only major indication for VVI is AV block associated with atrial fibrillation, in which synchronous atrial activation cannot be restored. In AAI pacing, the electrode is placed in the right atrial appendage and the atrium is sensed. Atrial contractions inhibit the pulse generator. It is the method of choice in patients with isolated sino-atrial (SA) disease, and normal AV conduction. In DDD pacing, two catheters are placed, one each in the right atrium and right ventricle. Slowing of atrial rhythm is sensed by the pacer, which is activated. Ectopic beats and normal AV conduction (evidenced by a ventricular contraction following the atrial) inhibit the ventricular pacer. DDD pacing is ideal for patients with AV block, with or without SA disease, but the pacing mode will have to be reprogrammed if atrial fibrillation develops. In DDI pacing both the atria and ventricles can be sensed and both can be paced. An exertional increase in the atrial rate will not trigger a similar increase in the ventricular rate unless specially programmed to incorporate rate responsiveness (DDIR). Rate responsive pacing (R) cannot be used in atrial fibrillation. The most widely used device senses physical activity from vibration and muscle noise. Others sense minute ventilation, body acceleration, temperature or adrenergic activity (as measured by the QT-interval).

During standard VVI pacing, the pacing stimulus triggers ESWL. For dual chamber devices, ESWL is triggered by the atrial paced event which may induce inhibition of the ventricular output. This can be eliminated by programming to a less sensitive setting [7]. Although programmable, the pacemaker is sensitive and could be affected by shocks, though some have subjected pacemakers to shock waves and found no damage [1]. Others using rate responsive pacemakers have noted shattering of the piezo-electric elements when placed at F2 [7]. The device should therefore be checked after ESWL therapy to the ipsilateral side in order to ensure no malfunction. If placed in the pathway of the shock waves, the device may discharge even when the shock waves are given at a speed below 100/mt [1]. If dual chamber pacemakers are not reprogrammed to single chamber then the lithotriptor will sense the atrial pacemaker stimulus and deliver the shock. The electromagnetic stimulus of the shock is sensed by the ventricular pacemaker sensing amplifier and this leads to a possibility of ventricular asystole [7].

If adequate transvenous pacing facilities are available, pacemakers, barring a few exceptions (see below), are no longer an absolute contraindication to ESWL [8]. A cardiologist well versed in pacemaker function and transvenous pacing must however be available to respond urgently to a call for help during treatment [9]. In such settings, ESWL is safe for patients with standard single chamber devices in a ventricular application [10].

However, ESWL remains contraindicated in patients with an abdominally implanted piezo-electric activity-sensing rate-responsive single chamber pacemaker. In general, any abdominal pacemaker should be at least 5 cm away from the blast path [9].

Patients with dual chamber and rate responsive pacemakers are at risk [10]. Dual chamber pacemakers should be reprogrammed to single chamber mode, and activity-sensing rate responsive single chamber pacemakers should have this feature programmed off during ESWL [10].

References

1. Vassolas G, Roth RA, Venditti FJ Jr. Effect of extracorporeal shock wave lithotripsy on implantable cardioverter defibrillator. PACE Pacing Clin Electrophysiol 1993;16:1245–8.
2. Hepp W. Electrical safety of the Dornier lithotriptor in ESWL for renal stone disease. In: Gravenstein JS, Peter K, editors. ESWL for renal stone disease. Boston and London: Butterworth, 1986:29.
3. Zeng ZR, Lindstedt E, Roijer A *et al.* Arrhythmia during extracorporeal shock wave lithotripsy. Br J Urol 1993;71:10–16.
4. Carlson CA, Gravenstein JS, Gravenstein N. Ventricular tachycardia during ESWL, etiology treatment and prevention in ESWL for renal stone disease. In: Gravenstein JS, Peter K, editors. ESWL for renal stone disease. Boston and London: Butterworths, 1986;119–24.
5. Vandeursen H, Tjandramaga B, Verbesselt R *et al.* Anesthesia free ESWL in patients with renal stones. Br J Urol 1991;68:18–24.
6. Timmis AR, Nathan A. Essentials of Cardiology. Oxford: Blackwell Scientific Publishers; 1993;207–27.
7. Albers DD, Lybrand III FE, Axton JC *et al.* Shock wave lithotripsy and pacemakers: Experience with 20 cases. J Endourol 1995;9:301–3.
8. Drach GW, Weber C, Donovan JM. Treatment of pacemaker patients with ESWL, experience from two continents. J Urol 1990;143:895.
9. Asroff SW, Kingston TE, Stein BS. Cardiac pacemaker in an abdominal location; Case report and review of literature. J Endourol 1993;7:189–92.
10. Cooper D, Wilkoff B, Masterson M *et al.* Effects of extracorporeal shock wave lithotripsy on cardiac pacemakers and its safety in patients with implanted cardiac pacemakers. PACE Pacing Clin Electrophysiol 1988;11:1607–16.

24. Safeguarding foetus and gonads

JAMSHEER TALATI

Because of the mutagenic potential of X-rays which are required for follow-up after extracorporeal shock wave lithotripsy (ESWL), even when the lithotriptor does not use ionizing radiation, lithotripsy is contraindicated in pregnancy. All female patients undergoing lithotripsy should be warned that they should use contraceptive methods during treatment. If it is discovered that the patient has become pregnant during lithotripsy, in spite of precautions, X-rays should be avoided, especially during the first trimester. The risks of foetal damage from already administered X-rays should be assessed, and suitable advice given.

Pregnant women with renal calculi who present with recurrent colic, or colic and fever, need to have a stent or nephrostomy [1]. All placements should be done without X-ray control. A single X-ray could reveal the cause of the obstruction, and definitive treatment given by, for example, ureterolithotomy, more safely in the second trimester than in the first where the risk of abortion is higher.

The mutagenic effects of shock waves are less well understood than those of X-rays. Shock waves (600–1200) given to the pelvis of female Wistar rats did not appear to affect the proportion of healthy to atretic follicles or produce long-term gonadal damage [2]. Whilst no recognizable foetal damage resulted when rats were subjected to shock waves in early pregnancy [3, 4], using an ultrasound imaged lithotriptor, foetuses located near F2 focal area showed lower mean weight than controls [3], and ESWL in the late stage of pregnancy in rats has caused cerebral haemorrhages and foetal death [5]. Healthy children with no chromosomal or congenital abnormalities have been born to patients who chose to become pregnant after ESWL, but three of ten such patients had miscarriages at least one year after ESWL [5].

Seminal parameters did not change 2–3 days and 90 days after ESWL given to adult male patients for pelvic ureteral stones on HM3, without shielding the testis [6]. Serum testosterone and semen analysis were unaffected by shocks delivered directly to the testes of non-human primates, but changes (which reverted to normal in nine months) were noted in the DNA histogram, especially the tetraploid cells [7].

Because of the fear of unknown effects of shock waves on gonads, we avoid lithotripsy of bladder stones in female children, and cover the testes with aluminium foil whenever treating male children with bladder stones

J. Talati et al. (eds) The Management of Lithiasis, 169–170
© *1997 Kluwer Academic Publishers. Printed in Great Britain.*

References

1. Eckford SD, Gingell JC. Ureteric obstruction in pregnancy – diagnosis and management. Br J Obstet Gynaecol 1991;98:1137–40.
2. Recker F, Jaeger P, Knonagel H *et al.* Does ESWL injure the female reproductive tract? Helen Chir Acto 1990;57:471–5.
3. Smith DP, Graham JB, Prystowsky JB *et al.* The effects of ultrasound-guided shock waves during early pregnancy in Sprague-Dawley rats. J Urol 1992;147:231–4.
4. Ohmori K, Matsuda T, Horii Y *et al.* Effect of shock waves on mouse fetus. J Urol 1994;151:255–8.
5. Vieweg J, Weber HM, Miller K *et al.* Female fertility following ESWL of distal ureteral calculi. J Urol 1992;148:1007–10.
6. Puppo P, De Rose AF, Pittaluga P *et al.* Evaluation of the seminal fluid in patients treated with ESWL of pelvic ureteral calculi. Arch Ital Urol Nephrol Androl 1990;62:65–8.
7. Hellstrom WJ, Kaack MB, Harrison RM *et al.* Absence of long-term gonadotoxicity in primates receiving extracorporeal shock wave application. J Endourol 1993;7:17–21.

25. Other high-risk patients

JAMSHEER TALATI

Patients with diabetes, hypertension, polycythaemia, neurological impairment or obesity; the elderly; nervous patients; and those with urinary infection, require special management. We treat all patients in these categories but take the precaution of bringing the patient into the best possible condition prior to extracorporeal shock wave lithotripsy (ESWL).

Deep venous thrombosis and polycythaemia

The minimal tissue injury produced by ESWL permits early mobilization and clinically detected deep venous thrombosis (DVT) is unusual. However, patients have to lie still on the lithotriptor for 30–45 minutes and this stasis may promote thrombosis in the calf veins. The ^{125}I-fibrinogen uptake test detects DVT in 1.4% of patients at no risk, 8.7% of patients with varices or obesity (above 20% ideal body weight) and 13% of high risk patients – those with major surgery within one week of ESWL, immobilization, congestive cardiac failure, previous thromboembolism, or post-thrombotic syndrome [1]. Heparin should be used for prophylaxis in the high-risk group, as many patients are asymptomatic.

Umekawa *et al.* [2] have studied sequential changes in thrombin–antithrombin III complex (TAT), alpha 2-plasmin inhibitor–plasmin complex (PIC), fibrin and fibrinogen degradation products (FDP) and D-dimer (D-D) before and after ESWL. Significant acceleration of TAT occurred on the first postoperative day, followed by acceleration of PIC on the third postoperative day. A transient acceleration was observed for FDP and D-D after operation. The levels of these parameters, however, returned to normal by the first postoperative week. These changes occur after ESWL for renal stones but not after ESWL for ureteral stones. Polycythaemia (a haematocrit over 50% not due to dehydration) increases the risk of DVT and pulmonary embolism in patients undergoing ESWL. We see a disproportionately larger number of polycythaemics in our stone patients compared to general urological patients, most often in heavy smokers. A haematological consultation, red cell mass determination, leukocyte alkaline phosphatase determination and bone marrow examination may be necessary. If no cause other than polycythaemia vera is found, we bleed the patient preoperatively and infuse saline to bring the haematocrit down to well below 50%.

J. Talati et al. (eds) The Management of Lithiasis, 171–173
© *1997 Kluwer Academic Publishers. Printed in Great Britain.*

Diabetes and hypertension

Diabetes is controlled prior to therapy. If it is difficult to control, admission prior to ESWL allows six-hourly blood glucose estimations and correction by insulin injections. As infection has serious consequences in such patients every effort is made to avoid obstruction, which together with the higher urinary sugar content, encourages multiplication of organisms and infection. A DJ stent is used more frequently in such patients in order to avoid the double hazard of infection and obstruction.

Hypertensives who are well controlled may be treated as day-care patients. However, for some, this involves waking up at 5 a.m. and travelling long distances (at times 90 miles by bus). This adds to the stress of ESWL and in some patients causes a sharp rise in blood pressure. Patients with poorly controlled hypertension and hypertensives living out of town, are best admitted overnight, given a hypnotic to ensure a good sleep, and midazolam premedication if anxious the next morning. Patients with a smooth course during lithotripsy may go home soon after. Hypertension is a more common cause of haematoma than bleeding disorder [3].

The obese patient

Body mass indices in excess of 25 cause problems as the stone may not come within the focus of the machine, since the subcutaneous fat increases the distance from the water cushion to the stone. Body mass index (BMI) may be calculated from the formula: BMI = weight in kg/[height in metres]^2. Patients with body mass indices up to 28 may yet be treated on the lithotriptor; beyond that, they compress the in-line scanner and this impairs image transmission. Excess fat refracts some of the shock waves, decreasing their concentration onto the stone at the second focus. In some patients it is possible to surmount this problem by using a oblique position. In others the fat distribution may be mainly anterior and the renal angle may be relatively depleted of fat.

In morbidly obese patients, stones beyond focus 2 (F2) have been treated very successfully by compressing the abdomen and utilizing the extended shock pathway beyond F2[3]. The stone-free rate at 3 months or longer was 68%, with another 10% having asymptomatic fragments of 4 mm or less in diameter. The re-treatment rate was 11% and the post-lithotripsy secondary procedures rate was 3% – results comparable to those obtained when treating patients weighing less than 136 kg. We do not use the blast path (see section on Factors determining need for two treatments) as the acoustic energy drops off sharply as one moves away from F2. The MPL 9000X has a special electrode which has a longer focal length (15 cm) and can be used for more deeply placed stones in obese patients.

The anxious patient

Anxiety produces restlessness, and such patients constantly squirm and fidget, thus moving the focus off target repeatedly during lithotripsy. These patients are prone to ventricular ectopics. Allowing the nervous patient to observe a lithotripsy being done without anaesthesia, often reassures them. If still apprehensive, the patient can be sedated, or treated under anaesthesia.

The paediatric patient

There are three concerns: the patient may be too short, and may therefore lie unsupported on the lithotriptor gap; his lung fields may receive shock waves with the possibility of pulmonary oedema; and the effects of shock waves on renal growth are yet uncertain. These concerns are addressed in Section VI.

The neurologically impaired patient

Such patients usually have complicating urinary tract infection, will have a higher incidence of struvite, bilateral and staghorn calculi, will require more ancillary procedures, have poorer clearance rates and rapid recurrence. The patient should be told of these possibilities prior to therapy.

The elderly patient

Elderly patients are more likely to have coronary artery disease. The natural history of the stone, whether the stone needs treatment, the general and ambulatory status of the patient, and the logistics of bringing the patient to hospital, all need to be considered in such patients.

References

1. Marx FJ, Gierster P, Rabini M *et al.* Role for prophylaxis against DVT from ESWL. In: Gravenstein JS, Peter K, editors. ESWL for renal stone disease. Boston and London: Butterworth, 1981.
2. Umekawa T, Kohri K, Yamate T *et al.* Studies on changes in parameters of the coagulation and fibrinolysis in association with extracorporeal shock wave lithotripsy. Urol Int 1993;50:159–63.
3. Thomas R, Cass AS. Extracorporeal shock wave lithotripsy in morbidly obese patients. J Urol 1993;150:30–2.

26. The role of ESWL in patients with leprosy and stone disease

GRACE WARREN

All who live in Pakistan have seen the disfigured faces, stumpy legs and neuropathic hands of leprosy patients. The sight is often aesthetically unbearable for non-medical people, and for centuries it was considered a stigma – a shame, a blot, and many were not allowed into churches.

Much of the fear about leprosy is unfounded. Only exceptionally have medical and paramedical workers contracted leprosy even when caring for such patients day in and day out, for years. Most of us are naturally immune to leprosy.

For those who are not immune, leprosy is contracted when infectious material from a diseased patient is spread by droplets. Fortunately, the infectivity of a patient drops so rapidly after commencement of effective therapy, that for all practical purposes, it can be said that the patient ceases to be infectious within 48 hours of the first dose of rifampicin.

In some patients, widespread deposition of immune complexes (the antigen from *Mycobacterium leprae* combined with antibody and complement) produces lesions – Erythema Nodosum Leprosum (ENL), similar to the erythema nodosum of other diseases. This is typified by rose pink nodular lesions, which appear in crops. Each crop lasts three to four days and then fades slowly. Crops occur at ten-day intervals and may be accompanied by fever, malaise, iritis and other localized inflammatory lesions. Exacerbated loss of neural function occurs as a result of the deposition of these immune complexes in nerves. All this in turn may cause marked deformity of the face, hands and feet.

ENL can be precipitated by any chronic infection, such as urinary infection, which may have as its root cause a urinary tract stone. ENL may continue intermittently until infection has been eliminated. It has also been noted that ENL will rapidly cease and not recur once urinary tract stones have been removed.

There is still much fear about the contagiousness of leprosy, so that many hospitals will not treat leprosy patients. Medical practitioners are hesitant to treat them for fear of becoming infected themselves, or from fear of losing patients because they do not like to sit in the same waiting area with them, or because word that leprosy patients were treated in doctor X's clinic, has spread.

Surgical and other patients do not wish to find themselves in a bed next to a leprotic patient with leonine facies, and whilst the doctor may be able to make them comprehend and become compassionate, they are embarrassed when relatives and friends visit.

J. Talati et al. (eds) The Management of Lithiasis, 175–176
© 1997 Kluwer Academic Publishers. Printed in Great Britain.

Treatment by extracorporeal shock wave lithotripsy (ESWL) avoids admission and the use of the operating room. Administrators and doctors feel more comfortable treating such patients by lithotripsy than surgery. Adequate and early therapy of stones therefore becomes possible by lithotripsy. As a corollary, urinary infection can be eliminated, ENL will cease to recur, neuritis and deformity can be circumvented and the severity of nephrotic syndrome resulting from widespread immune complex deposition is reduced.

Conclusion

The world is filled with prejudice stemming from ignorance. Few understand that leprosy cannot be transmitted once a patient is declared non-infective. Patients in a general ward do not want leprosy patients lying in the bed beside them. Hospital administrators have to pander to patients' sensitivities, and worry about spread of 'news' that in such and such a hospital, the operating theatres were used for operating on a leprosy patient. Urinary infections associated with stone disease can precipitate ENL. ESWL offers an effective treatment option, reduces risk of infection, ENL and other complications of leprosy.

Further reading

Pfaltzgraff RE, Bryceson A. Clinical leprosy. In: Hastings RC, editor Leprosy. Edinburgh, London: Churchill Livingstone, 1985:134–76.

27. Factors determining need for multiple treatments on the Dornier HM3

JOHN A. BELIS and GREGORY HALENDA

Extracorporeal shock wave lithotripsy (ESWL) may achieve a stone-free rate approaching 90%, but depending on the lithotriptor used, a significant number of patients require more than one treatment.

A number of factors including lithotriptor design determine the need for retreatment. In this chapter we identify these factors on the basis of our experience. A review of 1213 ESWL treatments performed in 1048 consecutive patients in a 4.5-year period by our urology faculty on a Dornier HM3 ESWL unit shared with community urologists, allowed us to characterize patients requiring two treatments. Differences in the post-ESWL course between those receiving one or two treatments were also noted.

These patients were treated with a shock wave force of 18–24 kV. A ureteral stent was used in 85% and epidural anaesthesia was used in 96% of patients. Calculus size was calculated as the sum of two largest dimensions, position and number were determined by KUB X-ray, IVP or CT scan. Major system disease was defined as a pre-existing medical condition corresponding to ASA classes II, III or IV. Urinary tract infections were defined as greater than 100 000 organisms per ml and were treated by appropriate antibiotics prior to ESWL. Retreatment was performed during the same hospital admission (with a short interval between treatments) in 54 patients, and at a later time in 43 patients.

Effect of lithotriptor design

Repeat treatments were required in only 97 (9.3%) patients. This is similar to the retreatment rates reported for the Dornier HM3 in other series [1–3], and is less than the retreatment rates of 25% reported for treatments on Dornier HM4 and MPL 9000 [4]. The difference compared to the report by Drach *et al.* [1] may be because of initial limitation of treatment to smaller stones. Using the piezolith lithotriptors, retreatment rates of 62% and 21% have been reported [5, 6] for stones, many of which would have been successfully treated in one session on the Dornier HM3. Lithotriptor design significantly influences retreatment rates.

J. Talati et al. (eds) The Management of Lithiasis, 177–181
© *1997 Kluwer Academic Publishers. Printed in Great Britain.*

178   *John A. Belis and Gregory Halenda*

Table 27.1   Comparison of patients having single vs. multiple ESWL

	One ESWL	*> One ESWL*
Number of patients (% of series)	951 (90.7)	97 (9.3)
Treatments	951	236
Calculi > 1 cm (%)	63	83*
Ureteral calculi (%)	8	17*
Urinary tract infection before ESWL (%)	10	29*
Age over 60 years (%)	37	45
Major system disease (%)	44	56
Average hospitalization (days)	1.3	5.5*
Average hospitalization (days)	1.3	5.5*

* Significantly greater than single treatment group.

Characteristics of patients requiring repeat treatments

Patients requiring repeat ESWL treatment had a larger average stone burden, a greater frequency of ureteral calculi, a higher incidence of urinary tract infection, older age and a greater incidence of a major system disease. Large stone size, ureteral location and urinary tract infection (UTI) predisposed patients to a significantly longer hospitalization (Table 27.1).

Urinary tract infections, most often with *Proteus* sp. and *Pseudomonas*, also predispose to a higher incidence of multiple ESWL procedures and consequent longer hospitalization. Thus, in a group of 28 patients with UTI requiring repeat ESWL, hospitalization averaged eight days. All patients with UTI who required repeat ESWL, had stones greater than 1 cm in size. Large struvite stones are the most difficult to treat; 80% require retreatment, a rate consistent with that reported in a series of similar patients [7] (Figure 27.2).

Retreatment is associated with higher auxiliary procedure rates

Patients requiring retreatment on ESWL also require auxiliary measures far more often than patients requiring a single treatment (Table 27.2). Auxiliary measures refer to percutaneous nephrolithotomy, percutaneous nephrostomy, ureteroscopy, or basket extraction of fragments under fluoroscopic guidance.

The greater incidence of auxiliary procedures in repeat ESWL patients compared to the single ESWL group generally reflected greater complexity of stone disease in

Table 27.2   Auxiliary procedures and final success rate

	Auxiliary procedure rate (%)	Final success rate (%)
Single ESWL	13	99
Multiple ESWL	22*	96
Immediate repeat ESWL	33*	92
Delayed repeat ESWL	12	98

* Significantly greater than single ESWL.

Table 27.3   Features of immediate and delayed repeat ESWL

	Same admission	Subsequent admission
Calculi > 1 cm (%)	90*	71
Ureteral calculi (%)	29*	9
Average days between treatments	3.6	98*
Average days of hospitalization	7.7*	2.4

* Significantly greater than opposite group.

the repeat ESWL group, although the single ESWL group contained patients who had percutaneous debulking of staghorn calculi followed by one session of ESWL, or impacted ureteral calculi having one unsuccessful session of ESWL followed by an auxiliary procedure. The great majority of patients having successful ESWL of small calculi kept the incidence of auxiliary procedures low in that group.

The influence of treatment spacing on results

The time interval between two ESWL treatments affects the need for auxiliary intervention. Delaying the retreatment dramatically reduced the requirement for auxiliary measures. The greater complexity of stone disease in the group receiving immediate repeat ESWL, led to aggressive multimodal therapy with 33% requiring auxiliary measures. Those receiving delayed retreatment required auxiliary measures only as frequently as the patients receiving one treatment.

Delaying treatment has a number of advantages: the initial hospitalization is reduced; retreatment can often be done as an outpatient; delay allows a number of fragments to pass spontaneously, resulting in smaller calculus burdens at the time of retreatment, and shorter hospitalization (Table 27.3); and the auxiliary procedure rate drops from 33% to 12%. Many patients (82%) have repeat treatments done as outpatients. Within the re-ESWL group, patients receiving two or more treatments during the same admission required hospitalization for periods three times longer than their counterparts (3.6 vs. 9.8 days). However, the presence of other risk factors, or the need for auxiliary procedures makes it necessary or practical to repeat ESWL during initial hospitalization in many patients. As an example, the higher frequency of residual fragments after ESWL monotherapy for struvite calculi and evidence for stone progression when large residual fragments remain support aggressive repeat ESWL in the initial treatment course [8].

When making a decision on the timing of retreatment, the size complexity and composition of the calculus is important. Similarly, the need for auxiliary treatment or risk of sudden calcular fragment movement which could obstruct the ureter, would dictate early re-ESWL or continued admission.

Treatment failures and final success rates

The final success rate is less in patients who have received multiple ESWL procedures than in those receiving a single procedure. For this study, the final success rate refers to the total of all patients who were stone free or had passable stones less than 4 mm in diameter. This difference was due to a lower final success rate in those patients treated within a short time (the immediate re-ESWL group). Patients in whom re-ESWL was delayed had a final success rate similar to patients receiving a single treatment.

In the single ESWL treatment group, most treatment failures were seen in patients with impacted ureteral calculi which were subsequently treated, successfully, by ureteroscopy or percutaneous nephroscopy and extraction.

Although repeat ESWL and a greater use of auxiliary procedures led to a successful result in many patients with complex calculi, the final success rate in the repeat ESWL group was lower. The retained fragments were usually in calyces and often found in patients with neurological impairment, or serious medical conditions where additional therapy to the fragment was not practical. The majority of patients with retained fragments were found in the group receiving immediate re-ESWL.

Conclusions

Retreatment rates are a function of the type of lithotriptor and are higher on the Dornier HM4 and the piezo-electric lithotriptors than on HM3.

Patients with calculi larger than 1 cm in diameter, ureteral calculi, and urinary tract infection before ESWL, have a greater chance of requiring a second treatment and a significantly longer hospitalization.

Delaying the second treatment allows a number of stones to pass spontaneously and reduces the auxiliary intervention rate.

Although the final success rate was higher and the need for auxiliary treatment lower, when repeat treatment was delayed, complex initial stone presentation and partial initial success with ESWL will define a group of patients where immediate re-ESWL is warranted. Retreatment should not be delayed unnecessarily if there are risk factors or unexpected sudden movement of fragments.

Stone characteristics, the method of application of shock wave, the total acoustic energy applied, and many other factors interplay in effecting successful therapy. These factors are discussed in Chapter 28.

References

1. Drach GW, Dretler S, Fair W *et al.* Report of the United States co-operative study of extracorporeal shock wave lithotripsy. J Urol 1986;135:1127.
2. Lingeman JE, Newman D, Mertz JHO *et al.* Extracorporeal shockwave lithotripsy: The Methodist Hospital of Indiana experience. J Urol 1986;135:1134.
3. Pettersson B, Tiselius H-G. One year followup of an unselected group of renal stone formers treated with extracorporeal shock wave lithotripsy. J Endourol 1989;3:19.
4. Tailly G. Experience with the Dornier HM4 and the MPL 9000 lithotriptors in urinary stone treatment, J Urol 1990;144:622.

5. Bowsher WG, Carter S, Phillip T *et al.* Clinical experience using the Wolff piezolith device at two British stone centers. J Urol 1989;142:679.

6. Miller HC. Initial EDAP LT-01 lithotripsy group experience in the United States. J Urol 1989;142:679.

7. Schulze H, Hertle L, Graff J *et al.* Combined treatment of branched calculi by percutaneous nephrostomy and extracorporeal shock wave lithotripsy. J Urol 1986;135:1138.

8. Beck EM, Rielhe RA Jr. The fate of residual fragments after extracorporeal shock wave lithotripsy monotherapy of infection stones. J Urol 1991;146:6.

28. Factors determining need for multiple treatments: Decisions based on stone bulk, composition and acoustic efficiency

JAMSHEER TALATI

An understanding of how stones fragment allows the physician to speed up fragmentation processes and reduce the number of repeat treatments.

The process of fragmentation

Shock waves, which are a type of acoustic wave, travel as alternate waves of compression and rarefaction. They are reflected to a varying extent when they meet an interface between two media with differing acoustic impedance. Acoustic impedance is the product of the velocity of sound in the medium and the density of the substance. The greater the difference in acoustic impedance, the greater the amount of sound waves reflected. Thus when sound waves travel through the abdomen, and meet air interfaces in the bowel, much of the sound is reflected. Similarly shock waves cannot penetrate bone and are mostly reflected by it. During the compression phase, the proximal face of the stone is compressed and energy is absorbed and converted into heat. As the wave proceeds to the distal face of the stone, it pushes it out causing the stone to bulge. Part of the wave is then reflected back from the inner aspect of the distal face. The returning wave creates tensile forces, which suck the main bulk of the stone away from the distal face of the expanded stone, causing the latter to shell off like an onion layer, in a process called spalling.

The tensile wave on exiting the proximal face of the stone produces cavities in the fluid surrounding the stone as the inherent strength of the liquid is exceeded. As the wave passes off, these collapse inwardly in the form of high speed liquid microjets [1], which erode and pit the stone. Pressures within the bubble may reach 10 000 bar and the temperature 20 000°K [2]. As the bubble collapses a new shock wave is generated which triggers early collapse of surrounding bubbles, thus augmenting the erosion of the stone by a cluster effect [2]. Fluid filled cracks also develop bubbles and eroding jets which contribute to effective fragmentation.

Gallstones are difficult to fragment: they are mobile (and part of the force of the shock wave is converted into kinetic energy); they are composed of organic matter which is difficult to break; and they are bathed in bile which is too viscous to penetrate the cracks, thus limiting the surface over which cavitation microjets can work.

J. Talati et al. (eds) The Management of Lithiasis, 183–190
© 1997 Kluwer Academic Publishers. Printed in Great Britain.

The efficiency of shock waves

The efficiency with which shock waves fragment the stone is affected by a number of factors.

Acoustic energy

Stone fragmentation ultimately depends upon the total acoustic energy delivered to the stone. The latter is determined by the energy (and hence voltage) delivered per shock and the number of shocks given to the stone. At a constant voltage, more shocks are needed to pulverize larger stones and the relation is linear. Experimentally, the volume of the crater produced by the shock wave is closely correlated to acoustic energy [3]. For a constant stone size, the number of shocks required to produce effective fragmentation rises exponentially as the energy (determined by the voltage) drops. This would imply that *in vivo* more effective fragmentation will result from high energy, high voltage shocks. Clinical experience however indicates better results with low energy shock waves.

Many have demonstrated that treatment on low energy piezo-electric lithotriptors produces erosion, advantageous in preventing *steinstrasse*, reducing the need for stenting and post-ESWL ancillary procedures. Even when treating patients on lithotriptors capable of delivering high energy (such as the MPL 9000) we recommend the use of lower energy [4], as higher energy shock waves produce larger fragments. Each of the larger fragments then requires a larger number of shocks and increases the chances of a fragment slipping into and blocking the ureter, causing type 2 and 3 *steinstrasse* and requiring ureteroscopy.

Using lower acoustic energy chisels away the stone. Large energies fragment it. The same total acoustic energy is better achieved through multiple shocks at lower voltage, which has the disadvantage of requiring more treatments, but which also reduces the need for unexpected interventional treatment.

Acoustic efficiency in relation to pressure characteristics

The efficiency of shock waves in fragmenting stones (acoustic efficiency) is not related to maximum pressure attained (Pmax), the steepness of the rise of pressure (time to pressure rise, Tr), half width of the pressure wave, or the negative pressure phase of the shock wave. Crater volume correlates poorly with pressure rise. Changes in Tr from 50–200% make only a 20% difference to the fragmentation [5].

Pressure readings have often been inaccurate and depend upon the sensitivity, response time, frequency, band width, and ability of the pressure graph to read high pressures and withstand shocks. Polyvinylidendifluoride (PVDF) membrane hydrophones do not loose their elasticity up to 10 000 shocks [6]. Pressure measurements by piezo-electric crystal transducers have a sensitive range up to 100 000 psi and a response time of not more than 1 m [7]. Pressures measured *in vivo* are lower by 100–300 bar than in water. Pressures drop dramatically as we move away from the centre of the focus and the wave form changes, with time to peak rise and negative phase being also dramatically different [8].

Factors interfering with acoustic efficiency

Repeating shock waves at a rapid rate reduces energy efficiency as the oncoming waves clash with the returning waves [9]. Additionally there is insufficient time for the charger to be fully charged before firing [10]. Clinically, fragmentation is more efficient at 1.25 shocks per second than at 10 shocks per second (when using a piezo-electric lithotriptor), but fragmentation of friable stones is independent of rate of repetition.

In experimental settings, accumulation of debris (produced by stone destruction) from the immediate vicinity of the stone within a latex membrane between the stone and the sieve holding the stone during fragmentation, decelerates stone fragmentation by a factor as high as 3.7, and which is dependent on the size of the stone [3].

In a clinical setting, the layer of the fragments surrounding the unfragmented remaining stone can reduce delivered shock wave energy to levels below the threshold energy required for stone disintegration. Administration of furosemide and consequent high urine flow rates washes away the debris. Large stones are best treated in sessions, allowing the debris to clear between treatments. Patients with multiple stones are also at a disadvantage, as the small stones act much as the debris produced after extracorporeal shock wave lithotripsy (ESWL).

Acoustic efficiency in the ureter

Fluid surrounding the stone assists cavitation and promotes efficient stone fragmentation. This suggests that ureteric stones pushed back to the pelvis will fragment more readily.

Though experimentally, synthetic stones fragment best when the stone is freely surrounded by fluid, and less so when impacted in a chamber [11, 31], we have noted that clinically, ureteric stones fragment quite well even when they have completely obstructed the ureter, and are not stented. However they require larger amounts of acoustic energy per equivalent stone burden (56 000 kV. shots/cm^2 compared with 33 100 kV. shots/cm^2) for the renal stone [12]. We use a higher voltage – 20 kV on the MPL 9000 as against 18 kV for renal stones.

Too heavy a shock burden can be detrimental. Increasing the shocks increases success only to a point: there is an optimal number of shock waves needed per mm^3 stone beyond which oedema becomes significant [13]; fragments of stone imbed in the oedematous mucosa, and do not clear.

The influence of stone characteristics on acoustic efficiency

Stone size and multiplicity are the most important determinants of success rates with ESWL, and hence of choice of treatment [14]. As stone size increases to more than 1 cm, stone-free rates with ESWL decrease from 90.6% to 77.8%, the number of shocks required rises from a mean of 2826 to 3066 and the number of secondary treatments rises from 9.9% to 29.4% [15].

Stone structure also affects fragmentability. Stones vary in their hardness and elasticity, and they vary in hardness in different parts of the stone. Stones which have a high elasticity modulus resist fragmentation, as shown by attempts to fragment synthetic stones composed of methylmetacrylate [2].

Calcium oxalate monohydrate, magnesium ammonium phosphate and cystine stones, without apparent structure pattern, show neither regional nor directional differences in their microhardness as tested by Knoop and Vickers indentors [16]. In contrast, calcium apatite stones, with distinctly concentric laminae structure, showed regional variations which were correlated with the chemical composition of stone constituents. Scanning electron microscopy of the indenter impressions showed that crystalline stones were isotropic within a layer and that the anisotropic Knoop hardness readings seen in the laminated regions were structural but not material-based.

Circumferential and radial lamenations in the stone, and interfaces between various crystals of differing composition, provide planes for cleavage. In calcium oxalate monohydrate and uric acid calculi the crystals are arranged in layers, and separate along the laminations. In struvite calculi the fragmentation occurs between calcium phosphate and struvite crystal masses. Cystine has no lamination and therefore resists fragmentation. Uric acid appears uniform but has concentric and radial laminations which produce interfaces for shock wave action [17].

Response by fracture, and retreatment rates therefore vary according to stone type. *In vitro*, the percentage of the original weight of the stone that had fragmented to 2 mm size after 200 shocks at 18 kV was 100% for calcium oxalate dihydrate (COD) and urate, 64% for calcium oxalate monohydrate (COM), 57% for struvite, 47% for brushite, and 16% for cystine [18]. Retreatment rates vary from 10.3% for COM to 2.8% for COD and 6.4% for struvite apatite stones [19]. COM has 64% of the fragility of COD.

Knowing the stone type, the physician can discuss the number of treatments required more efficiently with the patient, and choose between EPL and ESWL.

Can radiology predict the structure of the stone?

Patients like to be told the approximate number of treatments needed for their stone. Therefore it is necessary for a physician to predict fragility. Cohen *et al.* [20] have suggested electron microscopy scanning of the urinary sediments to predict stone type. Electron microscopy is however, not widely available.

The composition of stones can fortunately be gauged from their radiological appearance [19, 21] on high resolution mammographic paper. In a third world country, we compare the radiodensity ('whiteness') of the stone on an X-ray to that of the rib. Calcium oxalate monohydrate stones are very dense white. COD stones are less or equally dense and often have a sun-ray appearance; urate stones will vary in density (of the whiteness) according to the amount of urate in them. The majority of our urate stones contain less than 30% urate, and are therefore not totally radiolucent. A poorly radiopaque staghorn calculus in a patient with sterile urine is a urate calculus. COD rarely forms staghorns. Dense smooth stones are brushite or COM. Scalloped stones and those with reticulated edges are COD.

Magnetic resonance imaging, in addition to being expensive, does not differentiate stone composition [22], as all calculi have the appearance of a black hole which represent areas of decreased signal. *In vitro*, oxalate stones are light grey on T1 weighted and black on T2 weighted images; struvite and other stones appear dark grey on T1 and black on T2 weighted images [23]. A CT scan has occasionally proved that a filling defect in a calyx is a urate stone and not a tumour: uric acid stones are very dense white on CT scan. This is cost-effective only in a small percentage of patients in whom a real doubt exists about the nature of the filling defect.

Linear density of the stone assessed by single photon emission absorbitometry correlates with radiodensity [24]. The product of the stone area (length $\times$ breadth) [25] and dual photon absorbitometry (DPA) measurement correlates well with the fragility of the stone and the number of shock waves needed for full fragmentation [24].

Stones with a high attenuation on CT scan are resistant to fracture and stones with an attenuation below 600 HE can be successfully dissolved.

Targeting techniques that improve acoustic efficiency

Shock waves appear to be more effective when focused onto the front of the stone rather than the rear, when using electro-hydraulically (EH) produced shock waves or piezo-electric (PE) waves. Position of the focus does not make a difference to the amount of stone damage produced by shock waves produced electromagnetically [26].

Obese or heavily built individuals present difficulties in that the stone may be beyond the reach of the target point. At times a ureteric stone near the spine is difficult to reach. Dornier have developed a newer electrode with a focus depth of 155 mm for the treatment of ureteric calculi on the MPL X as compared to 120 mm on the conventional MPL. The focus is also larger and measures 6.5 $\times$ 45 mm.

In situations where stones are still beyond the reach of the focus, two techniques are suggested: blast path lithotripsy and high voltage lithotripsy. In blast path lithotripsy [27], the stone is kept in line with the shock wave but lies beyond the F2 focus. The blast path beyond the focus is sufficient to shatter the stone. *In vitro* experiments have shown that urate calculi can be shattered along extended focus pathways [27] and this principle has been used for treating stones in horseshoe kidneys.

Increasing voltage can increase the size of F2. This allows the stone to be treated by the tip of F2. More information regarding these two techniques is required before they can be generally recommended.

The importance of focal size when choosing the lithotriptor

A large focus treats stones with minimal need for intra-treatment targeting changes. The concentration of power on a large sized focus crushes everything in sight.

Hence in a few shock waves a large stone is pulverized; but in the process the kidney will also suffer damage. The MPL 9000 is an ultrasound monitored lithotriptor which utilizes electro-hydraulic technology for shock wave generation and has a very narrow focus reported variously as 34 × 4.2 mm [28] and 48 × 7 × 7 mm [29]. The fine focus requires accurate targeting and hence protects surrounding renal tissue. As a corollary, haphazard shock wave delivery will not be effective. Continuous visualization of shock wave targeting is necessary and made possible by continuous ultrasound monitoring. This results in safer treatment.

Rapidity of treatment must be balanced with minimizing repeat treatments with safety. There is one clear answer: safety comes first. Machines with smaller foci are preferable.

Fragmentation assists stone dissolution

As the stone breaks into smaller fragments, the surface area exposed to urine increases as a cube root of n times the original surface area, where n is the number of fragments [30]. Dissolution therapy becomes more effective as drugs have a larger surface area of the stone to act upon. When treating uric acid stones, we can capitalize on this by combining oral medication with alkali to change the pH and help dissolution, and with allopurinol to reduce the uric acid in urine, and hence increase the gradient from stone to urine.

Experimental materials for study of the physics of stone fragmentation

Calculi are unsatisfactory as material to test the effects of shock waves, because they vary in size, configuration, composition, orientation and distribution of lamellae, and susceptibility to fracture. Also, with the advent of ESWL it is becoming increasingly difficult to obtain stones. Dornier plaster stones are used in experiments in Dornier laboratories, and the resulting stones sieved through a 2 mm sieve. More recently, others have designed ingenious artificial stones.

Conclusion

Effective targeting techniques, correct choice of treatment mode (EPL vs. ESWL), voltage, power, and hence energy and judicious spacing of treatment, will result in better stone erosion with fewer complications.

References

1. Crum LA. Cavitation microjets as a contributory mechanism for renal calculi disintegration in ESWL. J Urol 1988;140:1587–90.

2. Sass W, Dreyer HP, Ketterman *et al.* The role of cavitational activity in fragmentation processes by lithotriptors. J Stone Dis 1992;4:193–207.

3. Lobentanzer H. The concept of acoustic energy in lithotripsy. Dornier User Letter 1991;7:22–6.

4. Talati J, Shah T, Memon A *et al.* ESWL for urinary tract stones. J Urol 1991;146:1482–6.

5. Folberth W. What makes a stone break up? New findings and technical implications. The Litholetter 1991;5:19–22.

6. Drexler B. Quality assurance in lithotripsy – a new pressure test unit. The Litholetter 1991;5:18.

7. Hunter II PT, Finlayson B, Newman RC, Drylie DM. Geometry of and pressures with ESWL. In: Gravenstein JS, Peter K, editors. Extracorporeal shockwave lithotripsy for renal stone disease. Technical and clinical aspects. Boston, London: Butterworths, 1986.

8. Lobentanzer H. The concept of acoustic energy in lithotripsy. Dornier User 1988;3:12.

9. Williams RH, Zhong P, Preminger GM. Maximizing shock wave intensity during piezoelectric lithotripsy. J Urol 1991;145:418A.

10. Coleman AJ, Saunders JE. A survey of the acoustic output of commercial extracorporeal shock wave lithotriptors. Ultrasound Med Biol 1989;15:213–17.

11. Parr NJ, Pye SD, Ritchie AW *et al.* Why are ureteral calculi more difficult to fragment in situ? J Urol 1991;270:23A.

12. Miyake O, Tsujihata M, Utsunomiya M *et al.* Extracorporeal shock wave lithotripsy for renal and ureteral calculi with MPL-9000. Correlation between stone burden and shock wave energy. Nippon Hinyokika Gakkai Zasshi 1991;82:1568–75.

13. Parr NJ, Ritchie AW, Monsa SA *et al.* The impact of extracorporeal pregoelectric lithotripsy in the management of ureteral calculi: Relation between number of shocks delivered and success. J Urol 1991;270A (abstract 23).

14. Politis G, Griffith DP. ESWL: Stone free efficacy based upon stone size and location. World J Urol 1987;5:255–8.

15. Preminger G. Shock wave physics. Am J Kid Dis 1991;17:431–5.

16. Zhong P, Chuong CJ, Goolsby RD *et al.* Microhardness measurements of renal calculi: Regional differences and effects of microstructure. J Biomed Mater Res 1992;26:1117–30.

17. Khan SR, Hackett RL, Finlayson B. Morphology of urinary stone particles resulting from ESWL treatment. J Urol 1986;137:1367–72.

18. Dretler SP. Stone fragility, a new therapeutic distinction. J Urol 1988;139:1124–7.

19. Dretler SP. Alternatives for the management of ureteral calculi. Pak J Surg 1989;5:50–61.

20. Cohen NP, Parkhouse H, Scott ML *et al.* Prediction of response to lithotripsy – the use of scanning electron microscopy and X-ray energy dispersive spectroscopy. Br J Urol 1992;70:469–73.

21. Prein EL, Dretler SP. Fragility and morphology of calcium oxalate calculi: Clinical significance. J Urol 1989;141:408A.

22. Angus DG, Webb DR, Doyle T *et al.* Magnetic resonance imaging of urinary duct calculi. Proceedings of the Australia Uro Society. Br J Urol 1988;61:79.

23. Cohen NP, Whitfield HN, Dolke G *et al.* In vitro magnetic resonance scanning of urinary calculi. In: Ryall R *et al.*, editor. Urolithiasis II. New York: Plenum Publishers, 1994:680.

24. Suzer O, Arikan N, Isikay L *et al.* Dual photon absorptiometry and scanning electron microscopic findings of stones having the same total stone load but different fragility indexes. In: Rao PN, Kavanagh JP, Tiselius H-G, editors. Vrolithiasis: consensus and controversy. Manchester, UK: Rao and Kavanagh; 1994.

25. Ackermann D, Dunthorn M, Newman RC *et al.* Calculation of volume and computer assisted staging. J Urol 1989;141:403A.

26. Zhong P, Chuong CJC, Preminger GM. Stone damage modes from three different lithotriptors. J Urol 1990;143:229A.

27. Whelan JP, Finlayson B, Welch J *et al.* The blast path, theoretical basis, experimental data and clinical application. J Urol 1988;140:401–4.

28. Ruchenwald M, Colombo Th, Mertl G *et al.* In situ treatment of ureteral calculi using Dornier lithotriptor MPL 9000 with X-ray localizing system. Dornier Newsletter 1991;7:16–21.

29. Mishriki SF, Cohen NP, Baker AC *et al.* Choosing a powerful lithotriptor. Br J Urol 1993;71:653–60.

30. Selli C, Carini M, Fiorelli C. The role of ESWL in the treatment of radiolucent and scarcely radio-lucent stones. In: Linari F, Marangilla M, Bruno M, editors. Contr Nephrol. 1987;58:266–9.
31. Parr NJ, Pye SD, Ritchie AW *et al*. Mechanism responsible for diminished fragmentation of ureteral calculi: an experimental and clinical trial. J Urol 1992;148:1079–83.

29. Prevention of *steinstrasse*

JAMSHEER TALATI

Steinstrasse is a term used to describe a ureter that is choked with stone debris. This term is derived from the German words *stein* (stone) and *strasse* (street), appropriate as the ureter appears like a cobbled street on an X-ray.

Steinstrasse (SS) are conveniently divided into three types, each requiring a different approach in management. Type I has fine gravel with no major particle hindering descent. This type will clear spontaneously on expectant treatment. Type II is also mainly composed of fine gravel, but there is a large stone fragment ahead of the rest which is preventing clearance (Figures 29.1a and b). Type III denotes a ureter choked with major stone fragments.

How can *steinstrasse* be detected?

SS are usually detected on a follow-up X-ray. They are often silent. Pain and fever do not always accompany obstruction or sepsis; 27–60% are asymptomatic [1, 2]. X-rays at regular intervals are necessary to detect SS which can occur even when a DJS is in place. An ultrasound is required to detect whether the SS is causing persistent obstruction [1]. Serum creatinine will detect impending failure in patients with solitary kidneys, and we have noted a rise in serum creatinine in patients with two functioning kidneys, if one is totally obstructed [3]. A white blood cell count will indicate impending sepsis and need for blood culture.

Treatment

Interventional treatment of SS is indicated if there is a lead stone or a type III SS which has little chance of spontaneous clearance. Multiple ureteroscopic extractions or an extended ureterolithotomy may be required for type III SS. Ureteroscopy will be more appropriate when there are a large number of calculi remaining in the kidney. At times, when extracorporeal shock wave lithotripsy (ESWL) has failed, a nephropyelo-ureterolithotomy may be justified to obtain immediate clearance.

If the lead stone in a type II SS is small, it may pass spontaneously. Expectant treatment is justified, but should be closely monitored with ultrasound and X-rays.

J. Talati et al. (eds) The Management of Lithiasis, 191–194
© *1997 Kluwer Academic Publishers. Printed in Great Britain.*

Dilatation of the urinary tract *per se* is not an indication for urgent intervention in ESWL treated patients. Judicious supervision is necessary: Cochrane *et al.* [4] have shown that 8%, 15% and 18% of calyceal, pelvic and ureteric stones had dilatation of the upper urinary tract. In 82% of calyceal, 68% of pelvic, and 84% of ureteric stones, the hydronephrosis disappeared spontaneously. In Fedullo's *et al.* [2] series,

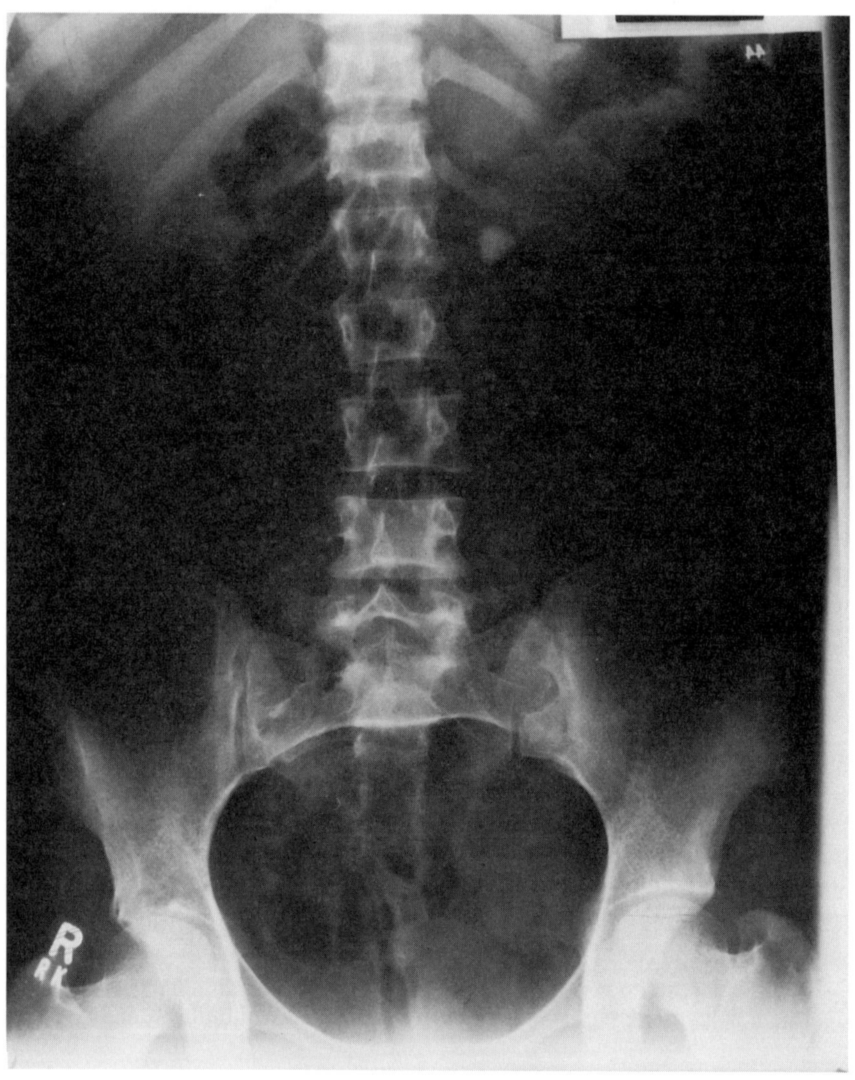

(a)

Figure 29.1(a) Left renal calculus

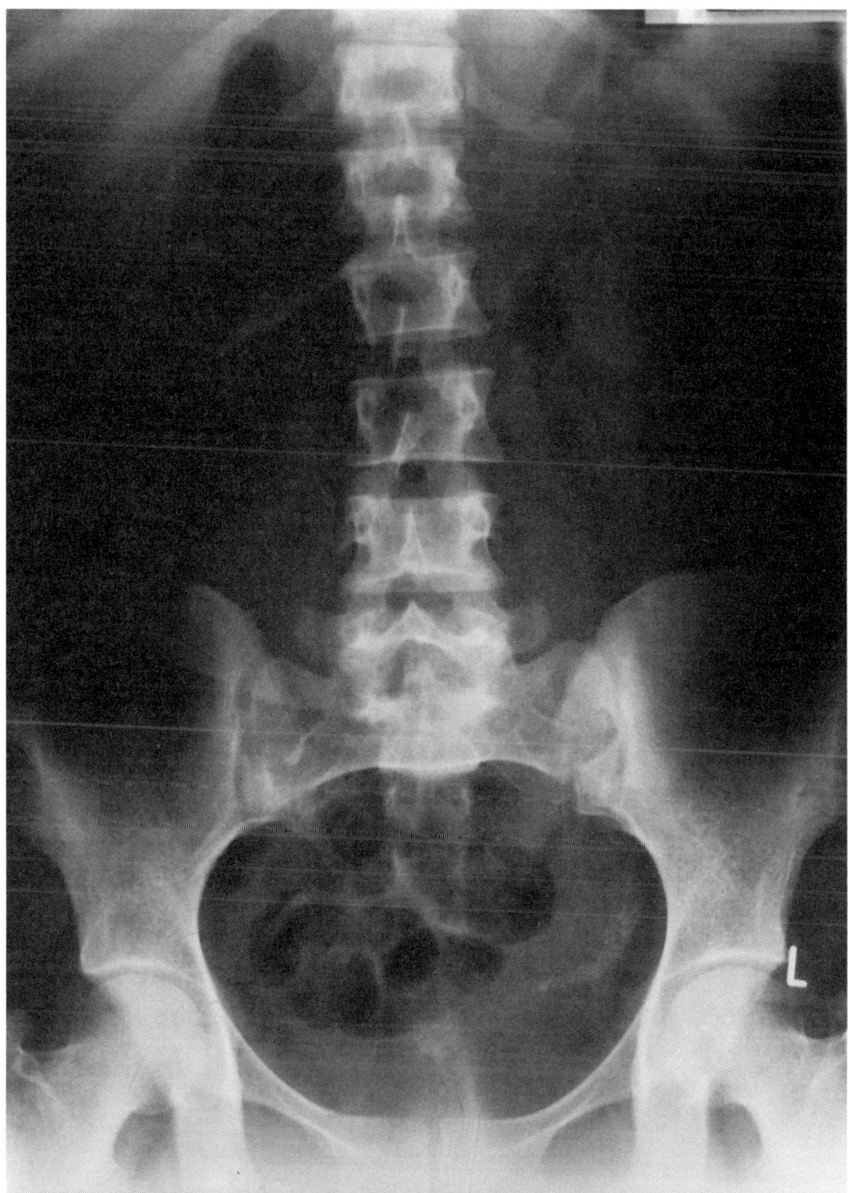

Figure 29.1(b) Steinstrasse with a small lead stone seen in the patient in Figure 29.1a

20% developed SS of which 65% passed spontaneously, 26% required endoscopic treatment, and 9% required radiological expertise for clearance [2].

Ten per cent of 25 mm stones treated on electromagnetic or electro-hydraulic lithotriptors are likely to need therapy for SS. Larger stones may require SS in 60% [1] unless care is taken to use shock waves with a lower power [5].

Large SS (in which a third of the ureter is choked with stone) occur in 3% of patients [6], especially in those:

- with large stones (especially staghorns);
- in whom the debulking was not possible or adequate; and
- in whom unexpected fragment movement occurred (when a large stone fragment moved into the ureter).

Alerted by the above conditions, one can expedite the second treatment if there is a suspiciously large fragment in the kidney, 'small' enough to enter into the dilated ureter (dilated because of the stent) to pre-empt unexpected fragment movement.

Prevention of *steinstrasse*

Prevention is easier and preferable to therapy. Stones treated by piezo-electric lithotripsy are less likely to develop SS, and if it does develop, it is usually type I. Learning from this experience, we recommend using low voltage shock waves to treat the patient. We feel that current rates of reported SS are unnecessarily high. Altered strategy for stone treatment, utilizing lower power shock waves does reduce SS rate and post-ESWL intervention [5].

References

1. David RM, Fuchs GJ. Management of steinstrasse after ESWL. J Urol 1989;141:242A.
2. Fedullo LM, Pollack HM, Banner MP *et al.* The development of steinstrassen after ESWL: Frequency, natural history, and radiologic management. Am J Roentgenol 1988;151:1145–7.
3. Talati J. Genitourinary surgery in Pakistan. In: Ahmed M *et al.*, editors. Surgery for all. Lahore: Ferozesons, 1992:369.
4. Cochrane ST, Barbarie ZL, Mendel HS *et al.* ESWL impact on the radiology department of a stone center. Radiology 1987;163:655.
5. Talati J, Shah T, Memon A *et al.* ESWL for urinary tract stones using MPL9000 spark gap technology and ultrasound monitoring. J Urol 1991;146:1482–6.
6. Weinerth JL, Flat JA, Carson CC. Lessons learned in patients with large steinstrasse. J Urol 1989;142:1425–7.

30. Urinary tract infection, stones and ESWL

JAMSHEER TALATI

Injudicious use of antibiotics escalates the cost of stone treatment, besides encouraging the development of resistant strains of bacteria, which then require third generation antibiotics for eradication. A course of injectable, third generation cephalosporins for seven days (US\$ 210) may cost approximately a third of the cost of lithotripsy (US\$ 500–600). Injectable antibiotics sometimes require admission, because of the lack of domiciliary services, which further add to the costs.

An understanding of the interrelation between stone and urinary tract infection (UTI), the common occurrence of sterile pyuria in patients with stone disease, release of bacteria from the stone during extracorporeal shock wave lithotripsy (ESWL), the effect of ESWL on the viability of bacteria, the incidence of post-ESWL bacteriuria and sepsis, the relation of infection to placement of stents, the relation between infection and stone recurrence, an understanding of the type of patients at risk for urinary infection, and above all the unit's audit of its work, will allow the evolution of an effective, rational policy for antibiotic usage.

Urinary infection as a cause of stone

Urinary infection with urease producing organisms results in production of ammonia and carbon dioxide. Ammonia (NH_3) hydrolyses to ammonium (NH_4) [1] which can raise the urinary pH to as high as 9, and precipitate phosphates and ammonium magnesium phosphate. The CO_2 hydrates to H_2CO_3, which combines with calcium to form calcium carbonate. Bacteria, obtained from the urine and stones of stone patients, form extracellular aggregates of crystals of bobierrite (magnesium phosphate). Their role in stone formation is not known.

Common urease producing organisms include *Proteus* sp., but a urease splitting organism that is usually not searched for is *Ureaplasma urealyticum* which was noted in 25% of infection related lithiasis, most often (in 70%) as the only urea splitting organism [2] in one series.

Urease activity can be inhibited by acetohydroxamic acid, which reduces stone recurrence [3]. However, the drug is seldom used now because of intolerable psychoneural and musculo-integumentary side-effects in up to 22% of treated patients.

The effects of urea splitting organisms are dependent on the initial pH of the urine and the amount of phosphate buffer in urine [4]. Lowering the pH of urine

J. Talati et al. (eds) The Management of Lithiasis, 195–199
© *1997 Kluwer Academic Publishers. Printed in Great Britain.*

and use of culture specific antibiotic, reduces the saturation of carbonate apatite and struvite [5] and hence lowers the rate of recurrence.

Pyuria and infection

In 1975, 60% of stones reported in Pakistan were associated with infection [6]. Stone patients at the Civil Hospital Karachi had infection due to *E. coli* (41%), *Pseudomonas* (10%) *E. coli* and *Proteus* (16%), streptococci (9%), *Proteus* (12%) and *Klebsiella* (8%) [7]. During the similar time period, at Jinnah Postgraduate Medical Center, also in Karachi, only 19% of 255 stone patients' urines were infected [8].

In our experience, pyuria is still a very common occurrence, but urinary tract infection (UTI) is present in only 6% of patients. Because of the large throughput from rapid treatment by the lithotriptor, far more stones are seen each year, and in an outpatient setting, stones are becoming the commonest cause of sterile pyuria.

The difference between our incidence of urinary infection and that of other units is reflected in the different stone composition. The vast majority of our patients have calcium oxalate stones, whilst in other units, up to 27% are magnesium ammonium phosphate or carbonate stones (see Chapter 1).

In Pakistani children, up to 19% of stones are related to infection [9]. In Japan, 6.5–9% were associated with infection [10, 11], which was due to *E. coli* in 43% and *Proteus* in 40% [8]. The incidence of bacteriuria is higher in ureteral compared to renal stones, with a preponderance in females [10]. Core culture of stones yielded organisms in 14 (70%) of 20 staghorn calculi; 65% of these isolates were the same as those found in the urine [10]. Bacteriuria may occur in non-infection stones [12].

Antibiotic policy for stone therapy

As patients with preoperative urinary infection do not fare well on any form of therapy, it is preferable to culture all pyuric patients first and treat the infection before definitive therapy.

The acutely septic patient in shock from UTI in a blocked kidney requires urgent nephrostomy and intensive antibiotic therapy and hydration.

For patients whose preoperative urine is sterile, a single dose of prophylactic antibiotic is justified. If at operation it is found that the urine pent up behind the obstructing stone is turbid, antibiotic can be continued until the culture report of the urine is obtained.

Infection rates as high as 50% after open surgery. Percutaneous nephrotomy 47% after (PCN) [13], and 21% after combined Percutaneous nephrolithotomy (PCNL) and ESWL treatment of staghorn calculi [14] have been noted, justifying the use of antibiotic prophylaxis and indicating the need for conducting a urine culture postoperatively.

Nephrostomy urine becomes infected despite prophylactic antibiotics. This can be eliminated by 2.5% noxythiolin irrigation through the nephrotomy [15] or even by irrigation with saline (A. Memon, personal communication).

Effect of ESWL on bacteria

Bacteria are killed by the shock waves. *In vitro* experiments in which *Proteus* organisms were coated with agar gel impregnated with calcium carbonate, have shown that 18% may however survive the shocks [16]. As there is a risk that the remaining organisms would multiply rapidly during the phase of partial obstruction from stone fragments, ESWL should not be undertaken without eradicating UTI.

In our experience, bacteriuria occurs in 6% of patients overall and is eradicated pre-ESWL, except in the occasional patient.

In infection-free ASA grade 1 patients, all ESWL is currently done without antibiotic cover in our unit. Initially we were concerned that the organisms in the centre of the stone may be released in urine after ESWL, and we treated all our patients with prophylactic antibiotics. It has now been shown that the number of patients with positive stone culture is small, unless the stone is composed of struvite or a mixture of calcium phosphate and carbonate [11], stones which (especially struvite calculi) are notorious for their association with ineradicable infection and which require persistent antibiotic therapy [17].

Some still express concern and require that prophylactic antibiotics should be used in view of the rates of post-ESWL bacteraemia and bacteriuria. Raz *et al.* [18] note that 4.8% of 145 patients who did not have pre-existing bacteriuria developed bacteriuria after ESWL and that bacteria is not dependent on stone size or number.

Bacteraemia has been noted in 4.3% of 22 patients who had 154 blood cultures [19], to 14.3% (of 49 patients) [20], and is explained on the basis of release of organisms from stone into an obstructed system, or obstruction of a previously infected system. Patients who have had a higher frequency of bacteriuria prior to ESWL, and those who have larger stones, are more prone to bacteraemia, and even fungaemia [21], and should be carefully monitored.

Fortunately the bacteraemia is transient, with 7.2% of patients having bacteraemia immediately after ESWL, but none having positive blood cultures at 1 hour after ESWL [22]. Such transient bacteraemia is not of importance to a healthy adult. However, patients at risk for bacterial endocarditis will require prophylactic antibiotic [20].

It is necessary to stop using antibiotics routinely. Petersen and Tiselius [23] noted a 6.7% incidence of urinary infection in all patients after ESWL, whether they had or had not received prophylactic methenamine hippurate or trimethoprim and sulphamethoxazole. Routine prophylactic use of antibiotics does not make a difference to the incidence of post-ESWL UTI.

It is sometimes necessary to perform ESWL to eradicate fragments of residual calculi in the presence of infection, and antibiotic therapy is indicated. Such a combined approach can eradicate infection in 76% patients [24].

Conclusion

The use of antibiotics should be discontinued before or during ESWL except when treating infection, or treating patients at risk for bacterial endocarditis, patients with struvite stones, and patients in whom UTI cannot be eradicated before ESWL; and perhaps in patients with *steinstrassen*. The interdependence of UTI residual recurrence is discussed in Chapter 41.

References

1. Coe EL, Favus MJ. Nephrolithiasis. In: Wilson *et al.*, editors. Harrison's principles of internal medicine. New York: McGraw-Hill, 1991:1205.
2. Becopoulos T, Tsagatakis E, Constantinides C *et al.* Ureaplasma urealyticum and infected renal calculi. J Chemother 1991;3:39–41.
3. Griffith DL. Struvite stones: Is chemoprophylaxis necessary? In: Giuliani L, Puppo P, editors. Controversies on the management of urinary stone. Basel: Karger, 1988:235–8.
4. Edin-Liljegren A, Grenabo L, Hedelin H *et al.* The influence of pH and urinary composition on urease enzymatic activity in human urine. Urol Res 1992;20:35–9.
5. Hess B. Prophylaxis of infection induced kidney stone formation. Urol Res 1990;18:45–8.
6. Rizvi SAH. The problem of urolithiasis in Pakistan. J Pak Med Assoc 1975;25:276–8.
7. Rizvi SAH. Calculous disease: A survey of 400 patients. J Pak Med Assoc 1975;25:268–74.
8. Farooqui S, Nasir A, Naqvi AJ. Analysis of 1423 new patients referred to the nephrourology department of the PMC Karachi. A 5 year study. J Pak Med Assoc 1975;25:286–8.
9. Parkash, Fayyaz, Farhat *et al.* Urolithiasis in children. Abstracts of the First International Symposium of the SIUT, Pakistan, Karachi 1995:F5.
10. Ohkawa M, Tokunaga S, Nakashima T *et al.* Composition of urinary calculi related to urinary tract infection. J Urol 1992;148:995–7.
11. Shigeta M, Yamasaki A, Hayashi M. A clinical study in upper urinary tract calculi treated with ESWL monotherapy with regard to bacteriuria before ESWL. Nippon Hinyokika Gakkai Zasshi 1993;84:866–72.
12. Oka T, Nishimura K, Tsujimura A *et al.* Influences of bacteria within stones on ESWL treatment. Hinyokika Kiyo 1992;38:999–1003.
13. Vogel E, Eusterbrock M, Leskovar P. Recurrence rates of phosphate stones after open surgery and PCN. Uro Res 1987;15:128.
14. Castillo-Rodriguez M, Larria-Masoidal E, Garcia-Serrano C *et al.* Staghorn calculi, combined treatment with PCNL and ESWL. Arch Esp Urol 1993;46:699–706.
15. Buck AC. The use of noxythiolin as an antiseptic agent in upper urinary tract drainage following percutaneous nephrolithotomy. Br J Urol 1988;62:306–10.
16. Reid G, Jewett MA, Nickel JC *et al.* Effect of ESWL on bacterial viability. Urol Res 1990;18:425–7.
17. Michels EK, Fowler JE. ESWL for struvite renal calculi; prospective study with extended followup. J Urol 1991;146:728–32.
18. Raz R, Zoabi A, Sudarsky M *et al.* The incidence of UTI in patients without bacteriuria, who underwent ESWL. J Urol 1994;32:30.
19. Gasser TC, Frei R. Risk of bacteraemia during ESWL. Br J Urol 1993;71:17–20.
20. Muller-Mathias VG, Schmale D, Seewald M *et al.* Bacteremia during ESWL of renal calculi. J Urol 1991;146:733–6.
21. Orenstein R, Bross JE, Dahlman M. Risk factors for urinary lithotripsy associated sepsis. Infection Control Hosp Epidemiol 1993;14:469–72.
22. Kattan S, Hussain I, El-Faqih SR *et al.* Incidence of bacteremia and bacteriuria in patients with non-infection related stones undergoing ESWL. J Endourol 1993;7:449–51.

23. Peterson B, Tiselius HG. Are prophylactic antibiotics necessary during ESWL? Br J Urol 1989;63:449–52.
24. Pode D, Lenokovsky Z, Shapiro A *et al.* Can ESWL eradicate persistent UTI associated with infected stones? J Urol 1988;140:257–9.

31. The judicious use of stents

JAMSHEER TALATI, MUNEER AMANULLAH and SALMAN ADIL

Ureteric stents are tubes of memory coded polymeric bio-inert material which recoil or angle at both ends after being straightened for insertion. Placed so that one end remains in the renal pelvis and the other in the urinary bladder, most stents contain a central channel, with multiple holes throughout its length. The Towers stent, an exception, drains through guttered channels on the outside of the stent, is little used, and is associated with more *steinstrasse* [1].

Stents are costly, do not always improve the effectiveness of ESWL, cause complications and are frequently ill-tolerated by patients. A stent should be inserted only if there is a clear benefit from its use.

Clearance of stones and prevention of obstruction

The stent is placed on the assumption that it ensures better drainage, and facilitates stone clearance. It is expected to protect the patient from obstruction of the ureter, and consequent renal damage and sepsis, which is especially important in patients with solitary kidneys [2, 3], diabetes and myocardial decompensation.

Stents dilate the ureter. Drainage occurs around stents, even in those with a central lumen which is blocked in a third of cases at the time of removal [4]. The dilated ureter eases subsequent ureteroscopy, if needed for persistent *steinstrasse*. As egress of particles through the ureter is mainly through peristalsis, the stent and consequent dilatation of the ureter do not help clearance [5–7] and we have seen patients in whom the kidney has been obstructed in spite of a stent.

Bierkins *et al.* [5] feel that the use of stents makes no difference to the incidence of *steinstrasse*, infection or fever, even for stone burdens greater than 200 mm^2. However their stone-free rate was lower (35%) in the unstented group as compared to the stented (44%). For larger stones treated on a lithotriptor with a powerful punch, such as the HM3, stenting reduces complications [8, 9] from 26% to 7%, and auxiliary procedure rates from 15% to 6% [6], especially the number of unanticipated percutaneous nephrotomies (PCN) for drainage of obstructed systems. In their early experience with lithotripsy, Cochran *et al.* [10] reported a need for PCN in 3% of 446 calyceal stones, 8% of 345 pelvic stones, 11% of 189 ureteral stones, 34% of 118 partial staghorns, and 56% of 61 staghorn calculi in the post-ESWL period because of fever and signs of obstruction. Stenting may have reduced the need for PCN.

J. Talati et al. (eds) The Management of Lithiasis, 201–213
© *1997 Kluwer Academic Publishers. Printed in Great Britain.*

Stents are unnecessary when treating patients with small stones [11], fragile calculi, especially when treated on piezo-electric lithotriptors, or by low power shock waves on any lithotriptor. The fine powder produced by gentle shock waves rarely causes *steinstrasse*. For other renal stones it is wiser to use stents when treating:

- 'hard' stones (such as urate and whewellite);
- radiolucent stones, which are difficult to follow up for obstructing particles;
- radiolucent stones on a radiologically monitored lithotriptor (when a flushing stent is used to perfuse the pelvi-calyceal system during lithotripsy to aid visualization for targeting of shocks);
- patients with diabetes, dubious PUJ obstructions, recently dilated strictures, or severe myocardial disease where sepsis (secondary to obstruction) would have disastrous effects;
- patients coming for lithotripsy from far away;
- patients with a solitary kidney; and
- patients requiring adjuvant chemolysis.

For patients with ureteric stones, stents are used:

- after push-up of the stone into the kidney;
- to bypass ureteric obstruction pending definitive treatment;
- as the first stage of a two-stage ureteroscopy, where the stent is inserted at the first sitting to allow the ureter to dilate and facilitate subsequent ureteroscopy;
- following traumatic ureteroscopy, where there have been multiple passes to remove stones;
- following recognition of perforation, mucosal erosion, or mucosal channelling/tunnelling;
- for treatment of a ureteric fistula following ureterolithotomy; and
- to bypass a stone in pregnancy. (Note: the stent will have to be placed without X-ray control).

Problems with stents

The most dangerous problem with stents occurs in the patient who gets best adapted to his stent and fails to appear for follow-up. This is problematic in countries where there is no family practitioner to remind and guide the patient. In a review of 56 patients stented at the Aga Khan University Medical Center (AKUMC), the average indwelling time was 89 days (Table 31.1). In our experience, 16% of patients with stents had not kept appointments for removal of stents. Discovered at monthly morbidity meetings, patients had to be specifically called in for removal of the stent. Without a review system, patients are at risk of retaining their stent for the rest of their life, with a possibility of encrustation, fragmentation and infections.

This is a problem common to all third world populations, but is worse in migratory populations: 1.9% of 299 patients with stents were lost to follow-up, 11.3% of

Table 31.1   Stent indwelling time

Stent removed in	n (%)
< 30 days	15 (26.8)
31–60 days	5 (8.9)
61–90 days	11 (19.6%)
91–180 days	18 (32.1%)
> 180 days	7 (12.5%)[a]

[a] Of these seven patients, two were removed in 181 days.

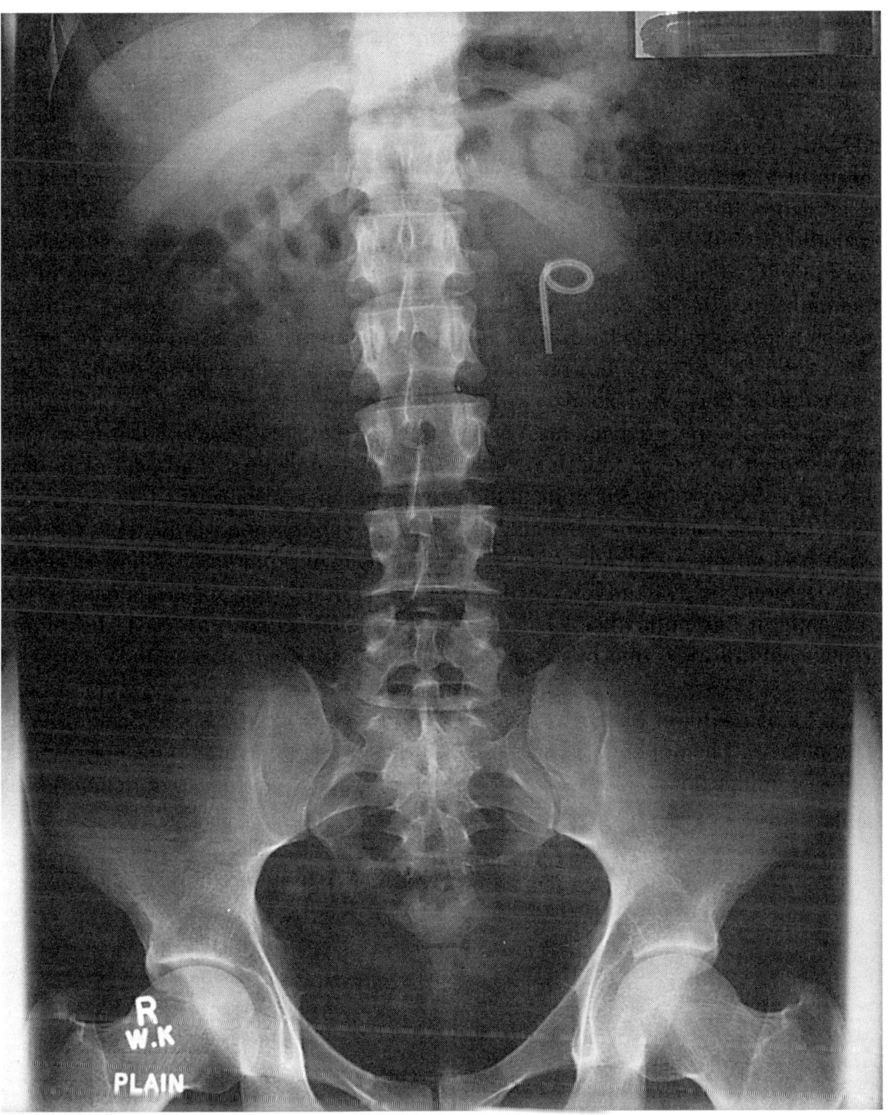

Figure 31.1   Fractured stent

stents remained inserted beyond their expiry date, and 0.3% fragmented *in vivo*, in a series from Saudi Arabia [4].

Complications during insertion

Guide wires used for stent placement can perforate the ureter and cause urinomas. They can tunnel submucously when negotiating obstructing stones with the threat that such submucous channels will fill with stone debris on removal of the stent.

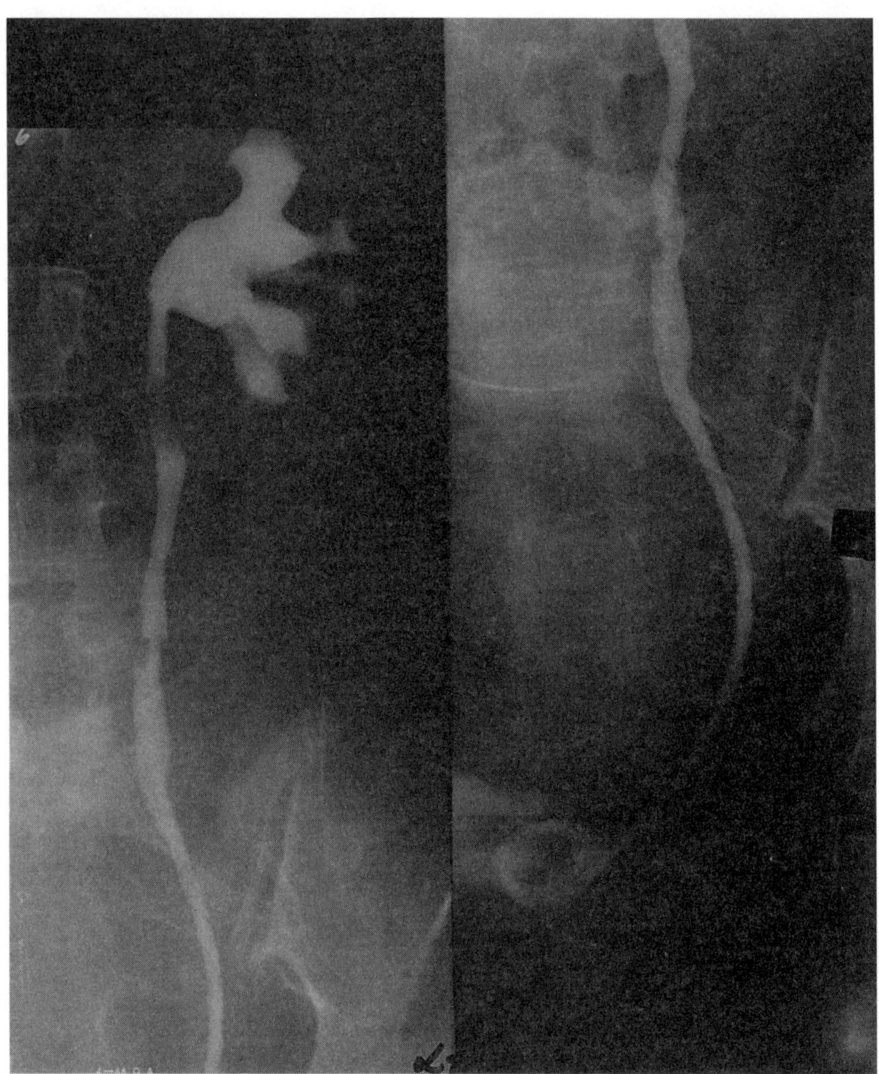

Figure 31.2 Intense ureteritis cystica in a patient with a stent

Stents can be pushed too far up the ureter so that they disappear from cystoscopic view because of rapid insertion by inexperienced operators.

Irritative symptoms, reflux, encrustation and blockage

Irritation by stents manifests as symptoms mimicking cystitis and can exceed patient tolerance and require early removal. Microscopic haematuria is common and innocuous. The stiffness and the coefficient of friction of the stent, the length in the bladder, and the indwell time, affect the degree of symptoms. Oxybutynin can relieve some of these. The histological picture is one of cystitis and ureteritis cystica and mucous metaplasia [12]. The latter leads to crystal aggregation and stone deposition even in the silicone stents [13], though to a lesser extent than in other stents. Hydrogel coating [14] reduces epithelial destruction, inflammatory reaction and encrustation.

Morbidity associated with stents is minimal in the first six weeks [4]; 9%, 48% and 76% of stents encrust if left for less than 6, 6–12 and more than 12 weeks respectively. [4]. Bierkins *et al.* [5] recommend removing stents in eight weeks, and reinserting them if necessary. This results in a high reinsertion rate and a high interventional rate for *steinstrasse*, which third world countries can ill afford.

In the Pakistan setting, 10.5% of stents become encrusted [15]. Encrustations severe enough to prevent removal without ancillary measures occur in up to 6.4% [4]. In our experience, encrustation is mostly at the lower end and can be nibbled away using biopsy forceps. Occasionally extracorporeal shock wave lithotripsy (ESWL) is required for upper end encrustations which have cemented the spirals of the stent into one solid ring (Figure 31.2).

Whilst we find polyethylene stents very stiff and difficult for patients to tolerate, others [16] found no difference in the short term in the symptoms produced by a variety of stents – Vanteck, Surgiteck, Siliteck, Uropas, Cook C Flex, and Cook polyurethane pigtail stent. Improper positioning from an incorrectly long stent causes irritation of the trigone. Readjusting a stent costs money and hence it is prudent to ensure that the correct length of the stent is chosen. Only one coil should lie in the bladder and the stent should curve up and away from the trigone.

Some patients complain of pain in the kidney on micturition, which may result from reflux or movement of the upper end of the stent when the detrusor squeezes the last drops of urine from the bladder.

Migration

Up to 2% of patients expel their stents, and 1.5% ascend up the ureter [17]. Stents with a full coil, compared with those with a simple J, migrate infrequently. Stents with round configuration migrate more often than those with a triangular cross-section [5]. Descent into the urethra produces incontinence and is seen more commonly in the tethered stents, which can become ensnared in the patient's clothes (zips or buttons). Straight ureteric catheters used as stents are liable to slide out:

multilength multiple coil stents seldom get displaced. Too long a stent can irritate the trigone and cause expulsion, because of repeated bladder spasms.

At times the so-called migration is due to inappropriate placement. Problems arise when the stent has been passed too high up into the kidney, and only a small curved portion of the stent lies in the bladder. There is a risk of the stent being pushed up into the ureter at the time that the pusher is being manipulated, or the guide wire is being removed, unless the position of the pusher/introducer is checked visually through the cystoscope.

During percutaneous antegrade stent insertion, the stent may coil up in the lower end of a massively dilated ureter. Subsequent cystoscopy may show no evidence of a stent in the bladder, suggesting upward migration incorrectly.

Colonization and urinary tract infection

Eleven (3.7%) of 295 patients receiving ESWL in our series and 5–6.7% [4, 17] of patients in other series develop urinary tract infection (UTI) post-ESWL. Of these 11, 63% had a stent. In a subgroup of 74 patients with a stent, 5.4%, compared with 3.7% in the whole group, developed post-ESWL UTI.

Stented patients may have an increased predisposition to infection, possibly due to incompetence of the ureteric orifices, and the presence of a foreign body [18]. The loss of the competence of the uretero-vesical junction may lead to a higher incidence of UTI, even after removal of the stent [18].

Colonization of the stent is seen more frequently, and though not accompanied by infection in the majority of cases, it does promote catheter encrustation and stent obstruction [19]. To avoid colonization, we do not stent a patient until pre-existing UTI has been eliminated.

Other problems with stents

Stents refract shock waves and reduce their efficiency. There are reports of the stent forming a knot at removal. Stents can fragment if left in beyond their indwell time.

Protocols, procedures and techniques for stent placement and removal

The most important step in stenting is the decision regarding its usefulness and need to insert it. Once that is made, discussions with the patient will lead to appropriate informed consent which requires an explanation of reasons for stenting, the procedure, possible complications and warnings, including an explanation of the following:

- insertion of DJS through cystoscope through the urethra, up to the kidney under general/local anaesthesia;
- expected indwelling time;
- advantages vs. probable risks if not placed;
- occurrence of haematuria after stenting and lithotripsy;

- the need to remove the stent as soon as a stone-free status is achieved, and within stent expiry time;
- importance of follow-up visits to detect any complication if it arises;
- the occurrence of renal pain (most patients complain of some pain in the renal angle on micturition and we selectively tell patients this, assessing which patient – most often the anxious patients – are likely to be bothered and troubled by this symptom).

As stent placement can and should be done by relatively junior surgeons, strict guidelines and helpful tips are needed. These are discussed below. Irrespective of whether the stent is to be placed under local or general anaesthesia, the patient should be thoroughly investigated prior to scheduling the procedure.

Timing the insertion of a stent

A stent should be inserted prophylactically, before the start of lithotripsy. Some authors suggest a non-stenting policy, with insertion of a stent if *steinstrasse* are troublesome. This policy is appropriate for units utilizing piezo-electric lithotriptors. Insertion of a DJS through a dense *steinstrasse* has a higher risk for perforation of the ureter and submucous false passages.

Noordzij suggests inserting the DJS prophylactically some time before ESWL, and removing it once the ureter dilates and before ESWL is started, on the principle that the stent is being used to dilate the ureter, and the stent itself is an impediment as it blocks part of the lumen (personal communication). Stone fragments at times do adhere to the stent and block egress of other stone particles.

Stent insertion at cystoscopy

The vast majority of our stents are placed retrogradely at cystoscopy. Expertise in stent placement builds up very rapidly and can be easily taught to residents. Antegrade placement will be required in up to 10% of patients [17] though difficulties in retrograde placement are encountered usually for reasons other than stone, as in patients with inoperable carcinomas producing ureteric obstruction. Stent placement even under local anaesthesia should never be considered a minor procedure. It is not without risk: cardiac arrest can occur in any patient at any time.

Protocols and procedures are described below.

- A review of the X-rays (which are left on the illuminator in the operating room) identifies the side for insertion and expected difficulties (the name and the number on the X-ray are checked against the name on the wristband of the patient).
- ECG electrodes are placed on the chest for continuous monitoring during the procedure.
  An IV line is established using a cannula, for infusion of Ringer's lactate.
- If the patient is a female, a female nurse or a female doctor should be available in the operation room to assist during the procedure, and reassure the patient.

This is especially important for procedures done under local anaesthesia in countries where culture demands this.

- The patient is placed in a cystoscopy (modified lithotomy) position after induction of anaesthesia, making sure that the thighs move up and out from the table at a gentle angle of about 45 degrees. Acute flexion of the hip as for haemorrhoid operations will result in the sacrum being lifted off the table, which will make ureteric catheterization difficult.
- All those present should wear a lead apron.
- The opportunity to look at the whole bladder and discover hidden pathology should not be missed at a preliminary cystoscopy.
- A DJS of appropriate length is selected and placed under fluoroscopic control using C-arm image intensification.
- At the end of the procedure, the position of the upper end is checked by C-arm, and the lower end visually to ensure minimal but adequate length (1 loop of the coil) in the bladder.
- Patients going immediately for ESWL have an indwelling Foley's catheter inserted as the irritation of the stent and the recent cystoscopy may make the patient restless, with a desire to void urine frequently during the subsequent ESWL.

Alternatively, instillation of 4% lignocaine jelly in the urethra will reduce the irritation. The patient is shifted to the recovery room under supervision of an anaesthetist. It is preferable to delay shifting the patient to the lithotripsy room until he/she is stable, and able to understand verbal communication clearly before starting lithotripsy. A restless, drowsy patient cannot be communicated with on the ESWL table, and patient co-operation will be difficult to obtain.

Determining the length of stent required

A short stent migrates up; one that is too long will irritate. The correct length of ureter is 0.83 times the length of the ureter measured by using a string on the intravenous urogram taken at our hospital. Smith and Lee [20] suggest that X-rays magnify by 10% and that if the stent is the same size as the ureteric measurement from X-rays, it will allow 2 cm of stent to lie in the bladder. Each unit should determine the amount of magnification in its X-rays. More accurate measurement can be made from peroperative measurement of the ureter by a ureteric catheter. Today, determination of the ureteric length is less important, as multilength stents are available, and it is more cost-efficient to stock these, rather than individual sizes, except for the odd, smaller, paediatric stents.

Local anaesthesia for stent insertion

Patients can tolerate insertion of size 5Fr stents easily under local anaesthesia; 6 Fr stents cause considerable discomfort. We feel that appropriate sedo-analgesia or anaesthesia is important, because the patient should not experience a painful procedure at the commencement of therapy. Discomfort with one procedure will produce a heightened sensitivity to pain and increase the analgesia requirements during ESWL.

Stent insertion under local anaesthesia is easier in females, but in our society, most conscious women object to the cystoscopy positioning and cystoscopy by a male, or in the presence of male nursing or anaesthesia attendants, from embarrassment and other considerations.

Measures to facilitate successful passage of stents

The entry of the ureteric catheter into the ureteric orifice should be very gentle. The catheterization channel with an Albarran lever should be used and the cystoscope kept close to the ureteric orifice. Care should be taken to avoid looping the catheter in the bladder, as correction of this often causes the top end of the catheter to slip down, out of the pelvis. Careless insertion of the catheter or the guide wire may result in a false passage and a mucosal flap especially just beyond the ureteric orifice. This can be avoided by assessing the obliquity of the ureter from the IVU. Many ureters end transversely, and need a rotation of the cystoscope so that the entry ports for the catheter are at 3 or 9 o'clock positions, pointing to the thigh on the side being catheterized. If a false passage has been formed, a ureteroscope is useful in identifying the correct channel to guide a guide wire into the upper ureter.

Difficulties in negotiating the ureteric orifices can be overcome by passing the ureteric catheter up to the ureteric orifice, protruding the guide wire from the catheter and into the ureteric orifice, and threading the ureteric catheter over it.

Once the ureteric catheter has bypassed the stone, a guide wire (floppy end first) is passed into the catheter, and threaded in up to the silver mark on the guide wire. This indicates that the guide wire has reached the end of the catheter. Under fluoroscopic control, the floppy end of the guidewire is pushed out of the catheter to coil in the pelvis. The catheter is then withdrawn, whilst pushing the guide wire in, making sure that the guide wire is not pulled out inadvertently, by intermittent imaging on the C-arm.

Though the radiation dose is small, cumulative radiation can build up to unacceptable, and unnecessary levels if the foot pedal switch of the image intensifier is depressed indiscriminately and for too long.

The DJ stent is threaded onto the guide wire which is held taut by the assistant, who must, at the same time, ensure that the guide wire is not pulled out. This can be ensured by asking the assistant to hold the wire taut, then fix his arm to his side with the elbow flexed, and plant his feet firmly and not move or tilt back. It is vital that the guide wire should not loop in the bladder. (When straightening such a loop, the top end slides out of the ureter.)

The DJS is gently guided into the ureteric orifice, and pushed up. The pusher propels the DJS further up the ureter. The pusher should be held against the stent as the guide wire is withdrawn. A short sharp thrust pushes the stent out of the cystoscope as the guide wire is withdrawn. The lower end should not be touching the trigone.

Special manoeuvres

In patients with impacted ureteral stones, and in large stones almost filling the pelvis of the kidney, the ureteric catheter should be led up to the stone and then introduced further only under constant gentle flushing with saline. This creates a space between stone and mucosa. Additionally the catheter tip should reach well beyond the stone before inserting the guide wire. (Also see section on treatment of ureteric stones, facilitating endoscopic manoeuvres complimentary to ESWL — Chapter 19, pp. 147–8.)

Bypassing kinks in the ureter, stent placement in a calyx of choice can be accomplished by the method described by Puppo [21], catheterizing the ureter with a 35-inch straight guide wire with a moveable core over which a cobra catheter is introduced. The cobra catheter is manoeuvred by rotation into the lower calyx, or past a kink. The soft moveable guide wire is advanced into the calyx and stiffened, the catheter removed and the DJS placed over the guide wire.

Confirmation of placement of stents by non-radiological means

At times, as in operative removal of large obstructing stones in the ureter or in patients with incomplete clearance of renal stones, a stent has to be placed intraoperatively. The correct placement of the lower end of the stent in the bladder can be confirmed by first filling the bladder with methylene blue so that the dye can be seen oozing out of the multiple holes as soon as the stent reaches the bladder.

Removal of stents

Stents should be removed as soon as one is sure that the stone fragments will pass spontaneously with little chance of blocking the ureter. A ureteric stent can be removed under local anaesthesia using a flexible cystoscope, by snaring it [22] in a loop of nylon glued onto a 5 French ureteric catheter or a Dormia basket [23], or tri-radiate forceps [24].

Upwardly migrated stents are best removed ureteroscopically. A percutaneous approach has also been used [25]. Alternatively, a Dormia basket with six wires can be passed up the ureter at cystoscopy, and the curved end of the catheter caught under fluoroscopic control within the wires and the basket withdrawn. Similar techniques may be used for retrieving broken stents.

The use of stents with an attached nylon suture obviates the need for cystoscopy for removal. The nylon wire is tethered to the penis or the abdominal wall with a piece of sticking plaster or tape. Sticking it to the thigh may cause an inadvertent pull out of the thread and stent. The stent is removed by pulling on the suture at an outpatient visit. No anaesthesia is required.

Upwardly migrated tethered stents can also be readjusted by a pull on the nylon suture.

These stents do not cause interference with intercourse [26] or incontinence unless the tip lies pulled out in the urethra. They can however be easily pulled out

[26], especially in women whilst drying the perineum, after micturition. A tethered or pull-out stent is well tolerated for 30 days, though most are made for 21-day placement. To reduce costs, any stent can have a 70 cm length of 4/0 monofilament nylon suture threaded through its terminal holes to convert it to a pull-through stent.

Measures to ensure follow-up

A card in duplicate is filled in by the urological or lithotripsy resident, detailing the date of placement of DJS, and the date by which it must be removed. One copy is given to the patient, the other is kept in a lithotripsy file. Each month the file should be reviewed. We have found a review of all DJ stent insertions (taken from the operating room registers) at periodic intervals useful and necessary to catch defaulters.

Reducing costs

An open-ended catheter can be used instead of a stent after push-up of ureteric stones, in those patients where the stone is likely to be crushed by a single sitting of lithotripsy. The open ended catheter is threaded through one of the eyes of a reasonable sized Foley catheter (size 20F) which is then inserted into the bladder through the urethra. Use of a smaller catheter causes blockage of the lumen by the 6Fr ureteric catheter. To produce a better lie of the ureteric catheter as it enters the eye of the Foley catheter, the eye should be slit in the direction of the tip of the catheter. Others [27] wedge a ureteral catheter with multiple side perforations (costing US$ 7) in the upper calyx, cut off the excess length protruding beyond the cystoscope, and push the catheter into the bladder with the obturator of the cystoscope. Such 'stents' can be retained in the bladder for 7–12 days.

Table 31.2   Costs in Netherlands and Pakistan of various procedures for treatment of stone

	Netherlands NHS[a] Guilders [$]		Netherlands private Guilders [$]		Pakistan private Pak Rs [$]	
Dormia basketing	89	[56]	276	[166]		
Ureteroscopy	302	[189]	553	[332]	2200	[73]
PCNL	415	[249]	827	[496]	5000	[167]
PCN	72	[43]	180	[108]	1500	[50]
ESWL	384	[230]	843	[506]	15 000	[500]
Antegrade stent	369	[221]	553	[332]	1500	[50]
Retrograde sent	66	[40]	159	[95]	550	[18]
Endo-lithotripsy	173	[104]	553	[332]	3000	[100]
Cost of stent					2000	[67]
Cost of silicone stent					6000	[200]

[a] NHS: National Health Service.
Figures from Netherlands courtesy Dr Joop Noordzig.
$ prices in US$ equivalent: $ = Pak Rs 30/-; Guilder = $.

Costs can be reduced by avoiding stenting. In the US, placing a stent will increase the cost of ESWL from US$ 600 to US$ 1000 [28]. In Pakistan, insertion of a stent under general anaesthesia will add US$ 50 in addition to the cost of the stent (US$ 67–200) to the patient's bill, if the procedure is done as a day surgery.

Silicone stents are costly, and are also prone to encrustation; they are not required in lithotripsy. Few stones should require stenting beyond three months.

Date expired stents lying unused in stock cost the hospital money. It is therefore best to stock one standard size (6F) of multilength (22–32 cm) stent. These uncoil to variable extent thus allowing a single size to fit all ureters from 22–32 cm long.

Stent placement under local anaesthesia or sedo-analgesia reduces costs. A DJS or ureteric catheter should never be reused. Encrusted stone or coagulated blood in the lumen makes cleaning impossible. If a packet containing a stent has been opened, but the stent insertion was not possible and the catheter has not been soiled by any body fluids, it may be resterilized.

We use a C-arm image intensifier. This is expensive. If it is not available, a portable X-ray can be used to confirm the positioning of the stent. There are some problems associated with passing the stent blind: at times the curve of the catheter cannot be seen. Furthermore perforation of the ureter cannot be assessed.

References

1. Kohri K, Yamate T, Amaski N *et al*. Characteristics and usage of different ureteral stent catheters. Urol Int 1991;47:131–7.
2. Ishii T, Imanishi M, Kohri K *et al*. Clinical study of ESWL for stones in a solitary kidney. Nippon Hinyokika Gakkai Zaashi 1991;82:1466–72.
3. Cohen ES, Schmidt JD. ESWL for stones in a solitary kidney. Urology 1990;36:52–4.
4. El Faqih SR, Shamsuddin AB, Chakrabarti *et al*. Polyurethane internal ureteral stents in the treatment of stone patients. Morbidity related to indwelling time. J Urol 1991;14:1487–91.
5. Bierkins AF, Hendrikx AJM, Lemmens WAJG *et al*. ESWL for large renal calculi: The role of ureteral stents. A randomised trial. J Urol 1991;145:699–702.
6. Libby JM, Meacham RB, Griffith DP. The role of silicone ureteral stents in extracorporeal shockwave lithotripsy of large renal calculi. J Urol 1988;139:15–17.
7. Preminger GM. Ureteral stenting during ESWL. J Urol 1989;142:32–6.
8. Shabsigh R, Gleeson MJ, Griffith DP. The benefits of stenting on a more or less routine basis prior to ESWL. Urol Clin N Am 1988;15:493–7.
9. Marberger MD. Retrieval of internal ureteral stents without cystoscopy. Endourology 1987;2:16–17.
10. Cochran ST, Barabric ZL, Mindel HJ *et al*. ESWL impact on the radiology department of a stone center. Radiology 1987;163:655.
11. Pryor JL, Langley MJ. Comparison of symptom characteristics of indwelling ureteral catheters. J Urol 1991;145:719–22.
12. Ramsay JWA, Miller RA, Crocker PR. An experimental study of hydrophobic plastics for urological use. Br J Urol 1986;58:70.
13. Rhind JR. Ureteric stents caveat. Br J Urol 1989;63:644–5.
14. Cormio L, Talja M, Koivusalo A *et al*. Biocompatibility of double J stent materials. J Urol 1995;153:494–6.
15. Nawaz H, Hussain M, Hashim A. Experience with indwelling JJ stent. J Pak Med Assoc 1993;43:147–9.

16. Langley MJ, Pryor JL, Jenkins AD. A randomized comparison of symptom characteristics of in-dwelling ureteral catheters. J Urol 1990;143:270A.

17. Zattoni F, Taska A, Favere DD. Personal experience using a double J ureteral stent. J Urol 1989;141:418A.

18. Franco G, De Dominicis C, Dal-Forno S *et al*. The incidence of postoperative urinary tract infections in patients with ureteric stents. Br J Urol 1990;65:10–12.

19. Gerber WL, Narayana AJ. Failure of the double curved ureteral stent. J Urol 1982;127:317–19.

20. Smith AD, Lee WJ. Characteristics and uses of the universal ureteric stent. Br J Urol 1983;(suppl):75–81

21. Puppo P. Use of cobra catheter for insertion of a ureteral stent. Br J Urol 1989;63:652 3.

22. Blandy JP. Lower urinary tract endoscopy. Br Med Bull 1986;42:279–83.

23. Upsdell SM. Removal of ureteric stents under local anesthesia. Br J Urol 1988;62:280.

24. Evans JWH. Removal of ureteric stents with a flexible cystoscope. Br J Urol 1991;67:109.

25. White PG, Evans C. Minimally invasive removal of retained ureteric stents. Br J Urol 1990;66:328–9.

26. Birch BRP, Das G, Wickham JEA. Tethered ureteric stents, a clinical assessment. Br J Urol 1988;62:409–11.

27. Kalash SS, Bezerdjian L, Bayer O. A simple non double J self retaining stent. J Urol 1989;141:33A.

28. Riehle RA Jr. Selective use of ureteral stents before ESWL. Urol Clin N Am 1988;15:499–506.

32. Protection of hospital personnel

JAMSHEER TALATI and SALAM KHAN

In this chapter, care in the use of X-rays, and protection of the eyes and hearing of personnel, are discussed.

Radiation from the use of X-rays

The surgeon's eyes, thyroid and hands receive radiation even when he is protected by a lead apron, both from the primary beam, and from secondary radiation scatter that emanates from the patient or is reflected off the table. The primary beam comes from a point source. The X-ray intensity around it is proportional to the inverse of the square of the distance from the beam, and falls rapidly to 5% of the primary beam within a few cm, and to 1% at 1 metre from the edge of the beam. The intensity of scatter radiation does not obey the inverse square law because the effective source is large.

The primary beam from an image intensifier is attenuated as it is intercepted by the patient and the table. The beam intensity and scatter is 10 times greater at entry compared to when it leaves the patient. An under-the-table position of the tube therefore will reduce irradiation risks to personnel. The average radiation dose from 25 m of fluoroscopy by C-arm, for percutaneous access and stone removal has been calculated, per case, as 10 mrem (0.10 mSV) for the radiologist, 0.04 mSv for the surgical nurse and 0.03 mSv for the anaesthetist [1]. Radiation levels can be as high as 3000 mrem per hour at the edge of the table, and the annual permissible limits may be exceeded after 10 cases of percutaneous nephrolithotomy (PCNL) requiring 30 m of screening time [2]. With an under-the-table position, the surgeon could safely do 30 procedures per week [3] but he must keep his hands and face away from the beam. This is easily remembered during a ureteroscopy, but in a PCNL, the left index finger receives the most irradiation, as it steadies the scope during screening.

During lithotripsy on radiologically monitored lithotriptors, the scattered radiation is approximately 0.5 mR per hour at 90 cm from the centre of the HM3 tank [4]. Radiation dose to personnel in the lithotripsy room averages less than 2 mrem (0.02 mSv) per case [5]. Persons working with radiologically monitored lithotriptors over a long period of time should therefore wear dosage badges. Many suggest there is no need for a lead apron.

J. Talati et al. (eds) The Management of Lithiasis, 215–218
© *1997 Kluwer Academic Publishers. Printed in Great Britain.*

Amongst the more recent lithotriptors, the mean annual dose to staff using the Storz modulith SL 20 lithotriptor [6] is 4.8 mSv. The projected annual dose equivalent to the eyes has been calculated at 6.1 mSv for the surgeon and 3.5 mSv for the radiographer; the mean absorbed dose (per patient) is 4.7 ± 0.5 mSv to the eyes for the surgeon, and 2.7 ± 0.3 mSv for the radiographer [6].

Irradiation exposure to patients was higher when unskilled surgeons moved the gantry to position the patient for lithotripsy. Inexperienced surgeons exposed their patients to 3.38 ± 0.86 rad entry exposure, compared to an exposure of 2.64 ± 0.97 rad when the procedure was done by skilled surgeons [7]. Consequently, inexperienced surgeons will increase their own exposure to radiation.

Radiation to patient, staff and surgeon can be reduced by:

- minimizing exposure time;
- minimizing beam width;
- using an under-the-table position for the X-ray tube;
- wearing lead aprons or standing behind lead shields;
- increasing skill at using the gantry; and
- removing the hands from the path of the primary beam during ureteroscopy and PCNL.

The addition of radiation goggles and thyroid shields needs to be considered when doing PCNL.

Because of the spread of the lithotriptor equipment, the walls of the room are at a distance from the radiation source in most radiologically monitored lithotriptors. Hence walls do not require additional lead shielding.

Proper use of lead aprons

Lead aprons are not designed to stop primary radiation coming from the X-ray tube. Their sole purpose is to provide protection against scattered radiation reflected from or passing through the patient's body or equipment being exposed, e.g. X-ray cassette, operating table, instruments and accessories. The thickness of lead (lead equivalence) of the apron should not make the surgeon complacent. The duration of the radiographic exposure should be minimized to protect the areas of the body not covered by the lead apron.

Diagnostic X-ray apparatus does not allow usage of over 120 kV in the main X-ray department. In portable/mobile equipment, the radiation dose does not exceed 100 kV for fluoroscopic work and rarely goes to 105 kV for radiographic work (and that only for special procedures such as lateral hip X-ray of an obese patient). The scattered radiation produced in operating rooms can be adequately absorbed by lead aprons of 0.25 mm lead thickness equivalence.

The procurement and replacement of lead aprons for operating rooms should be the responsibility of one person – the operating room manager. All aprons should be examined for holes and cracks which reduce their efficiency. Healthy aprons are essential for the health of the users. They crack easily and are expensive – US$ 200 each. They should be hung carefully from hangers, or kept flat, and must never be folded.

In third world university settings, where there are a large number of observers during operative procedures, the number of lead apron users can be minimized by having observers leave the room during X-ray exposure; or alternatively stand behind a mobile lead screen.

Noise and vestibular exhaustion

The lithotriptor produces sudden bursts of sound – impact noise – against which normal protective reflexes are ineffective. Dampening of continued noise is effected by the acoustic reflex in which contraction of the stapedius, which occurs at levels beyond 85 dB, limits ossicle movement and reduces damage to the cochlea. This reflex cannot protect the ear from impact sound, as the protective mechanism comes into play after the sound has subsided. Sound levels are of the order of 95 [8] to 112 dB [7] near the patient's ear, and 110 dB near the console – probably from reflection of sound [9]. To measure levels of the 'impact' noise a very sensitive linear impact sound meter is required. Acceptable levels for a work-place are 60 dB, with occasional periods with a maximum of 90 dB. Though opera-tors are subjected to intensities of sound below this limit, their exposure is over a longer period. It is therefore essential that lithotripsy personnel wear protective ear muffs, even when operating at a distance from the machine. Some of the sound is conducted through the ground, and cannot be eliminated.

Unfortunately, lithotripsy staff perceive only the loudness of sound (the psycho-logical correlate of intensity) and not its real intensity. The ear appreciates loudness as a ratio of increase, in a way similar to our appreciation of motion: we feel accel-eration but cannot appreciate the constant speed (400 mph) of an aeroplane when in the air. As they become accustomed to the sound, staff tend to avoid using ear muffs, especially as they are cumbersome, and cause sweating and a feeling of being cut off from the surroundings. Where the movement of the table for position-ing the patient is through automatic gears, ear muffs dampen the accelerating sound which normally warns the operator that the table is moving faster. We insist that personnel wear protective head gear, but compliance is poor.

Hazards from reflected light and ultrasound monitors

Reflection of bright light from air bubbles or near objects during cystoscopy pro-duces a glare. Whilst it has not been proven that this can cause macular damage, it is preferable to use lower intensities of light or a video camera. The level of blue light transmission also appears to be within the safe limits but the use of blue filters has been suggested, as long-term effects are not known [10].

Continuous ultrasound image tracking can cause monitor watching eye fatigue. Operators need to relax accommodation from time to time.

References

1. Bush WH, Jones D, Brannen GE. Radiation dose to personnel during percutaneous renal calculus removal. Am J Roentgenol 1985;145:1261–4.
2. Kelsey CA, Lane RG, Somers JW. Radiation exposure during fluoroscopically controlled percutaneous lithotripsy. J Urol 1984;132:1254–5.
3. Inglis JA, Tolley DA, Law J. Radiation safety during PCNL. Br J Urol 1989;63:591–3.
4. Lin PP, Hrejsa AF. Patient exposure and radiation environment on an ESWL system. J Urol 1987;138:712–15.
5. Bush WH, Jones D, Gibbons RJ. Radiation dose to patient and personnel during ESWL. J Urol 1987;138:716–19.
6. Baldock C, Greener AG, Batchelor S. Radiation dose to patients and staff from Storz Modlulith SL 20 lithotriptor. J Stone Dis 1992;4:216–19.
7. Saunders JE, Cleman AJ. Physical characteristics of a Dornier shock wave lithotriptor. Urology 1987;29:506–9.
8. Lusk RP, Tyler RS. Hazardous sound levels produced by extracorporeal shock wave lithotripsy. J Urol 1987;137:1113–14.
9. Chen WC, Lee YH, Chen MT *et al.* Factors influencing radiation exposure during extracorporeal shock wave lithotripsy. Scan J Urol Nephrol 1991;25:223–6.
10. Briggs TP, Parker C, Miller RA *et al.* Blue light emission from urological equipment. Can it damage the eyes? Br J Urol 1992;70:491–5.

Section IV
High Technology at Affordable Cost

33. Introduction: High technology at affordable cost

JAMSHEER TALATI

Technology is here to stay and it will continue to be used extensively. Many accepted technologies such as extracorporeal shockwave lithotripsy (ESWL) provide innumerable benefits but are costly. Consequently, in the third world, ESWL is available only to those poor patients who can access their government facility. The district surgeon in a government hospital has to perform open ureterolithotomies as he has no machine, no choice. Six lithotriptors may be available in a single town, 90 miles south of his hospital, whilst the surrounding towns to the north, east and west within a 200-mile radius have none.

Technology is expensive

ESWL is expensive because the machine is expensive and because of ancillary costs such as building and air-conditioning modifications, image intensifiers, nurses, paramedics and engineers required as support staff, bad debts, replacement and maintenance contracts.

ESWL was invented in a country that spent freely on research and development (R&D). To ensure further research, the costs incurred during development of the machine have to be recovered. Health care costs for industrial workers in advanced countries have also to be recovered. This makes the instrument cost more than its components and construction costs. In contrast the lithotriptor made in China is cheaper because it is less sophisticated and because of lower R&D costs, and the lower cost of living and medical expenses of its workers.

Achieving equity by government–private sector co-operation

Resources are limited and technology is expensive but health care can extend to more people through a combination of private and government participation in health care. In the third world, the national government must increase the spending on health and for stone disease. It should be responsible for distributing lithotriptors strategically all over the country. The private sector has the responsibility for running its programmes cost-effectively. Both have a responsibility to limit unwarranted use of the lithotriptor, and reduce purchase and maintenance costs.

J. Talati et al. (eds) The Management of Lithiasis, 221–224
© *1997 Kluwer Academic Publishers. Printed in Great Britain.*

Lack of technical expertise can hamper equitable health cover

Equitable health cover is impossible today because of factors other than costs. Specialized skills e.g. ureteroscopic skills (when required for post-ESWL *steinstrasse*) are available to a variable extent even in the most advanced nations. Today, at the brink of the twenty-first century, ureterolithotomy still remains the most common way of removing ureteric stones throughout the world. What is talked of in journals is not available to every person.

Increasing resources for health

Pakistan spends 2.5% of its government budget on health, India 3% and Indonesia 2.5% [1]. By comparison, it is projected that America will spend 20% of its GNP by the year 2000. The developing countries spend too much on defence. Using only half of the 120 billion dollars that they spend on military hardware, a 100 million lives a year could have been saved [2]. The cost of one F-16 jet could finance 25 000 to 27 000 lithotripsies. In 1992, the world spent US$ 700 billion (in 1993 dollars) on wars, some 30% more than in 1970 [2]. Many wars are avoidable and if we work towards global peace by concentrating on education, enfranchisement and democratic governance, a more sensible disbursement of available resources can occur [3].

Resource allocation for stone disease

In authoritarian states in third world countries resource allocation for expensive equipment is based more on the thrust, power and influence of the requesting person than on the basis of a rational analysis of the need in that population. Capital funding for major equipment is supported and facilitated in corrupt societies because of the kick-backs obtained. In the first world, lobbying by financially powerful sectors influences decisions.

Resources should not be allocated on the basis of machines. Resources should be allocated to programmes according to need [4], which has to be decided jointly by government, economists, the public and health professionals.

A cost–quality analysis should be given to the government, taking into consideration the cost to patients if their disease was not treated, the cost in terms of pain and suffering, the benefits that result from saving of hospital beds, and from reduced absenteeism from illness. The improvement in quality of life (life without dialysis, because the stone can be treated early in the course of the disease) is also an important consideration. The freeing of consultant time and his availability to look after other sick patients, and the freeing up of expensive operating room time should also be brought to the attention of the government.

Unfortunately, lobbying for funds becomes easy when projects are politically effective and appealing to the public (such as those affecting children). Programmes such as diarrhoea control, which can easily obtain support from external funding agencies, obtain government support more easily than lithotripsy programmes. Few are ready to realize the destructive power of stone disease. In Pakistan, unfortunately there is more sympathy for patients on dialysis than for patients who have a disease (stone disease), the treatment of which will prevent a significant number of cases of renal failure.

Resource distribution throughout the country and controls to prevent overcapacity

Strategic towns easily accessible by surrounding areas where stone disease population density is maximal should be the sites for placement of lithotriptors and ureteroscopes. Accessibility by road and subsidized flights by air (if the roads are unsatisfactory) will be required to assist the poor. In the third world, the national airline can (and in Pakistan does) provide subsidized air fares (e.g. US$ 6 for the flight from Gilgit to Rawalpindi, a 17-hour journey by road).

The government, through a democratic process, should control the number of lithotriptors in any area, and in the whole country. Australia faces an overcapacity in technology because of failure to do so [5]. Currently there is an uneven distribution of lithotriptors in Pakistan.

Reducing the costs associated with ESWL

Costs can be reduced by reducing the cost of the machine, and reducing the costs accrued as a result of using the machine. Judicious buying, advantageous maintenance contracts, second-hand lithotriptors, cheaper lithotriptors from, say, China, leasing and loan agreements, lithotriptor sharing, careful maintenance to prolong machine life, training local talent for maintenance, and refurbishing electrodes are some ways of reducing costs.

Uncritical use in a 'free treatment' setting adds to costs for the government. Patients hear about the latest treatment on television or read about it in *The Times* and demand 'nothing but the best'. To them the word 'latest' is synonymous with 'best'. Patients whose medical costs are covered by insurance, insist on obtaining the most expensive treatment as they wish to maximize benefits of their premiums which they have paid – something psychologists and economists call 'sunk costs'. Doctors are often pressured by threat of litigation and at times comply with the patient's wishes. In the east, many patients with staghorns insist on treatment by ESWL. Over use and uncritical use push up total costs for governments.

The costs incurred by government and private institutions can be reduced by providing lithotripsy only to small stones under 1 cm in size. This will reduce the number of patients accessing the lithotriptor, reduce repeat treatment and hence allow more patients to be treated, produce more stone free patients in a shorter time, and allow fewer lithotriptors to serve larger populations.

Another more appropriate method of reducing costs is to use technology only after careful critical analysis for its need, which we have covered in Section II.

Conclusions

Technology dependent procedures must be considered when working out the best treatment for a patient. If the patient needs technology because it is the only way of treating the stone, some way of making this available is needed. If technology is not available, the individual should not be subjected to an operation; if he has no insurance or cannot pay, he should not be treated in a less than appropriate way. Costs can be reduced by outpatient treatment and by reducing the use of antibiotics and stents. The following chapters address some of these issues.

Treatment must be disbursed equitably. But how can one practice equity in a setting where a farmer cannot travel to town for treatment and where no technology is available? The physician will have to define equity in his own terms in the interests of his patient.

For the third world country, equity may be achievable only to the extent of saving a kidney. Every effort has to be made to preserve renal function by removing ureteric obstruction promptly. The question of whether this is done by operation endoscopically or by ESWL is secondary. All patients must have access to treatment for removal of obstruction.

Equity will be more easily achieved when there are fewer stones to treat. Technological and surgical manipulations are half-measures for disease processes analogous to situations where the thief is caught after the act. The correct approach to health is to prevent the stone. Until prevention is achieved, specialty surgery, allowing refinement of surgical and endoscopic skills and application of sophisticated technological masterpieces, will play an important part, together with epidemiological studies, aetiological research, and preventive measures in the community at large.

References

1.   Administrative Committee on Co-ordination, Subcommittee on Nutrition (ACC/SCN). Country trends. In: Second report on world nutrition situation, Vol. 2. Geneva: United Nations, 1993.
2.   Francis D. Dawn Karachi. 26 November 1993.
3.   Russet, B. Peace among democracies. Sci 1993;269.
4.   Drummond MF. Resource allocation decisions in health care: A role for quality of life assessments. In: Dowie J, Elstein A, editors. Professional judgement, a reader in clinical decision making. Cambridge: Cambridge University Press, 1988:436–55.
5.   Hirsch NA. Diffusion of new technologies to treat renal stone in Australia. J Publ Health 1993;17:384–7.

34. The economics of stone disease therapy: An economist's views

SARFARAZ KHAN QURESHI

Economists are trained to manage scarcity. The physician is concerned with how best to manage the patient. Both are concerned with how to manage limited resources most efficiently. Both willingly accept the challenge of finding ways to provide economical care for stone disease therapy.

The economist looks at problems arising from scarcity from two angles: equity and efficiency. For 100% efficiency, economists advise stone treatment only for those who can pay. This becomes one way of rationing scarce resources, in this case the services of a lithotriptor. If more patients require the service than can be provided by the limited number of machines (available capacity), the price will rise. Consequently, more patients will not be able to afford therapy and only those willing to pay the market clearance price would get the service.

This is similar to the supply of water in towns: the poor are neglected. Such a solution is callous and inhuman, and unacceptable for health care related services, but from an economist's point of view it provides 100% efficiency and is self-financing. It is unacceptable to the clinician, and we reiterate the need to have physicians on the panel when resource allocations are made by government so that essential services are not left to self-financing schemes.

Considered from the equitable or egalitarian aspect, the limited resource, for example the lithotriptor's service, would be available regardless of the patient's ability to pay. Here too, not everyone who needs the service will get it, but the criterion (for receiving the service) will be the need of the patient and not his ability to pay. Two issues result from this: physicians must evolve needs-based criteria, and the economists must devise methods to subsidize the treatment costs which may overrun the revenue accrued.

The efficient model described above is financially more sound, but should be and will be rejected by physicians. Because of the financial risk of the egalitarian model, physicians must critically think through every treatment need, and the government or a non-governmental agency must step in to support the programme in order to provide services for the poor.

Finally, the lack of means of transportation and deficient infrastructure which may prevent people from benefiting from the provided service (the lithotriptor) for logistic reasons must be mentioned. Economists tend to pay little attention to such factors and have a habit of 'assuming them away'. However, such factors play a

J. Talati et al. (eds) The Management of Lithiasis, 225–226
© *1997 Kluwer Academic Publishers. Printed in Great Britain.*

crucial role as a binding constraint in the ultimate on-site provision of life-saving medical services to patients who need them. In practical terms, the problem of bad roads and poor transportation should be considered a 'structural hindrance' to easy access to the service. Providing better communication facilities – road, rail and air – results in a multitude of benefits and is best handled by the government who can justify the use of taxpayers' money to overcome the problems.

The problems associated with providing lithotripsy to all are more complex than stated above. The options are: government funding from tax sources; free enterprise; or a combination of the two which could be elegantly designed, but usually arises by accident, as in the city of Karachi, in Pakistan.

35. Selecting a lithotriptor: Hospital perspectives

NADEEM MUSTAFA KHAN and MANSUR DHANANI

In a rapidly changing environment, an investment decision involving millions of rupees represents a major milestone in the life of an institution and is fraught with risks. Such decisions require a thorough review and a careful analysis of all impacting factors, in order that the investment will be beneficial to the institution.

Current trends in technology for health care show rapid innovations with respect to material-based, laboratory-based or computer-based technology. While such medical advancement in technology has helped improve medical care, costs have increased disproportionately and so have risks. The highest risk factor is obsolescence occurring at different times for different machines. The higher the costs, the greater the risk, as the value of the machine decreases by 30–35% immediately upon purchase. The life of the machine is also a strong determining factor. The more stretched out the life cycle, the less risky the option. Therefore, the following questions must be addressed: does it make sense for us now to invest in such a high cost item, and does it make sense overall strategically for the institution to do so at this point in time?

This chapter deals with the decision process involved in the purchase of an extracorporeal shockwave lithotriptor (ESWL) but the analysis used is applicable to all expensive capital equipment. Whilst we are describing an approach developed for our hospital locally, it is an effective approach and can be applied by any institution evaluating any programme which requires the purchase of expensive equipment.

The decision process: An overview

A wise initial step is the review of the strategic plan and goals of the institution. If the capital investment is for a service which fits into the stated goals, the programme can be considered. Further planning can then identify the threats and opportunities to the institution as well as the potential barriers to investment such as capital requirements, affordability, human resources, etc.

The next step is to assess how lithotripsy as a methodology for removing kidney stones is 'going to fare' over a period of time. This can be achieved by discussions with suppliers, urologists, individuals who know, understand and can predict trends in technology and lithotripsy, and a review of relevant literature. At this stage, it may be useful for some key members of the surgical (urological) faculty as well as the purchasing department to visit relevant ESWL centres and manufacturers to

J. Talati et al. (eds) The Management of Lithiasis, 227–233
© *1997 Kluwer Academic Publishers. Printed in Great Britain.*

gain further knowledge about the programme, its strengths and weaknesses, benefits that can be derived and the internal and external risks. This helps in the selection of a lithotriptor. In third world countries, it is preferable to select tried and tested technology in order to avoid unknown risks involved when dealing with new and untried equipment.

Given the knowledge gained from such trips, a preliminary programme statement and a financial feasibility can be worked out. This will show whether the programme is financially feasible and whether it is likely to generate enough cash to plough back into the programme for ongoing training of staff, research and capital replacement when the equipment becomes obsolete or out-of-date.

A preliminary report is made to the Board for approval and guidance on how to proceed further. If everything is approved on a preliminary basis, media announcements could be made stating that the programme would commence in 6 to 12 months so that the target population is made aware that a new programme is in the offing. A working group can now be formed to give practical shape to the approved programme.

Formation of a work group

The work group initiates the programme, works out all the details and leads the programme to its successful implementation. Terms of reference, timetable, responsibility, authority and membership need to be defined.

For the ESWL programme at the Aga Khan University Medical Center (AKUMC), the work group consisted of four key members: the Director of Materials Management; the Professor of Urology; the Director of Finance; and the Director of Facilities Management. At a later stage, other members of the AKUMC team joined the work group, such as the Nursing Manager (Operating Rooms), Marketing Manager, etc. A one-year timetable with benchmark dates was also laid down to ensure progress with proper feedback to senior management and the Board. Detailed terms of reference were defined which were broadly as follows:

1. To specify requirements for a lithotriptor and AKUMC's expectations/needs.
2. To evaluate the lithotripsy equipment thoroughly. To include visits to manufacturers as well as other hospitals, to ensure full awareness of the capabilities of the machines being considered and to recommend a 'state of the art' lithotriptor at the most cost-effective prices and to ensure that the necessary support and personnel are available and trained to commence the service on schedule.
3. To identify and recommend space for the machine and ensure that all necessary changes are made to the identified space to install the machine.
4. To ensure that all necessary back-up facilities such as maintenance, spares, warranty coverage, technical staff, nursing, supplies, etc. are ready for operation on 'day one'.
5. To negotiate the most cost-effective rates and credit facilities.

6. To evaluate the operational viability of this service including the need for patient welfare (see Chapter 37) and the recommended charges for various procedures.

Defining needs and expectations

The needs and expectations from any programme must be defined so the future direction, aims and objectives are clear from the start. As the majority of cases will be genitourinary stones, attention and priorities should focus on perfecting fragmentation of all urinary tract stones choosing a lithotriptor which will:

- fragment stones irrespective of site (whether in the kidney, ureter or bladder);
- be able to visualize and treat both radiopaque and lucent stones;
- pulverize the stone down to the finest powder so that ancillary procedures are minimized (between 5%);
- minimize patient costs, professional time (including urological expertise) and hospital stay; and
- ensure that the programme is declared an unconditional success, with patients not going away unhappy or to another institution for further treatment.

Technical evaluation

The technical evaluation of ESWL equipment should concentrate on:

- the modality used for localization;
- energy output; and
- the ability to retrofit new developments.

These are discussed in detail below.

Localization techniques

Either X-rays or ultrasound can be used to localize the stone. The lithotriptors, therefore, fall into two categories: those which localize by ultrasound and those through X-rays. Ultrasound technology has progressed very rapidly and is likely to improve further. It is believed that ultrasound is the localization system of the future and will gain further importance over the next few years. X-ray localization may still be required for mid-ureteric stones.

The advantages and disadvantages of each localization technique must be considered in the selection process. X-ray localization gives a radiation dose to both the patient and the operators. However, X-ray localization modality has a distinct edge over ultrasound modality in producing the best image of ureteric stones and also for small stone particles. At the same time, with ultrasound, the process of treating stones in real time is an added advantage. The quality of the ultrasound picture needs to be assessed.

Energy output

Lithotriptors are currently available with three different types of energy source: spark gap; piezo-electric array; and electromagnetic. Each of these types must be evaluated for the force of the punch. Apart from different force/punch of the various energy sources, the number of shocks per second is also extremely relevant to the treatment of stones in the body. The ability to deliver a very rapid series of shock may not be an advantage as emitted shocks may be interfered with by returning reflected shocks if the speed is very fast. However the ability to reduce the rate of shock wave delivery will be of value in patients who experience pain in rapid-fire delivery.

The selection process should consider the maximum 'punching-ability' of each machine as well as the ability to vary power.

Ability to retrofit developments in the future

Research and development of new technology continues after its introduction. It is, therefore, of the utmost importance to discuss new developments in programme with the suppliers and also select equipment in which it is easier to retrofit new developments on the same machine. This is likely to be cheaper than replacing an obsolete machine with another costly machine in the future in order to avoid becoming out-of-date due to advancements in technology.

Supplier evaluation

The purpose of supplier evaluation is to consider the following:

- The supplier's experience in lithotripsy equipment in particular and medical equipment in general.
- The number of units sold and to whom.
- Experience of users (by direct contacts with some of them).
- Strength of the company (balance sheets, assets, income, personnel, life of company, ability to withstand economic down-turns).
- Strengths and weaknesses of equipment.
- Ability to extend maintenance and technical development support.
- Cost of equipment.

Evaluation of space, maintenance and other factors

A proper space plan, review of maintenance arrangements and a total care approach are the requirements in the evaluation and later successful implementation of any programme.

Space

Proper space needs to be allocated not just for the lithotriptor but also for patients' reception, waiting and recovery. The lithotriptor room requirements are not as stringent as those for MRI, but even so, the size of the room to 'house' the machine and all the accessories, the weight of the equipment (this is particularly important for equipment housed on higher floors), the ceiling support (if some equipment is to hang from the ceiling), voltage power to the machines, water supply, compressed air, nitrogen and the need for noise control and acoustic designs must be considered. In square footage, a lithotriptor room of about 300 sq.ft and ancillary spaces of about 600–700 sq.ft should be reasonable for a compact designed unit.

Maintenance arrangements

These should be considered in detail during the purchase process. Some form of arrangement to maintain the machine directly or provide training/basic spare parts with back-up support should be negotiated at the outset. This is crucial for sophisticated equipment such as a lithotriptor, because if it is not done at this stage, it can cause problems later. These may be due either to breakdown with no chance of recovery, or alternatively, the supplier charging a higher price later than is bearable by the purchaser. Furthermore, there may be some particular consumables such as electrodes which can be obtained from the supplier alone. These should be negotiated for three to five years during the purchasing process. Training of biomedical staff responsible for technical maintenance (if such staff exist at the purchasing institution) can also be considered and is a useful investment.

Development of para-ESWL skills at ureteroscopy and PCNL

While the rapid development of ESWL has been viewed with great excitement since it has obviated the need for open surgery and the resultant long hospital stay and a longer period off work, this non-invasive procedure should be practised with caution and care and should not be used as monotherapy for all types of stone (i.e. ESWL being used as the single means to treat the stone). Facilities for percuta-

Table 35.1   Comparative analysis of equipment

Criterion	Suppliers	Rating
Localization		
Energy force		
Ability to retrofit newer developments		
Total costs per patient/maintenance capability		
Company profile		
Overall		

1 = Highest rating
4 = Lowest rating

neous nephrolithotomy (PCNL) and ureteroscopy (URS) are therefore also required.

Comparative analysis

Based on the detailed analysis of each piece of equipment (its technical supplier evaluations and cost), the lithotriptors can be evaluated against each other. A point system, 1 to 4, could be used where 1 represents the highest rating and 4 the lowest. It should be noted that the rating is a relative measure – a comparison of one lithotriptor against another – and a rating of 4 does not necessarily mean an undesirable machine. It could mean that, on a particular criterion, the said lithotriptor came out the lowest against the other three vendors. Table 35.1 describes a sample scheme for rating each vendor which could be followed by detailed explanations of each criterion. The final rating will be a judgmental decision and should not be based on a summation of the individual scores.

Developing plans for the programme's success

It is important for the success of any programme that it is properly projected to patients in the different constituencies which it will serve, that the physician/technical resources are properly trained and available, and that the service delivery process is smooth and efficient so that the patients feel that they are deriving an 'added value' from the service.

Marketing plan

In the private sector, a proper, well-thought through marketing plan is a 'must' for any programme's success. The marketing plan should strike a balance between marketing the programme based on patient care and education on the one hand and financial success on the other. The latter approach is important if the programme is to sustain itself and provide support for ongoing training of staff, research and monies for replacement capital when the equipment becomes obsolete or out-of-date. A detailed action plan should be prepared with time frames and responsibilities for action which should be closely monitored on an ongoing basis.

Training

Proper training in the use of ESWL is essential for both physicians as well as technicians if the maximum benefit is to be derived from the equipment. In this regard, the physician urologist should be trained initially at an off-site location where the selected equipment is installed. He/she can then impart training to the other physicians/ technicians in the initial breaking-in period, i.e. the first month after installation. The training should also be negotiated with the supplier during the purchasing process.

Administration

A good administrative support is essential to the success of the programme. Screening patients through clinics, scheduling them, following-up appointments, carrying out the procedure, discharge, follow-up in clinics, etc. is a meticulous process requiring close attention to detail. The administrator must ensure that the process is efficient and easy to use, and ongoing patient feedback is used as a method of catering for patient needs and improvement of the system so that it is a service that patients derive 'added value' from.

Programme evaluation

Ongoing evaluation of any programme is crucial if the maximum benefits as originally envisaged are to be derived from the programme. The purpose of this evaluation is to re-examine the actual derived benefits versus those originally envisaged and to evaluate the programme needs and expectations and consider how the programme has fared. This evaluation process can take place annually.

Conclusions and recommendations

Using the analysis given previously AKUMC followed the highlighted methodology; the resultant comparative analysis showed that the Dornier MPL 9000 was the machine that met most of the required criteria and AKUMC purchased it in November 1988. The programme has been evaluated each year and some changes made in the strategies. Further notes on development of lithotripsy services are included in Chapter 38, p. 253.

Our advice to all institutions considering investments in major pieces of equipment is to approach the decision scientifically – marry the programme with the strategic plan, visit sites and discuss the plan with outside users of ESWL, carry out a feasibility study and evaluate risks. Then follow through the detailed work group process outlined above. A comprehensive check-list for evaluation of the equipment can be used. It is our view that by meticulously following such a thorough process and involving several knowledgeable sources, the decision, almost inevitably, will be a sound and effective one.

36. Lithotriptor sharing

R. VLEEMING, JOOP W. NOORDZIJ, TH. M. DE REIJKE and NOSHIR
F. DABHOIWALA

**Mobile extracorporeal piezo-electric lithotripsy in The Netherlands;
European experience and applicability to the third world**

The first commercially available extracorporeal shock wave lithotripsy (ESWL)
machine, the Dornier-HM3, introduced in 1980 [1, 2], was a huge machine which
had a large focal area (9.0 $\times$ 1.5 cm) and high energy density at skin level which
caused pain, necessitating general anaesthesia and hospitalization. It is still the
most effective machine in terms of stone disintegration with a success rate of
70–90% [3–5]. However its associated morbidity [6–11], high initial investment,
running costs, and hospitalization costs prompted further research. As a result the
second generation lithotriptors replaced the large tub with a waterbag system or a
small water bath confined to the treatment area only.

These machines were compact and therefore easy to transport. In The
Netherlands financial constraints limited the procurement of a number of lithotriptors. The two university hospitals in Amsterdam and the academic hospital in
Leiden therefore decided on a joint venture to exploit a mobile Wolf 2200 lithotriptor in June 1987. In this machine the shock waves were generated by 3500 piezoceramic elements incorporated in a small waterbath of 50 cm diameter
(extracorporeal piezo-electric lithotripsy, EPL). This method offers several advantages: a more precise focal area (1.2 $\times$ 0.4 cm) and reduced loss of shock wave
energy through scatter. A lower energy level per shock wave and a higher frequency of firing is thus achieved. This technique results in slow erosion and pulver-
ization rather than explosion of a stone. The treatment is almost painless and
neither general anaesthesia, sedation nor hospitalization are required [12–14]. Real-
time 4.5 MHz ultrasonography is employed to locate the stone and focus the shock
waves as well as to monitor disintegration of the stone during treatment. Expensive
X-ray adaptations are not required for the lithotripsy room since no fluoroscopy is
employed. The big disadvantage, however, is that localization and treatment of
ureteric calculi is extremely difficult in these cases and only very limited success
can be achieved.

Within the first six months no technical transport related failures occurred and
two other hospitals in the western part of The Netherlands joined the venture. A
total population of 3 million inhabitants in an area of approx. 1000 sq. km was thus

J. Talati et al. (eds) The Management of Lithiasis, 235–243
© *1997 Kluwer Academic Publishers. Printed in Great Britain.*

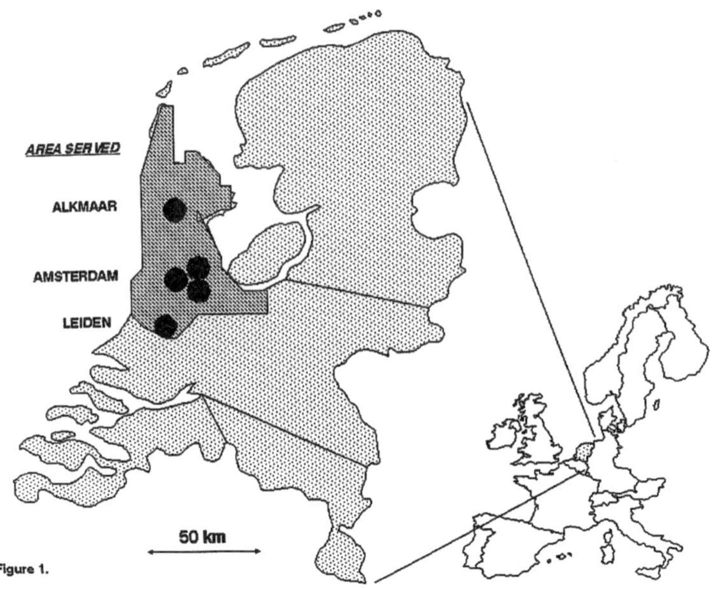

Figure 36.1 Area of The Netherlands served by one mobile lithotriptor

covered by one mobile lithotriptor (Figure 36.1). To exploit the piezolith in all five participating treatment centres a separate foundation was created. Depending on the expected number of patients to be treated in each participating centre, a pre-planned schedule of transport is agreed upon after periodic mutual discussion between the centres. The machine is thus rented from the foundation by each treatment centre for a specified limited period of one or two weeks at a time. It is transported by road from one centre to the other, using a specially adapted vehicle to accommodate the machine (Figure 36.2). The installation procedure and a routine check-up at a centre usually take less than one hour. The lithotriptor is operated by the local urologist or a resident under supervision after undergoing a short EPL introduction course. A specially trained EPL nurse accompanies the machine to all hospitals, and takes care of installation and routine check-ups as well as assisting in operation and handling of the machine.

Pretreatment assessment of a patient includes a careful medical history with special attention to urological pathology and possible haemorrhagic disorders. Laboratory investigations include urine culture, haemoglobin, platelets, serum creatinine, urea, prothrombin test and an intravenous urogram or a plain X-ray of the abdomen and ultrasound check-up of the kidneys and bladder. In case of a positive urine culture, appropriate peri-treatment antibiotic cover is provided. Anticoagulant therapy, if any, is temporarily interrupted.

Treatment sessions usually last one hour and 2500–4000 shock wave pulses are applied in one session depending on stone load, location and rapidity of disintegration. In the daily treatment planning (6–8 patients) at least one place is reserved for urgent EPL therapy (e.g. obstructive ureteric stone with a potential danger of renal

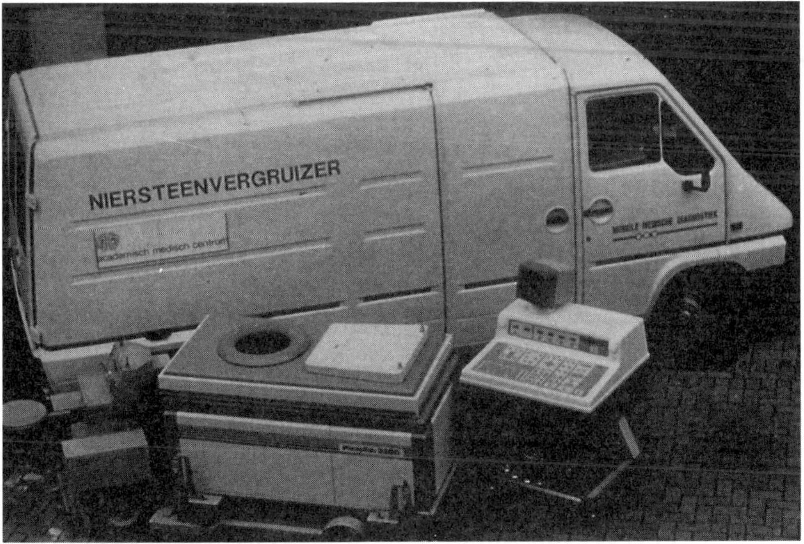

Figure 36.2 Vehicle for transport of the lithotriptor

function deterioration, recurrent severe renal colic or repeat therapy sessions for large stone burden). For such urgent indications the patient is referred for treatment in the centre where the lithotriptor is stationed at that time. In February 1988 the Wolf 2200 machine was automatically upgraded by the manufacturers to a 2300 version with an improved waterbath, a dual ultrasound scanner and an improved degassing system. These improvements resulted in an increased shock wave energy and easier localization of the renal stones. Even calculi in the proximal and distal part of the ureter could now be localized by ultrasonography, albeit still with difficulty.

The Wolf 2500 lithotriptor, purchased by the foundation in January 1991, combines both fluoroscopy and ultrasound localization in an integrated system, thus permitting localization and treatment of virtually all renal and ureteral stones *in situ*. The use of fluoroscopy, however, restricts the handling of the 2500 lithotriptor to a room adapted for radiological applications, while the use of the machine is in principle a joint operational responsibility of the urologist and radiologist at the centre concerned.

The registration of patients, their medical history, the type of treatment and the follow-up data are all collected and stored in a database on a laptop computer, which is transported together with the lithotriptor. A data manager is appointed by the foundation to oversee collection and analysis of all data from the various centres.

Patients and methods

From June 1987 to June 1992 a total of 2488 patients were treated by EPL on the three different lithotriptors used. The results of 2292 patients were eligible for

Table 36.1   Stone localization, number of calculi and mean size

Stone location	Wolf n	2200 Size (mm diameter)	Wolf n	2300 Size (mm diameter)	Wolf n	2500 Size (mm diameter)
Renal stones						
Upper pole	21	9.8	194	11.1	69	10.1
Middle pole	41	9.0	297	10.1	78	9.3
Lower pole	79	10.4	685	0.4	220	11.0
Pelvis	42	13.9	400	15.0	114	15.4
Partial staghorn	6	22.4	28	29.8	7	28.4
Ureteral stones						
Upper ureter	15	10.1	88	10.5	85	10.3
Middle ureter			3	6.7	22	9.3
Lower ureter	1	10.1	18	10.6	95	9.0
Total	205	11.1	1713	11.8	690	11.2

analysis, whereas patients treated on two different lithotriptors successively (n = 196) were excluded. In 316 patients (14.8%) more than one stone was present and 0.8% of patients were younger than 12 years of age. On the Wolf 2200, 182 patients with 205 stone fragments were treated (189 treatments). On the 2300 lithotriptor, 1462 patients with 1713 stones were treated (1654 treatments). On the piezolith 2500, 648 patients with 690 calculi have undergone therapy (704 treatments). The number of treatments on each lithotriptor is demonstrated in Figure 36.3; stone localization, number of calculi and mean size are listed in Table 36.1.

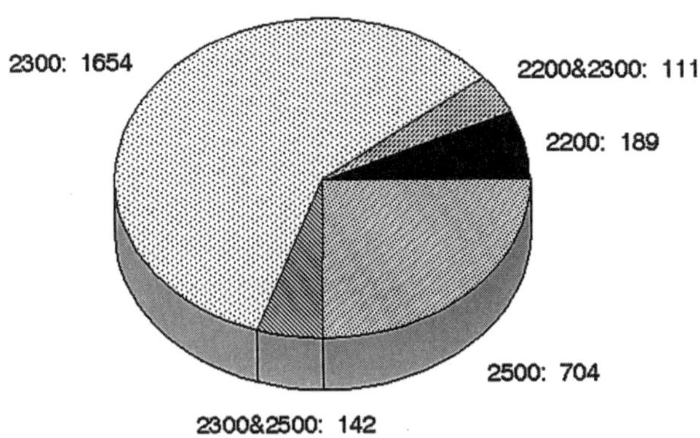

Figure 36.3 Total number of treatments and type of Wolf lithotriptor (1987–92)

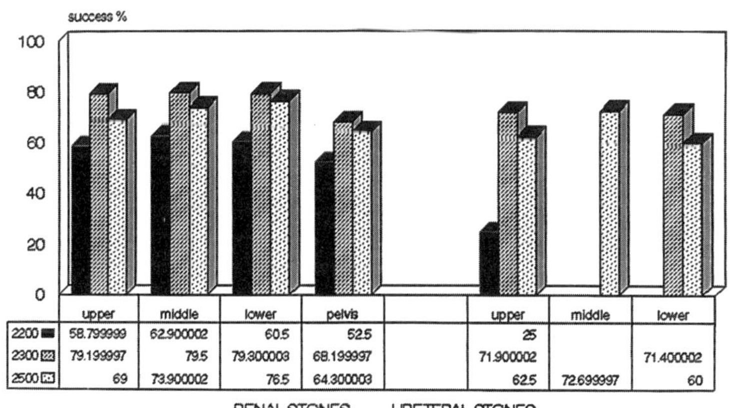

	upper	middle	lower	pelvis		upper	middle	lower
2200 ■	58.799999	62.900002	60.5	52.5		25		
2300 ▨	79.199997	79.5	79.300003	68.199997		71.900002		71.400002
2500 ⬚	69	73.900002	76.5	64.300003		62.5	72.699997	60

Figure 36.4 Success rate versus stone location and lithotriptor type

Success is defined as stone freedom on plain X-ray and/or ultrasound or residual stone fragments whose total diameter is less than 3 mm at three months posttherapy. More than 80% of these residual fragments are expected to pass spontaneously [4, 15, 16].

Results

A total of 2608 renal units have been treated. Multiple sessions are often required for larger (greater than 2 cm) calculi, so that a total of 4097 treatment sessions have been performed.

The relationship between the success rate of EPL treatment and the location of the stones is graphically demonstrated in Figure 36.4. A total of 32.8% of patients required a second treatment session and the retreatment rate per stone was 1.41. Ancillary measures were required in 10.9%: an indwelling ureteric double J stent in 9.3% and nephrostomy drainage prior to lithotripsy in 1.6% of patients. Treatment for pain was necessary in 1%. Diclofenac suppositories were generally sufficient. Antibiotics were prescribed in 19.8% of patients either as therapy (13.3%) or prophylaxis (6.5%). The incidence of side-effects and complications was low (Table 36.2) and in no more than 0.5% of patients was hospital admission and

Table 36.2 Complications and side-effects

Fever	1.4%
Haematuria	0.5%
Renal colic	7.3%
Steinstrasse	9.8%

Table 36.3   Urological procedures after EPL

Double J Stents	2.3%
Nephrostomy	0.5%
Open procedure	8.5%
Percutaneous nephrolithotripsy	4.2%
Endourological procedure	1.6%

additional urological management needed. Only stone-related urological complications were observed. Operative procedures after ineffective EPL treatment were performed in 15.6% of patients, primarily in the early learning stage. Additional urological procedures after EPL (double pigtail catheters or nephrostomy) are today only required in 2.5% of patients and inpatient EPL therapy is now undertaken in about 8% of cases (Table 36.3).

Discussion

The success rate of the Wolf 2200 is relatively low, mainly because of a low energy level of the shock waves but also due to the learning curve phase in our series. The results of the Wolf 2300 and the 2500 lithotriptor are however in accordance with other series using various similar types of lithotriptors [12, 14, 17–22]. In a Dutch multicentre trial the efficacy of five different types of lithotriptor, including our 2300 machine, has been compared. Differences were found only in the location of the stones treated relative to the imaging system used, the need for anaesthesia, the application of auxiliary procedures and the need for hospitalization. While the overall success rates of all compared second generation lithotriptors were similar, they were however generally lower compared to success rates obtained using the Dornier-HM3 [3]. The fact that the mobile lithotriptor is operated by several different urologists in five different treatment centres does not seem to affect the overall treatment results obtained.

Initially most patients were treated as inpatients (96%), but as soon as it became evident that the morbidity of EPL was very low, treatment policy was reviewed and currently most EPL sessions (more than 90%) are performed on an outpatient basis. Our present indications for inpatient EPL treatment are staghorn calculi, multiresistant infections of the urinary tract, a compromised immunological, haematological or haemostatic status, or obstructive ureteral stones with a high risk of precipitating urosepsis.

The need for auxiliary measures is in our series low in comparison to other series [19] and is still diminishing. Initially, double J stents were inserted in cases of large stone bulk to prevent ureteral obstruction by stone fragments (12.9%). This auxiliary measure seemed however to be overcautious [23–25] and has been subsequently abandoned by us, except in stones larger than 4 cm diameter. The use of ureteral stents prior to treatment now accounts for only 6.5% of cases and is essentially restricted to cases of solitary functional kidney, severe infection in an obstructed system, severe repeated renal colic not responding to spasmolytic drugs, or severe long-standing ureteric obstruction and partial or complete staghorn. The financial aspects of sharing a mobile lithotriptor are favourable. In the past five years only 2.5% of the operational time was utilized for transport, maintenance service and repairs. The total costs for transport, maintenance and repairs are less than 7% of the yearly financial turnover. In comparison the staffing costs in The Netherlands are quite high: about one-fifth of the yearly turnover or about 10% of the original purchase price (approx. US$ 1.3 million). Hospital stay in The Netherlands is however also quite expensive (approx. US$ 500 per day) and outpatient EPL treatment is therefore comparatively cheap (approx. US$ 750).

In conclusion, our overall results of treatment using the Wolf 2300 and 2500 mobile lithotriptors are similar to data from other series. The low incidence of side-effects and the ease of treatment make EPL a safe outpatient therapy, resulting in a significant saving of costs. The convenience of relatively painless EPL treatment results in high patient compliance. Thorough pretreatment assessment and patient education remain extremely important to prevent serious complications and maintain a low hospitalization rate.

The only negative factor is the greater need of repeated treatment sessions for the same stone.

The regular transport of the lithotriptor unit has in our experience not resulted in a higher incidence of technical failures. Sharing a mobile lithotriptor makes EPL available to several hospitals in a cost-effective manner within the setting of the Dutch health system.

Acknowledgements

Dr A.A.B. Lycklama à Nijeholt, Academic Hospital Leiden; Dr S. Rep, Medical Centre Alkmaar; Dr Th. J. M. Schlatmann, Onze Lieve Vrouwe Gasthuis Amsterdam; Dr E.A.J.M. de Jong, Academic Hospital Vrije Universiteit Amsterdam; and C. van Galen, Stichting Mobiele Steenvergruizer Amsterdam, for providing data and their valuable assistance.

Comment by Dr J. Noordzij

I consider myself fortunate to have had both the opportunity to take part in the mobile extracorporeal lithotriptor scheme in The Netherlands and to gain some experience on the urological situation in Pakistan.

The success of the Dutch mobile lithotriptor scheme is based on several requirements:

- The distances between the hospitals which take part in such a scheme must allow the possibility for urgent cases to obtain treatment within an acceptable time limit.
- The urologist must be prepared to learn how to use the machine and co-operate with his colleagues in a 'lithotripsy team', treating 'foreign' urgent cases when necessary.

- Patients are treated on an outpatient basis, but hospital beds should be available and additional treatment possible.
- The method of transport must be comfortable, causing no damage to the lithotriptor, which should be small and easily transportable.

The reasons for embarking on such a joint venture are valid in any clinical setting in which the cost of the lithotriptor is not justified by its medical, social and financial yield. The Dutch study shows the mobile lithotriptor scheme to be a very acceptable solution for all parties concerned. Furthermore, it enables other urologists to take advantage of advanced, but costly treatment techniques, while encouraging professional discussions among colleagues and enhancing the quality of care.

As a third world developing country, Pakistan has several infrastructural problems, one of which concerns the quality of the roads. Although the machines used in this study did not seem to be susceptible to transport-related malfunctioning (the truck used has standard shock absorbers), transport by rail and treatment on a sidetrack could perhaps be an alternative in areas with an acceptably dense railway system. Other forms of treatment, including percutaneous, transurethral and open surgery can still be employed instead of EPL/ESWL in urgent cases, although quick and safe transportation to the lithotriptor location at a reasonable cost should remain the first choice option.

The good treatment results in the Dutch study are comparable to that of stationary lithotriptors, while the mobility of the machine does not add to repair and maintenance costs. Unless the number of patients sufficiently justifies the purchase of such a machine for a single hospital, it seems worthwhile to consider joining a lithotriptor club.

References

1. Chaussey CH, Brendel W, Schmiedt E. Extracorporeally induced destruction of kidney stones by shockwaves. Lancet 1980;ii:1265–8.
2. Chaussy CH, Schmiedt E, Jocham D *et al.* First clinical experience with extracorporeally introduced destruction of kidney stones by shockwaves. Urology 1982;127:417–20.
3. Bierkens AF, Hendrikx AJM, de Kort VJW *et al.* Efficacy of second generation lithotripters: A multicenter comparative study of 2206 ESWL treatments with the Siemens Lithostar, Dornier HM4, Wolf Piezolith 2300, Direx Tripter x-1 and Breakstone lithotripter. In thesis: Extracorporeal shock wave lithotripsy for urinary calculi. Nijmegen, 1991
4. Drach GW, Dretler S, Fair W *et al.* Report on the United States cooperative study of extracorporeal shock wave lithotripsy. J Urol 1986;135:1127–33.
5. Fetner CD, Preminger GM, Seger J *et al.* Treatment of ureteral calculi by extracorporeal shockwave lithotripsy at a multi-use center. J Urol 1988;139:1192–4.
6. Davidson T, Tung K, Constant O *et al.* Kidney rupture and psoas abcess after ESWL. Br J Urol 1991;68:657–8.
7. Higashihara E, Asakage Y, Aso Y. The effect of shockwave application on kidney. In: Berichte aus der Urologie. Baden Baden, Germany: Druck Roland Steinbrück, 1991.
8. Knapp PM, Kulb TB, Lingeman JE *et al.* Extracorporeal shockwave lithotripsy-induced perirenal hematomas. J Urol 1988;139:700–3.
9. Lingeman JE, Woods J, Toth PD. Blood pressure changes following extracorporeal shock-wave lithotripsy and other forms of treatment for nephrolithiasis. J Am Med Assoc 1990;263:1789–994.

10. Sofras F, Delakas D, Vlassopoulog G *et al.* Renal tissue damage following ESWL. Int Urol Nephrol 1990;22:125–7.

11. Zwergel Th, Millée K, Rassweiler J. Moderne steintherapie. Urologe [A] 1990;29:21–7.

12. Marberger M, Turk C, Steinkogler I. Painless piezo-electricextracorporeal lithotripsy. J Urol 1988;139:695–9.

13. Philip T, Kellett MJ, Whitfield HN *et al.* Painless lithotripsy: Experience with 100 patients. Lancet 1988;2:41.

14. Rassweiler J, Gumpinger R, Mayer R *et al.* Extracorporealpiezoelectric lithotripsy using the Wolf-lithotriptor versus low energy lithotripsy with the modified Dornier HM-3: A cooperative study. World J Urol 1987;5:218–22.

15. O'Flynn JD. The treatment of ureteric stones: Report on 1120 patients. Br J Urol 1980;52:436.

16. Ueno T, Kamamura T, Ogawa A *et al.* Relation of spontaneous passage of ureteric calculi to size. Urology 1977;10:544–9.

17. Eisenberger F, Fuchs G, Miller K *et al.* Extracorporeal shockwave lithotripsy (ESWL) and endourology: An ideal combination for treatment of kidney stones. World J Urol 1985;3:41–7.

18. Rajagopal V, Bailey MJ. Mobile extracorporeal shockwave lithotripsy. Br J Urol 1991;67:6–8.

19. Riehle RA, Fair WR, Vaughan ED. Extracorporeal shock-wave lithotripsy for upper urinary tract calculi. J Am Med Assoc 1986;255:2043–8.

20. Vallancien G, Aviles J, Munoc R *et al.* Piezoelectric extracorporeal lithotripsy by ultrashort waves with the EDAP LT 01 Device. J Urol 1988;139:689–94.

21. Wilbert DM, Reichenberger H, Noske E *et al.* Second generation shock wave lithotripsy: Experience with the lithostar. World J Urol 1987;5:225–8.

22. Zwergel U, Neisius D, Zwergel T *et al.* Results and clinical management of extracorporeal piezo-electric lithotripsy. World J Urol 1987;5:213–17.

23. Bierkens AF, Hendrikx AJM, Lemmens WAJG *et al.* Extracorporeal shock wave lithotripsy for large renal calculi: The role of ureteral stents. A randomized trial. J Urol 1991;145:699–702.

24. Cass AS. Ureteral stenting with extracorporeal shock wave lithotripsy. Urology 1992;39:446–8.

25. Preminger GM, Kettelhut MC, Elkins SL *et al.* Ureteral stenting during extracorporeal shock wave lithotripsy: Help or hindrance? J Urol 1989;142:32.

37. Cost factors in equitable care

JAMSHEER TALATI

Finding a reasonable charge for lithotripsy for patients paying for their treatment

In order to remain a caring institution treating the rich and the poor, difficult decisions have to be made when fixing a charge for lithotripsy. The major factors that affect the decision include: costs the hospital incurred in procuring, setting up, and running the lithotriptor; the ability of the patient to pay; the expected number of patients per year; the expected life of the machine; and competition.

The hospital may wish to offset costs against specific benefits which elude mathematical formulae. The hospital may feel it is essential to be seen as a total care provider and may want to avoid the cost of loss of image (as a provider of a total urological service) and may, therefore, want to reduce the total charge and absorb the loss.

Keeping the charges low will allow more patients to access the machine but then the recovery of the cost of purchase will take longer. Moreover, rich patients who would spend in excess Rs 300 000 (US\$ 10 000) on treatment abroad would get treatment at low charges. There is, therefore, a need for a differential charge for persons with differing incomes, not easily introduced when the service is mainly provided to outpatients (in our experience in 85% of patients). It is difficult to construct differential charges as the patient does not choose a private or semi-private room or a general ward bed; his address does not indicate his income (he may be a *chowkidar* (security guard) in an expensive locality); and patients do not like to disclose their income. For inpatients, most hospitals charge general ward occupants at a lower rate than private wing patients for operations and operating room use.

Acceptable total revenues would result even when the charges are low, if there are larger volumes. But volumes must exceed the capacity of the service to provide quality care. One possible solution is to fix a reasonable but not too low a charge and support the poor through welfare funds, social security or insurance.

Covenants with self-paying patients

Patients charged on the basis of each treatment are distressed when they are told unexpectedly that an additional sitting or treatment is required and that they need to

J. Talati et al. (eds) The Management of Lithiasis, 245–251
© *1997 Kluwer Academic Publishers. Printed in Great Britain.*

Table 37.1   Predicting the number of lithotripsies needed for 100 patients on the basis of proportions of small, large and staghorn calculi

Percentage of patients with different stone bulk	Number of treatments per patient	Total of treatments
60%	1	60
20%	2	40
10%	3	30
10%	4	40
	100%	170[a]

[a] This equates to 1.7 treatments per patient, an inaccurate (low) prediction of the reality; many patients with long-standing large stones presented for lithotripsy as knowledge of the capabilities of the 'machine' spread.

pay more. They prefer to know the total cost at the start, as a predetermined package. Success in running packages and covenants with patients, however, requires an ability to predict accurately the number of treatments on the lithotriptor and for post-ESWL complications.

We expected 1.7 treatments per patient, gauged from our knowledge of the types of patient, the size of their stones and the proportion of patients with staghorn calculi consulting us for surgery (see Table 37.1). Accordingly a cost per treatment was calculated. At the start of our lithotripsy programmes, patients were charged according to the number of treatments received.

For the patient with large stones, costs built up rapidly, and patients requiring additional treatments, especially those requiring it unexpectedly, were either unable or unwilling to pay the extra costs. This posed a serious problem when a stone fragment which was small but greater than 5 mm was seen remaining in the pelvis, threatening to escape into and block the ureter. We felt it advantageous to treat this by lithotripsy but the patient shied away from therapy because of costs.

We therefore developed a package which then became a covenant between the patient and the hospital: even if the patient needed more treatments, he would not have to pay any additional costs. The covenant excluded procedures such as unexpected ureteroscopy, in which the physicians waived 60% of their fees.

Patients expected to require one or two treatments were charged a single consolidated cost. Similarly those needing more than two treatments were charged differently. A review of our initial experience allowed us to predict the numbers of patients requiring ancillary procedures, DJS insertion etc., and it was possible to assess the proportions needing two versus more than two treatments. With this information in hand, an average cost was easily worked out. This system of two-tier charges worked well, until our experience allowed us to extend lithotripsy to staghorn calculi and expertise attracted larger stones. This necessitated the introduction of a third tier of charges. The percentage differences in charges were A for the first tier (up to two treatments), B ($A + 50\%$) for the second tier, and C ($A + 80\%$) for the third tier (more than four treatments).

The package system worked well for the patient, as he/she knew the total charges for lithotripsy at the start of therapy.

As more lithotriptors appeared on the scene, the relatively small stones were rapidly eliminated and the mix of cases changed. Patients now needed an average of 2.2 treatments (up from 1.7).

Yet another compounding factor was the physicians' inability to predict treatments accurately. A review over two months of the accuracy of the physicians' assessment of expected numbers of treatments showed that underestimate was made in 40 treatments which needed 58 extra treatments, and resulted in a major loss, which, if projected to a year, would have cost 2.8 million rupees. Patients charged at tier 1, on average needed only 1.2 treatments. Patients at tier 2 needed 1.6 treatments. Patients at tier 3 needed 1.9 treatments. In spite of the average number of treatments appearing appropriate, 13% (43 of 331) estimated to complete their treatment within two treatments exceeded two treatments; 30% (52 of 177) exceeded four treatments when they were expected to complete treatments in four sessions. Tiers 1 and 2 were therefore problem areas.

Unfortunately the result of the miscalculation of package 1 tiers resulted in major losses in revenue, reducing the revenue per procedure to nearly 50% of the expected level. The patient was happy but was replaced by unhappy budget specialists and administrators. In order to refine the system and give as accurate a prediction and maximum benefit to the patient, definitions of the tier were made more objective.

Until then many of the decisions were judgmental and all welcomed more rigid criteria. As experience in UK, Germany and India had shown that 1-cm sized calculi are easily treated within one treatment, tier one was now restricted on the basis of size. Even within this group the physician was given the option to alter staging if he thought that obesity or the hardness of the stone would require more than two treatments. At the other end of the scale, all partial staghorn calculi and multiple calculi were classified with staghorn calculi as tier 3 stones.

Lithotripsy is an expensive treatment. Patients can budget and plan for a procedure, but are unable to bear additional unexpected costs. It is therefore better to have a package price as a covenant between hospital and patient.

This price will have to be worked out carefully, keeping in mind the patient mix, type of stone, average number of treatments, and risk of additional procedures. Criteria for charging for one or other levels of treatment should be objective so as to decrease financial loss.

Welfare and financial assistance

There needs to be a balance between economic viability of the lithotripsy programme (essential for the viability of the hospital – perhaps more so in the private and trust hospital settings) and the cost of treatment (important to the patient). Welfare programmes need to be developed with the co-operation of the financial adviser, administrators, clinicians and social welfare officers. Extracorporeal shock wave lithotripsy (ESWL) will be used throughout as a model.

The need for welfare

ESWL is required for treatment of most stones. If it is appropriate technology it should reach out to all. Stone disease is a disease of the poor in the socioeconomically poor countries, and of the rich in the well fed industrialized nations and the affluent towns of the poor nations. The majority of stone patients in Bombay came from the slums [1]. Eighty-nine per cent of the stone population visiting a teaching government hospital in Punjab in 1975 [2] earned less than Rs 500 per month (US$ 41, at 1975 rates). Stone patients are poorer than the general population admitted to hospital – 39% earn less than Rs 100 per month, compared with 24% of patients without stone disease who utilize the same hospital facility. Bladder stone disease is rampant in the poor child in the villages of Sindh (see operating room statistics from Sujjawal Taluka level hospital, Table 3.2) and Hazara division (see Chapter 3). Khan [2] has shown that bladder stones constitute 65% of all stones in the lowest income groups compared with 39.18% overall.

Therefore, provision must be made for free or subsidized treatment for patients with all types of stones, especially bladder stones. If treatment is not provided to the masses at charges that they can afford the machine does not justify its existence. Low volumes will not allow financial viability and the programme would eventually draw revenues away for other important areas in the hospital.

Sources of funding for indigent patients

Sources that could be tapped to assist patients include third party payers (insurance, social security, corporate employers) government funds, *Zakat* funds (see below), philanthropists, and self help from a proportion of revenues generated for the hospital by lithotripsy.

Third-party payers
Health insurance does not exist to any appreciable extent in Pakistan. The worker in a factory is covered by social security. As a result he and his dependants get free treatment. However, lithotriptors are not available in the social security hospitals in Karachi. Companies negotiate suitable fees for lithotripsy with the hospitals which have the lithotriptor, and consider treatment at their own hospital, often by operation, if charges are not competitive.

When developing pricing strategies for corporate clientele, provision must be made for the number of patients requiring ancillary procedures; the cost of these must be spread over the entire population. Corporate budgets do not permit unexpected large additional bills resulting from ureteroscopy, etc. Hospitals owning a lithotriptor therefore need to come up with a package price that allows financial viability to the hospital, and is suitably priced at not much above the hospital bill of a patient receiving alternative treatment.

Free treatment
It could be provided by government hospitals (for example the Larkana General Hospital and Mayo Hospital Lahore) and this would lessen the burden on the

private hospitals. In reality this does not occur. The government does not have unlimited funds at its disposal. Patients receive treatment only if they bring in various
drugs, catheters and stents which they have bought on the open market.

Zakat funds
These are funds donated as a religious obligation for welfare of the needy. Many
patients who are offered *Zakat* funds would not use them as they are not indigent.

Donations
The entire cost of the machine and maintenance could be borne by a philanthropist
who helps install the machine and hence all treatment would be free. Experience in
the UK warns that donor funded equipment often has no provision for maintenance,
the burden of which then falls on the government and National Health Service. All
donations should be made to endowments and used judiciously for both capital and
running costs. Donations must cover various programmes to cover all diseases and
will be swayed by the emotional pull of the request. Donations may suddenly dry
up. It is preferable not to rely on donations.

Funding from within
A welfare system which recycles a proportion of revenues (e.g. 10%) from
lithotripsy permits a share of the earnings to be utilized for the poor.

Who should receive welfare?

Should one aim at maximum benefit to some or a little benefit to many? The first
step in welfare programme development is to reach a consensus on the mechanisms
for eligibility and distribution. When disbursing welfare funds:
- The distribution should be equitable, and be seen as being so.
- Funds should not be utilized for disbursement of discounts to sensitive cases or
  tax or government officials.
- The welfare budget should not be exceeded.
- Welfare should be proportional to the need of the patient.
- Priorities should be established, with non-urgent patients receiving welfare in
  the next month and urgent cases borrowing money from the next month's
  welfare.
- Monies should be set aside for patients requiring large amounts for financial
  support.

A review of our experience has shown that welfare expenses may vary from as
little as 24% to as much as 78% of the total cost of lithotripsy for that patient.
Some control measures may need to be instituted to prevent overrunning the fixed
percentage of the revenues dedicated to lithotripsy. Non-urgent cases may be post-
poned until the following month if welfare funds are exceeded. Even so, in 1991,
12.7% of all patients treated on the lithotriptor were assisted with (on an average)
45% (10–78%) of the total costs of their treatment by lithotripsy.

Through welfare the poor were able to receive ESWL. Lithotripsy welfare patients
are poor and have complex stones as a result of long-standing neglect. Hence the cost

of their treatment is higher than the average cost of treatment. The disadvantage of using this mechanism to help the impoverished is that a few patients, supported by up to 70% of their bill, utilized a large volume of the welfare, resulting in a smaller number (12.7%) of patients being helped. An alternative method of financial assistance could restrict welfare to a percentage of total costs, say 20%, instead of allowing the welfare component to rise to 78% of costs. In that way many more patients would be helped. In such a system, one has to be wary of the sharp small-business owner out for a concessional discount or bargain. No person should expect totally free treatment; they must put in as much as they can, even if it is only a little.

Whatever the mechanisms, the margin for welfare as a proportion of income should be maintained. We have found that 10%, though an arbitrary figure, works well. No person qualifying for welfare was turned away because of lack of funds at any time.

Optimized provision of health cover for all is a responsibility to be shared by the government and private sector. The patient also has a responsibility in this system: a patient requesting welfare should be ready to disclose their real income and assets, and there should be a mechanism to help detect fraudulent welfare requests. This is easier said than done. When the sensitive issues of income are broached in a society which avoids tax, the truth may not be stated.

The institution must include a cut-off level of income above which welfare will not be provided.

Whatever mechanism is used to detect the financial stability of a family it must be done with great sensitivity and understanding of human dignity. No one should be asked to sell off a truck in order to pay for lithotripsy. The truck may be the sole means of the family obtaining their livelihood, and the one truck may be supporting a large extended family.

Reducing costs

Costs can be reduced by using refurbished electrodes, modifying operating room tables, and reducing the use of DJ stents and antibiotics, and admissions.

As the electrode is used up during a treatment, the spark generated across the inter-electrode space wears down the points of the electrode, and consequently increases the spark gap and therefore the focus size at F2. This results in loss of focal integrity with potential for causing damage to larger areas of the kidney. Additionally the larger spark gap weakens the energy delivered to F2.

Maintenance contracts usually ensure that used electrodes are returned to the company and are not refurbished by the purchaser. However, when the purchaser has access to the physics department of a university or other appropriate commercial concern with the ability to refurbish the electrode, considerable savings result. Focal integrity and energy delivery of these electrodes must achieve appropriate standards.

Costs can be brought down by eliminating the need for special tables. Universal operating room tables can be modified to have a radiolucent Formica top. This will reduce the cost of buying separate tables for use with a C-arm image intensifier.

Careful selective use of antibiotics and DJ stents will reduce the overall costs, and were dealt with in Section III.

Day-care lithotripsy

Outpatient treatment can reduce costs. We treat 85% of our patients on an outpatient basis. Many of those treated from the wards were because of emergency admission for obstructing stones. Admissions for lithotripsy are for patients with:

- hypertension in whom blood pressure has been poorly controlled;
- high-risk cardiac conditions;
- arrhythmias;
- poorly controlled diabetes;
- ureteric stones who need two treatments over two days and live out of town;
- severe ureteric colic post-treatment;
- fever post-ESWL;
- benign prostatic hypertrophy due to undergo TURP following ESWL of bladder calculi;
- bleeding disorders requiring correction;
- persisting infection with Pseudomonas which requires dual chemotherapy including aminoglycosides (these require drug dose monitoring by peak and trough levels) in patients who have no accommodation in Karachi, no accompanying relatives, and live far from Karachi; and
- complex stones requiring operation or percutaneous nephrolithotomy procedures with ESWL.

We regularly treat patients coming from Hyderabad, 90 miles from Karachi, on an outpatient basis, and they return on public transport on the same day.

Conclusion

A combination of judicious choice of treatment, considered and concerned, and perceptive use of shock waves, cost-conscious selection of technology, and welfare support of patients unable to afford therapy, will provide an excellent service for all categories of patient.

References

1.   Hussain F, Billimoria FR. Some biochemical observations on urinary stone formation amongst slum dwellers in North Eastern Bombay. In: Nath R, Thund SK, editors. Urolithiasis research. New Delhi: Ashish Publishing House, 1989:187–94.
2.   Khan F. Stone bladder in children. Prog Med 1974;3;116–21.

38. Commencing and expanding lithotripsy services

JAMSHEER TALATI

Successful growth of lithotripsy programmes requires carefully planned, staged expansion of the programme with a controlled patient load. This is necessary in order to prevent breakdown of follow-up services which would have disastrous effects on patient care.

Careful selection of patients, heavy consultant involvement at the start of programmes, diligent follow-up, and rapid intervention by ureteroscopy (URS) or Percutaneous nephrotomy (PCN) when required will ensure success.

At all times lithotripsy should remain a quality service, capable of dealing with all complications. Prior to acquiring a lithotriptor, the unit must have the skills required to perform all ancillary procedures such as ureteroscopy, percutaneous nephrostomy and nephrolithotomy. A consultant can then be identified to be in charge of the lithotripsy programme, and sent to a unit for training on the type of lithotriptor to be purchased. In the initial phases of the programme, selection of patients and treatment should be done by this individual, who assesses the results and modifies protocols. Once these are established, referring physicians can be educated as to which patients are suitable for extracorporeal shock wave lithotripsy (ESWL) or other forms of treatment, and a larger number of consultants and residents can be trained in lithotripsy. Discussions at morbidity conferences will refine treatment protocols.

Early stages

In the early stages, it is preferable to treat calculi in the kidney only, choosing the 'easy' stone: the thin patient, resident in the same town, who has easy access to the lithotriptor, with a single stone under 2 cm in size, no outflow obstruction and no need for a DJ stent; a stone with a coralliform appearance, which needs only one treatment, and which will clear from the kidney within 2–3 weeks. It is necessary at this stage to limit treatments to three or perhaps four patients a day. As expertise develops, larger stones, ureteric stones and out-of-town patients can be treated. The latter have special requirements – they need to be accommodated at short notice, require treatments to be completed quickly and put extra demands on a service.

At a later stage, out-of-town filter clinics can be developed so that patients need not travel all the way to the tertiary centre for evaluation, only to learn that their

J. Talati et al. (eds) The Management of Lithiasis, 253–255
© 1997 Kluwer Academic Publishers. Printed in Great Britain.

stones are not suitable for lithotripsy. A further extension of the programme could include a roving lithotriptor service. This is well established in Europe, with mobile lithotriptors visiting various towns. However, the roads in Europe are safe, and smooth; not so in Pakistan. Currently therefore, mobile lithotripsy is not feasible in Pakistan unless it is mounted on a rail carriage and utilizes railway stations. Chapter 36 documents the experience of a European centre with a shared lithotriptor.

Effect on other services

Programmed expansion is important and should take into consideration the ability of the urologists, radiologists, nursing services, clinics, and emergency and operating room, to keep pace with the numbers of follow-up visits for patients that will rapidly build up. Each patient may need five or six visits before being declared stone free, and may need operating room time for the push-ups, DJ stent insertion and anaesthetic time for these procedures, and return operating room time for removal of the DJS. With the increased number of patients and increased number of post-ESWL visits, lithotripsy clinics can grow exponentially. It is useful to develop a separate operating room for lithotripsy ancillary procedures.

Lithotripsy services can swamp out all other urology care if the flow of patients is not controlled. Fifty per cent of the increase in urological work in a unit (1981–87) in France was attributed to ESWL. When the ESWL service is an outpatient service, the natural ceiling on work done that occurs when beds are not available is not there, and one can go on increasing the lithotripsy volumes to a point that exceeds the ability to look after them postoperatively. An idea of the impact of ESWL on radiological work load can be gauged by a report from Cochrane. Patients required an average of 6.3 KUB and 1.2 ultrasound studies per treatment session and 0.6 post-ESWL intravenous pyelograms and 0.1 nephrostomies per patient. In all 8478 radiological procedures were required for 955 patients.

At the Aga Khan University Hospital, the projected increase of work by 10% increment per year was outstripped by actual volumes (see Figure 38.1), which were three times the projected volumes.

Development of dedicated lithotriptists

Quality care can be better delivered by persons dedicated to doing lithotripsy than when it is performed by staff rotated through the department. Who should this permanent staff be? Lithotripsy can be taught to paramedical staff, but the decision as to whether they should be the major lithotriptists or whether a doctor should be performing the procedure is a point to be determined by each country and each hospital. The advantage of having a doctor present is the prompt response in case of bradycardia or cardiac arrest. The doctor is better equipped to make decisions which improve the quality of care during lithotripsy. His participation in lithotripsy

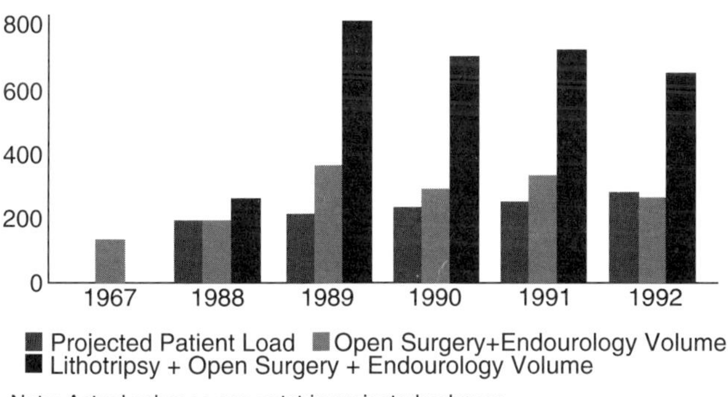

Figure 38.1 Projected patient load for lithotripsy and surgical procedures for urinary tract stone disease

as well as the pre-assessment and post-ESWL clinics ensure continuity of care. The same doctor sees the patient in lithotripsy clinics, treats him on the lithotriptor and follows him up. Having worked on the lithotriptor and experienced the difficulties of localizing stones in the very obese for example, the doctor enhances his expertise in selecting appropriate treatment modalities for his patients. The doctor can assess the effects of sedation, and if excessive drowsiness and consequent respiratory depression ensue, can assess the need for supplemental oxygenation. He can better judge the anxiety level of the patient; decide what kV power will be used during lithotripsy, and increase sedo-analgesia if higher kV is to be used; and identify the patient with previous surgery and anticipate that he will experience more pain, and so will be able to determine the appropriate dose, and what is more important, judge when to give the analgesic.

Pakistan has an excess of unemployed doctors. For these reasons it is appropriate, beneficial and expedient to utilize their services.

39. Financing the lithotriptor

MEHER KAKALIA

In developed economies such as the US, health care may consume up to 14% of the GNP. The State and private health insurance provide for the higher levels of expenditure required for costly medical equipment such as the lithotriptor. In developing economies health care is very much the responsibility of the private sector. Given the prevalent low income levels, health care equipment which requires high capital expenditure cannot be commercially viable if the charges for therapy are to be kept reasonably within the reach of the common man. Some form of financial assistance for purchase of the lithotriptor is therefore required.

Lender's risks

Before committing finance, the lender will want to assess the commercial viability and risks of the project. The risks of lending money to the 'sponsor' will depend on the purchase price, maintenance costs, resale value, availability of expertise for repair, the sponsor's operational know-how, availability of suitable manpower, the sponsor's equity stake in the company, his credit record and reputation, and form of security agreements.

   The commercial risk will be assessed by a feasibility study with cash flow projections and profitability. An analysis of the demand and supply for the service and an industry analysis which includes existing competitors, threat of new entrants, political influence on the project and future prospects will be required. Financial statements audited by a chartered accountant are required for loans in excess of Rs 10 million.

Choosing a financier

Just as the lender is careful in selecting whom he will loan money to, the purchaser (sponsor) should select the financier carefully. The size of the loan (price) is the most important criterion in evaluating different financing options and should include, in addition to the purchase price, fees, maintenance contracts, costs of structural changes, and other charges.

J. Talati et al. (eds) The Management of Lithiasis, 257–262
© *1997 Kluwer Academic Publishers. Printed in Great Britain.*

Since the income from the use of a lithotriptor is generated over a period of time, a 'net present value' (NPV) analysis (which predicts returns from the project) should be used to determine the structuring of the loan repayments.

If a project is set up with a social purpose in mind, the lenders should know this from the start so that the financial institution may be in a position to assist or advise the sponsor on suitable lines of credit or government grants for such purposes.

Most borrowers seem little concerned about anything other than the ability to obtain the loan. However, several other factors should be considered when choosing a financial institution.

The size, flexibility and experience of the lending institution are of importance. Large institutions have the capacity to disburse larger sums of money and can withstand reduced repayments if unforeseen adverse events occur during operations. The level of their assets and the diversity of their portfolio allow them a greater degree of flexibility, as compared to smaller institutions, who may not be able to assist at the time of need.

Organizations which have prior experience in funding medical equipment are to be preferred as these firms are familiar and comfortable with the nature of the project and the requirements for its viability. As health care projects differ from commercial business ventures (in that the level of demand for the service may be dependent on variables other than commercial economics) the lender should be flexible and creative in developing financing options best suited to the nature of the project.

The organization should be honest, give correct advice to the client, approve loans quickly and respond to the physician's or hospital's needs promptly.

Financing options often have different loan covenants all of which favour the financial institution. In most cases the clauses are standard and the lender may not agree to alter them. However in cases where the institutions do not have proven track records it pays to negotiate with the financier and eliminate covenants which give him undue advantage.

A natural query at this point would be, 'But how will I know which institution will be best for me?'. Unfortunately in Pakistan, institutions are not rated on different areas. The sponsor may have to do so by filling in the grid as shown in Table 39.1. The key is first to identify what is most important to the hospital, and then choose a lender who can best serve these needs.

Table 39.1   Grid for evaluating institutions

	Weightage	Institution	Product
Speed of credit approval	1.5	7	10.5
Size	0.6	9	5.4
Pricing	1.5	9	13.5
Flexibility	2	5	10.0
Creativity in structuring	2	5	10.0
Good working relationship	0.5	6	3.0
Professional work environment	1.4	6	8.4
Previous experience	0.5	0	0
Total	10		60.8

A hypothetical institution is related here as an example.

The weightage for various characteristics may be arranged according to the needs of the hospital, but should total 10. Each institution can then be ranked according to its strengths. The product of the first two columns gives the actual value of each lending institution. The institution scoring the highest points will be the most suitable.

Financing options

The sponsor traditionally has two major sources of funds, i.e. debt and equity. Only one of these options has actually been used to finance a lithotriptor in Pakistan (deferred payment letter of credit).

Equity usually creates creditor confidence and acts as a security for the creditor. Equity is the investor's own investment in the asset and gives the investor the right of ownership of the asset/project. In Pakistan, financial institutions can lend only to those companies which have at least a 40% stake in the project (i.e. 40% of the long-term debt).

To supplement equity, the investor can borrow funds from other institutions to acquire the asset. Debt may be subordinated or senior, the latter being repaid first in the event of a liquidation. This is the most common form of debt as it is the most secure from the point of view of the lender.

Sources of funds

Loans may be obtained from the World Bank, export credit agencies, the host government, commercial banks, or development financial institutions. World Bank loans have lower costs, finance large amounts, and have longer repayment periods. However, approval procedures are cumbersome and finance is given for projects rather than individual pieces of equipment.

Export credit agencies (financial institutions in the country of the exporter who take on the risk and advance money to the importer) provide financing to the importer through a letter of credit.

In a supplier's credit, the loan is made to a supplier who quotes the financing terms. In most cases when the supplier is in a country other than the buyer's, in order to cover his/her risks, the supplier asks for a bank guarantee shifting the risk assumed to the local bank. When the goods are imported, such credits in Pakistan are structured through a usance letter of credit (LC) whereby the risk of default is borne by the local bank opening the letter of credit.

This source of funds has been used in Pakistan for financing the lithotriptor through commercial banks. It is a very useful mode for financing one-off items such as a lithotriptor. Its major advantage is speed of processing and relatively lower financing costs. However, a supplier's credits is in foreign currency and therefore the sponsor has to pay for the foreign exchange risk cover and LC charges to the bank. Moreover all suppliers may not be in a position to give credit. Commercial banks are the largest and the most common source of funding. Banks offer a wide range of services to the borrower, allowing them the convenience of dealing with only one institution. For an asset such as a lithotriptor, a borrower can open the LC, issue guarantees, take a loan under the LC and obtain short-term working capital financing from the same bank. The borrower can also maintain an account and use various other facilities offered. Very often commercial banks also provide leasing facilities, are quick in project approvals, provide a one-window service, and are generally professional. However, commercial banks are traditionally not inclined towards project financing and therefore may require additional security, and usually prefer shorter financing periods. Longer-term loans are generally routed through a syndicate of banks.

Development finance institutions (DFI) in Pakistan have access to various foreign financing lines through world agencies or foreign government subsidies, and have the capacity to finance large projects at comparatively lower costs. The disadvantages of dealing with DFIs are lengthy approval processes, binding loan covenants and some level of management control depending on the risk assumed by the DFI.

Leasing is a form of financing where the lessor (leasing company) owns the asset and allows the sponsor to use the asset for a predetermined rent. Depending on whether the lease is an operating or finance lease, the lessee has the option to repurchase the asset at the end of the lease terms.

Financial instruments

Long-term loans

Such loans usually have a payback of one year and may involve one or many lenders (syndication). The repayment is usually in the form of instalments over the life of the loans. Some commercial lenders may require submission of bank guarantee as security. Long-term loans may be based on a fixed or floating interest rate. (Long-term loans from commercial banks may carry a floating interest rate, which is a certain percentage above the Treasury Bill rate.)

Usance letter of credit

When the foreign supplier is providing financing, a local bank opens a letter of credit to import goods. A 10%–20% down payment is required with the remaining amount being paid over a period of two to five years. Although the cost of credit may be comparatively low, the additional costs in terms of foreign exchange cover and LC fees increase the overall cost which must be factored in when evaluating the proposal (the approximate added cost is 17–18% per annum).

Lease

Under the leasing option, ownership of the lithotriptor remains with the leasing company (lessor) for the lease period (3–5 years). Lease can be either operating or finance. Under a pure operating lease, all costs of maintenance and repair are borne by the lessor. As the lessee does not contribute towards the ownership of the asset, this form of leasing is almost akin to hiring and the instalments received are called rents. Based on the technical nature of the lithotriptor and its limited resale value in Pakistan, most leasing companies would not be willing to enter into a lease of this nature.

Under a finance lease, ownership vests with the lessor; however the economic ownership lies with the lessee who has a purchase option at the end of the period at a predetermined price. Although the accounting treatment for both these types of lease is different, the tax treatment in Pakistan is exactly the same, which allows significant tax savings in leasing compared to a loan.

Working capital financing

For the day-to-day running and maintenance of the equipment and the clinic (if any), the sponsor can take a working capital loan from a commercial bank. Such loans are usually short term in nature, i.e. for a period less than one year. Although not suitable for the purchase of the asset, such financing is important for the daily operation of the clinic or health centre.

Debt with equity kickers

Debt and equity combinations, although relatively uncommon in Pakistan, are effective financing techniques for risky transactions. The equity element is usually a small part of the package and acts as a sweetener for high anticipated gains. Under such transactions, the downside for the lender is limited to the return on the debt while the upside is unlimited in terms of returns on equity through dividends or capital gains.

Conclusions

Financing a lithotriptor or any other medical equipment is really no different from normal project financing. As the capital outlay is fairly substantial, in most cases the need for financial support other than equity will be necessary. This chapter should be used as a guideline to try and investigate all possible options, no matter how unusual, and not to discard any possibilities.

Acknowledgements

The assistance of Mr Savak Talati and Mr Maruf Ahmed in the preparation of this manuscript is gratefully acknowledged.

Appendix: Regulatory requirements

In the context of Pakistan, prudential regulations govern loans, advances and leases extended to clients. It is therefore imperative for the borrower to need these requirements in order to be eligible for financing from financial institutions. The three most important requirements are:

1. Borrowed amount:

Less than Rs 500 000	– No financial statements required (only in the case of a loan)
Less than Rs 2 million	– Financial statements signed by the proprietor or director of the company and countersigned by a chartered accountant
Rs 2–10 million	– Financial statements countersigned by chartered accountant
Greater than Rs 10 million	– Financial statements audited by a practising chartered accountant.

2. The current ratio (current assets/current liabilities) should be at least 1 by January of the year.
3. The long-term debt to equity ratio should be 60:40. Therefore the sponsor should have at least a 40% equity stake (40% of capital cost) in the organization or project.

Section V
Prevention of Urinary Tract Calculi

40. Introduction: Prevention of urinary tract calculi

JAMSHEER TALATI

Physicians managing stone disease need to anticipate and prevent recurrence of stone formation. Can they reach out further – can they predict the person who is going to form his first stone? Prevention of both the first stone and recurrence is important if the physician is to reduce the incidence of stone related end-stage renal failure.

The prevention of recurrence in stone patients

Stone patients come to our attention as a result of symptoms. For such patients who have formed a stone, preventive measures can only thwart recurrences. Nevertheless, they safeguard the patient against future obstructive uropathy from stone. Stone disease is recurrent in up to 75% of patients, with 10% recurring in two years [1] and 60% in five years [2]. Patients who have formed a stone within the last year, or whose stone grew in the preceding year, or who have documented passage of stone or gravel in the preceding year should be considered active stone formers even though a biochemical abnormality cannot be detected. Such patients are at greater risk for stone recurrence.

Each recurrence anticipates the arrival of the next at ever shortening intervals [3]. If four or five stones have been formed, the stone-free interval may be less than two years [3]. Recurrence is a better predictor of future recurrences than 24-hour urine studies [4].

Not all who have recurrences will have specific abnormalities [5, 6], but when abnormalities are detected, their correction through attention to water and dietary intake aided by medication, may reduce new stone formation. To plan such regimes effectively, knowledge of the type of stone, dietary intake and urinary excretion rates are necessary. Persisting infection in patients with a past history of urinary infection, may have a role in recurrence. Diligent eradication of infection will reduce recurrence.

Prevention of stone disease in the person at risk before he forms his first stone

Prophylactic measures are instituted after the patient has formed a stone. There is enough evidence to indicate that brothers of stone patients are at higher risk for

J. Talati et al. (eds) The Management of Lithiasis, 265–267
© 1997 Kluwer Academic Publishers. Printed in Great Britain.

stone than the general population. Perhaps this population subgroup could be kept under surveillance and asked to maintain a high fluid intake, in the hope that stone formation will be prevented or at least detected at an early stage. If a metabolic abnormality is detected in the family all affected members could receive prophylactic treatment. Currently there is no test that will categorically identify persons at risk for stone.

For a disease that is so prevalent, it is worth attempting prevention in the population at large. Advice on increasing water intake can be given to the entire population through newspaper articles and informal talks with various socially conscious groups such as rotarians etc.

Prevention of damage from undetected stone

Many patients have undetected asymptomatic stones. Screening by ultrasound and X-ray can pick up the asymptomatic patient with a small stone before it slips into the ureter and causes obstruction.

Mass screening of the population, even in endemic areas, by these methods will not be cost-effective. Though Scott [7] picked up a prevalence rate of 3.5% in Scotland, a 10% life-time incidence gives a rate of 1 stone per 50 000 patient years. The chance of picking up a stone on any particular day will be very small and cost-ineffective as many small stones pass spontaneously. Even given a prevalence of 3.5%, ultrasound screening (US) alone will cost Rs 350 per ultrasound, or US$ 1200 per 100 screened patients and hence US$ 342 per detected case.

One could increase the effectiveness of screening by concentrating on the families of stone patients. In our survey, 22% of patients have an affected sibling (in 16% a brother is affected), and whilst only 1.6% of all the brothers of stone patients have stone, if in a family two brothers are affected, then 26% of all brothers will have stone. Selective screening will increase the yield.

Is it useful to pick up small stones in asymptomatic patients? What will be the benefits? Having picked up a small stone, should it be treated on the lithotriptor? (See section on asymptomatic stones, Chapter 9, p. 77). Will the asymptomatic relative be able to afford treatment? Ethical questions then arise. Another more cost-effective approach to this problem would involve focusing on educating the public on preventive measures against recurrence and detection of remediable causes.

Reducing risks of stone disease in the unborn child

Consanguinity is seen at a high level (18%) in populations in which stones occur frequently. In some northern areas of Pakistan, up to 60% of marriages may be within the tribe and hence consanguineous. Though easier said than done, consanguineous marriages and marriages between stone formers should be discouraged.

Such efforts are unlikely to be successful at the present time in Pakistan. Attention should be given instead to eliminating all residual calculi and urinary tract infections; detecting and treating hyperparathyroidism; advising suitable diets; and encouraging fluid intake. These issues are addressed in the following chapters.

References

1. Sandlow JI, Winfield HN, Loening SA. Does ESWL augment stone recurrence? J Urol 1989;141:407A.
2. Schneider HJ. Epidemiology of urolithiasis. In: Schneider HJ, editor. Urolithiasis, epidemiology and etiology. Berlin: Springer-Verlag, 1985:137.
3. Ala-Opas M, Lehtonen T. Recurrence of urolithiasis. Ann Chir Gynaec 1990;79:50–3.
4. Ryall RL, Marshall VR. Value of a 24 hour urinary analysis in the assessment of stone formers attending a general hospital outpatients' clinic. Brit J Urol 1983;55:1–5.
5. Leskovar P, Huber J, Piendal J. An improved discrimination between stone formers and controls. Urol Res 1987;15:117.
6. Wong SY, Slater SR, Evans RA *et al.* Metabolic studies in kidney stone disease. Quart J Med 1992;82:47–58.
7. Scott R. Prevalence of calcified upper urinary tract stone disease in a random population survey. Report of a combined study of general practitioner and hospital staff. Br J Urol 1987;59:111–17.

41. The residual calcular fragment: A risk factor for recurrent stone disease

JAMSHEER TALATI

Calcular fragments (residuals) left behind after initial therapy of stone may grow with time, especially in patients with metabolically active stone disease [1]. Each fragment can become a nidus for a new stone [1] which grows in size by as much as 25% over two years [2]. Many so-called recurrences, especially those seen soon after extracorporeal shock wave lithotripsy (ESWL), may be due to growth of residuals which had not been detected on post-treatment X-rays. Observed 'recurrent stone' formation is three times more common when a residual stone is present and the higher rate of recurrence seen in patients with multiple stones (16% vs. 5% in simple stones) may result from the more frequent residuals left in such patients. Residuals encourage recurrent urinary tract infection (UTI), when they occur in patients with pretreatment UTI and consequently new stone formation.

Though residual calculi are a major problem with all forms of treatment, residuals and recurrences after ESWL have been more widely studied than after pyelolithotomy. This is because ESWL is expensive and comes under greater scrutiny in this era of cost-consciousness. Additionally, residuals left after ESWL pose a problem if they are too small to warrant further active therapy. In contrast, residual stones after percutaneous nephrolithotomy (PCNL) and surgery can often be treated with ESWL.

Residuals after ESWL

Earlier reports claimed clearance rates after ESWL of 90% [3] to 84% [4] at three months after ESWL. Today, reported stone-free rates vary from 50% [5] to 80% [6, 7]. Large stones will leave behind more residuals, even if more shocks and greater power is used. Clearance at six months was 89% for stones smaller than 1 cm but only 79% for stones greater than 2 cm [4].

Initially many ignored calcular fragments less than 4 mm, assuming that these fragments would pass spontaneously. This does not always happen – up to 60% of these may be in an inferior calyx which is difficult to clear of stones [8]. A recognition of this has resulted in more accurate reporting and it is recognized that residuals may be seen in up to 25% of patients. In comparison, residual stones remain after PCNL in 1–8%, after pyelolithotomy in 8–20% and after atrophic nephrolithotomy in 5–28%.

J. Talati et al. (eds) The Management of Lithiasis, 269–273
© *1997 Kluwer Academic Publishers. Printed in Great Britain.*

The higher residual rates and recurrences seen after ESWL are not due to change in the metabolic parameters after ESWL [9].

Factors favouring residual stones

Banner [10] has listed conditions favouring residuals: stone burden (multiplicity and size); location (e.g. in a calyx or a calyceal diverticulum); composition; quality of stone disintegration; ambulation and hydration potential of the patient; urinary tract abnormality peculiar to the individual; previous ureteral or pelvic ureteral surgery; and fixation of the ureter. Additional factors are:

- obesity which reduces shock wave effectiveness because of refraction;
- excess shocks causing mucosal damage, ulceration, and consequent fibrinous binding of stone to mucosa;
- the use of high voltage – detrimental because it produces large fragments;
- treatment of large volume of stone in one sitting without diuresis;
- obstruction of the ureter by calcular fragments; and
- special calyceal configurations.

Accurate detection of residuals

Inaccurate detection will mislead the physician into declaring a patient stone free. Poor quality X-rays and poorly interpreted X-rays or ultrasounds and the limits of resolution of these two modalities affect whether the patient will be declared stone free. In stones with admixture of uric acid, stone fragments may be missed.

The ability of KUB X-rays and ultrasound to detect particles will vary according to the nature of the equipment, the user, and degree of obesity and bowel preparation of the patient. Conventional X-rays may at times be unable to detect 1 cm sized stone particles [11]. The same observer or different observers may report differently on the stone free status on KUB 25–52% of the time [12].

More residuals will be detected if two different exposure angles are used [5]. Conventional film screen and digital tomography imaging are better than standard KUB. Digital tomography appears to be the most effective method but there is a 24% interobserver and a 16% intraobserver difference in reporting tomograms, and false positive interpretations are frequent. Therefore it is not recommended routinely [13], but justified in patients with infection, those who have frequent recurrences, and persistent metabolic abnormalities resistant to intelligent dietary control.

Ultrasonography (US) will detect radiolucent and radiopaque fragments and is superior to X-rays when there are overlying gas shadows which interfere with the interpretation of the X-ray. US, will, in addition, detect hydronephrosis. However stones in the ureter, and stones hidden by a rib or in close proximity to the spine, are difficult to visualize. Smudged well fragmented calculi may appear as dense as a stone on static images (image taken when the kidney is not receiving shock waves). Radiology is generally superior to sonography when detecting ureteral fragments and the completeness of stone fracture [14]. In patients after ESWL, an intravenous pyelogram does not add significant information to that obtained from a KUB X-ray and ultrasound.

Is a radiologist's interpretation of X-rays and ultrasound necessary?

The urologist in a non-tertiary centre in Pakistan will have to read his own X-rays and ultrasounds. There could be no more motivated person to do so, because the urologist has to determine whether his patient is stone free, or needs further treatment. However, some studies have shown the superiority of radiologists in interpreting ultrasound, which is operator dependent [14].

Residuals and recurrence in patients with urinary tract infection

Whilst persistence of infection accelerates recurrence, elimination of infection alone does not protect the patient against recurrence if residuals are left behind, because residuals encourage recrudescence of infection. There is a 13-fold increase in post-ESWL UTI (84% vs. 6%) if residual fragments persist in patients who had pretreatment UTI. Infection in turn causes the residual fragment to grow and new stones to form. Where the residual fragment has remained undetected, this will be recorded as a new growth.

The majority of recurrences occur in patients with infection, or with stones indicating an infection related aetiology [15]. Struvite stones recur in 30% of patients within five years [16] unless rigorous attempts are made to eradicate residuals.

Measures to facilitate the clearance of detected residuals

Because recurrence is linked with residuals, it is cost-effective to use all possible means to ensure elimination of residuals. Heroic measures, including percutaneous dissolution or PCNL are justified when residuals are associated with upper UTI or struvite stones. Aggressive therapy of the residual is not indicated if there is only lower urinary tract infection [17].

Liberal percutaneous hemiacridine irrigation, even in the absence of demonstrable residuals after surgery for struvite stones, has yielded long-term stone-free status in some hands [16] though not in all. Percutaneous catheters for irrigation are placed close to stone fragments. Pfister's *et al.* [18] explicit recommendations should be reviewed, and chemolysis temporarily discontinued if there is fever, serum Mg greater than 3.5 mg/dl, a rise in creatinine greater than 1 mg/dl, or a serum phosphate rise to 1.5 times normal. Infusion is permanently discontinued when there is failure to reduce size by 50% in two weeks, a failure of serum creatinine to return to normal within three days after temporary cessation, resistant UTI or urosepsis.

Stone analysis of fragments passed after ESWL will allow a choice of irrigating solution. Hemiacridine or Suby's solution G (both with a pH of 4.0) should be used for phosphate stones, sodium bicarbonate for urate stones, and EDTA for calcium oxalate stones. Hemiacridine and Fe EDTA have been found to be very toxic to renal cells in culture [19] and recommendations about discontinuing use should be strictly adhered to. In the future, cystine stones may be treated by ESWL to enlarge their surface area (see Section III) and then dissolved by acetylcystine percutaneous irrigations [20]. Chemotherapy with very dilute (0.5%) acetic acid has been used cautiously by us to dissolve phosphate residual calculi.

Calyceal stones clear only in 20–30% of patients [5]. Whilst in normal calyces, urine and stone can be easily expelled by contraction (systole), a calyx in which a stone has resided for months may have lost its expulsive power as a result of fibrosis. The angle at which the lower infundibulum joins the pelvis (in 74% it is at an angle of more than 70 degrees), and the size of the infundibulum (in more than 40% it was smaller than 4 mm) can additionally hamper stone clearance [21]. Calyceal stones are a problem even in percutaneous clearance of stones. Obsitnik *et al.* [22] have identified stones left behind a narrowed infundibulum of a minor calyx as a major cause of residuals after PCNL.

Vibration and gravity assist drainage and facilitate stone clearance from inferior calyces. We suggest that the patient lies in a knee chest position whilst a relative performs tapotement, or thumps the renal angle on the affected side with a fist. A commercial hand held vibrator will loosen out clot held debris from the lower calyx.

We do not contest the well-known fact that urine drains from the pelvis by peristalsis and not gravity, but stone fragments appear to remain in dilated calyces until assisted by gravity, especially when their musculature has been made ineffective either by destruction, or paralysis by presence of stent.

Oral therapy can also be used to dissolve resistant urate calcular fragments [23]. Patients are required to increase urine volume to 2500 ml daily; reduce dietary purine and protein intake; and alkalinize urine to a pH of 6.5–7.0. Of all these changes, a change in urinary pH alone may be equally effective. A higher pH is likely to deposit calcium apatite. The pH should be adjusted to between 6.4 and 6.8, but the commercially available pH sticks are graduated at intervals of 0.5. Of all these measures, a change in pH alone may be adequate. Allopurinol is advised for those persons unable to conform to a diet. All patients should be warned of the possibility of ureteric obstruction as the stone may slide down into the ureter when it becomes smaller in size. Potassium salts are used in addition to sodium salts, to alkalinize the urine to reduce sodium intake (important in cardiac patients) and prevent sodium urate deposits on the surface of the stone (as this is less soluble than monopotassium urate) and as sodium bicarbonate may increase the urinary loss of potassium.

In patients with normal renal function, a recommended starting dose is 25 mEq of a potassium alkalinizing salt 3–4 times a day. In addition sodium bicarbonate tablets may be added: there are roughly 12 mEq of base in each gram of sodabicarb; or roughly 7.5 mEq in each 10-grain tablet of sodium bicarbonate. Therapy should continue until the stones dissolve. How long this takes will vary from patient to patient, as will the dose required to reach a certain pH.

Because of the suspected relation between residuals and recurrence, every effort must made to detect and eliminate residuals, especially when associated with infection.

References

1. Segura JW. The role of percutaneous surgery in renal and ureteral stone. J Urol 1989;141:780.
2. Eisenberger F, Rassweiler G, Bub P *et al.* Differential approach to staghorn calculi using ESWL and PCN; an analysis of 151 consecutive patients. World J Urol 1987;5:248.
3. Chaussey C, Schmeidt E. ESWL for kidney stones, an alternative to surgery? Urol Radiol 1984;6:80.
4. Liedl B, Joacham D, Schuster C, Haupt G. Prognosis of residual calculi after ESWL. Urol Res 1987;15:128.
5. Miles SG, Kandi JV, Newman RC *et al.* ESWL, prevalence of renal stones 3–21 months after treatment. Am J Roentgenol 1988;150:307–9.
6. Rielhe R A Jr, Fan W R, Vaughan E D Jr. ESWL for upper urinary tract calculi. A one year experience at single center. J Am Med Assoc 1986;255:2043.
7. Drach GW, Dretler S, Fair W *et al.* Report of the US cooperative study of ESWL. J Urol 1986;135:1127–33.
8. Neils Peter, Bucholz N-P, Meier-Padel S, Rutishauser G Minor residual fragments after ESWL, spontaneous clearance or risk of recurrence? Abstract 391, p. 180, Société International d'Urologie, 23rd Congress, Syndey, Australia; 1994.
9. Brown RD, Pak CYC, Preminger GM. Effect of lithotripsy on stone forming risk factors. J Urol 1989;141:207A.
10. Banner MP. ESWL: Selection of patients and long term complications. Radiol Clin 1991;21:543–56.
11. Pfab R, Kloiber W, Kropp W *et al.* The endoscopically radiologically non recognizable residual fragment. Urol Res 1987;15:127.
12. Jewett MAS, Bombardier C, Caron D *et al.* Potential for interobserver and intraobserver variability in X-ray review to establish stone free rates after lithotripsy. J Urol 1992;147:559 62.
13. Sachs EM, Fajardo LL, Hilman BJ *et al.* Prospective comparison of plain X-ray abdominal radiography with conventional and digital tomography in assessing ESWL patients. J Urol 1990;144:1341–6.
14. Abernathy BB, Wilson WT, Morris JS *et al.* Evaluation of residual stone fragments after lithotripsy: Sonography vs KUB. J Urol 1989;141:176A.
15. Sandlow JI, Winfield HN, Loening SA. Does ESWI augment stone recurrence? J Urol 1989;141:407A.
16. Silverman DE, Stamey TA. Management of infection stones: Stanford experience. Medicine (Baltimore) 1983;62:44–51.
17. Huggoson J, Grenabo L, Hedelin H, Petersen S. Residual concrements and UTI, Abstracts of the 13th Urolithiasis Symposium. Uro Res 1987;15:127.
18. Pfister RC, Dretler SP, Yoder IC. Percutaneous catheter dissolution of renal stones. Br J Urol 1983; Supplement: 69–74.
19. Vogel E, Schultz W, Lehmer A *et al.* Toxicological studies of stone dissolving solutions. Uro Res 1987;15:126.
20. Schmeller NT, Kersting H, Schuller J, *et al.* Combination of Chemolysis and shock-wave lithotripsy in the treatment of cystine renal calculi. J Urol 1988; 131: 434–8.
21. Sampio FJB, Afonso HMA. Inferior pole collecting system anatomy. Its possible role in ESWL. J Urol 1992;147:322–4.
22. Obsitnik M, Skutil V, Lutter I *et al.* Cause of the residual stone in patients with complete staghorn calculi treated by nephrotomy or percutaneous litholapaxy. Urol Res 1987;15:127.
23. Rodman JS, Williams JJ, Peterson CM. Uric acid calculi can be dissolved by prolonged oral therapy. J Urol 1984;131:1039–43.

42. Primary hyperparathyroidism in urinary tract stone disease in Pakistan and the West

J. TALATI and S.R. BIYABANI

Overview: Screening for primary hyperparathyroidism is pertinent in the developing world

TIMOTHY S. HARRISON

In Oman, we determined serum calcium in over 5000 subjects – randomly drawn blood samples in eight different locations. This was an extension of a WHO approved diabetes survey. The logistics of finding patients in the top 2 percentile of serum calciums in remote villages is formidable but potentially worthwhile.

Patients with occult persistent hypercalcaemia probably need to be protected from the effects of hypercalcaemia, no matter what the cause. Some will have primary hyperparathyroidism.

The physician may think it worthwhile to try and feel adenomas preoperatively and commit him/herself to a side before surgery. We have experience with palpable and even visible glands overlooked by ultrasound and computerized tomography. The physician will often be wrong but it 'lightens the air' for concerned patients to enter the game. The patient should be asked where the adenoma is.

The current dreary preoccupation with preoperative localization is best avoided in the developing world and elsewhere.

Suppressed glands should always be biopsied. There is no reason to make a patient hypoparathyroid by doing so.

There are patients who, though 'asymptomatic', feel improved after successful parathyroid surgery; 'Doctor, I never realized that I was not feeling well'.

Definition of primary hyperparathyroidism

Primary hyperparathyroidism (PHPT) is a syndrome characterized by elevated serum calcium, low or low normal serum phosphorus, and elevated parathyroid hormone (PTH). Urinary calcium excretion is normal in 30% of patients [1], because PTH increases reabsorption of calcium. The prefix primary denotes that the changes result from autonomous hypersecretion of PTH and are not secondary to vitamin D deficiency, renal failure or other causes.

J. Talati et al. (eds) The Management of Lithiasis, 275–287
© *1997 Kluwer Academic Publishers. Printed in Great Britain.*

Epidemiology, aetiology and prevalence

In the West, PHPT is commonly discovered by screening populations biochemically for hypercalcaemia, and is discovered in up to 25 per 100 000 persons [2]. In menopausal females, as many as 0.19% [1] to 1% [3] may have the disease. Stone disease by comparison is seen in 1.2–4.6 per 10 000 in the UK [4] and more commonly in males [5].

In Pakistan, PHPT is twice as common in females. Fifty-seven per cent of our patients are less than 40 years old (mean age 38 ± 13 years). PHPT is the responsible aetiological factor in 1.25% of our stones [6], a situation similar to that in the West in the years 1961–79 [7, 8], when 1–5% of stones were due to PHPT. Now, only 0.17% of stones are due to this disease [9], as early detection and therapy reduce the possibility of long-standing disease. In Taiwan, in contrast, 7.8% of stone formers have PHPT [10].

In the West, units operate on as many as 75 patients a year [11]. In Pakistan, PHPT is less common, rarely detected, and seldom reported. Few units would operate on more than five patients a year. In our unit, 0.075% of the surgical operating output is for PHPT, with 35 operations done over a period of nine years. This is comparable with a personal series from the West [12] and from India [13].

In the normal gland, an increase in serum calcium is the chief signal for decrease of PTH secretion. In the presence of the normal calcium-ion-sensing cell-surface protein, extracellular calcium ions stimulate phospholipase C, leading to the accumulation of inositol 1,4,5-triphosphate, which in turn elevates the cytosolic calcium concentration by release of calcium ions from intracellular stores [14] which then lowers PTH excretion.

Not much is known about the reasons for development of PHPT, except in the rare neonatal fulminant form of hereditary hyperparathyroidism which occurs in families with idiopathic familial hypocalciuric hypercalcaemia (IFHH). These two diseases are caused by a genetic mutation (homozygous in neonatal hyperparathyroidism, and heterozygous in IFHH) in the gene for the calcium-ion-sensing cell-surface receptor, which is situated on the long arm of chromosome 3 [14]. The mutation results in inactivation of the protein receptor, and hence a failure of parathyroid secretion to be suppressed by high serum calcium levels. Isolated cases of adult hereditary hyperparathyroidism (autosomal dominant or recessive inheritance) are rare, as is PHPT as part of multiple endocrine neoplasia syndromes (autosomal dominant inheritance). Atomic bomb survivors from Hiroshima and Nagasaki have a higher incidence of PHPT [15], but the genetic mutation involved is not known.

Lithium increases the tritiated-thymidine uptake by abnormal parathyroid glands [16] and it may be a trigger mitogen promoting and accelerating the development of PHPT. Patients on lithium stand a higher risk of becoming hypercalcaemic, as lithium alters the set point of parathyroid cells.

In some patients it has been possible to lower PTH levels by administration of calcitriol (dihydroxy-vitamin D_3), as it down-regulates the expression of the PTH gene in the parathyroid gland, suggesting that vitamin D can alter the set point of PTH secretion [17]. The role of vitamin D, if any, in pathogenesis is not clear.

Parathyroid hyperplasia, adenomas and carcinomas

Hyperparathyroidism can result from hypersecretion of adenomatous, hyperplastic or carcinomatous glands. In the West, 90% are due to adenomas. In our experience, 88.6% are due to adenomas, 5.7% due to hyperplasia, and 5.7% due to carcinoma. Yoshioda [18] noted a similar incidence of carcinoma (4.6%) in asymptomatic patients. The incidence of carcinoma is higher in series from the East as compared to the West, where only 0.26–0.4% have carcinoma [19–21].

The clinical picture

In general, patients with PHPT can present with a variety of symptoms which reflect the diverse actions of PTH: bone pains; renal colic; symptoms of pancreatitis or peptic ulcer; psychiatric symptoms; or polyuria, constipation, and renal failure. Some will have hypertension, which maintains the normal circadian rhythm, [22] with a fall in blood pressure at night. This hypertension is not secondary to renal failure; serum renin is normal and the hypertension is related to serum calcium. Polyuria results because calcium has a diuretic action on the proximal tubule, and inhibits the action of antidiuretic hormone.

When such symptoms occur in stone patients, they alert the physician to the possibility of PHPT. In most stone patients PHPT does not produce symptoms (other than those produced by the stones). Therefore, if PHPT is to be detected as a cause of stone, all patients with stone disease will have to be screened biochemically by a serum calcium test for PHPT.

In our series, 34%, 31% and 28.5% of patients had bone disease alone, stone disease alone, or bone and stone disease, respectively. Bone disease was identified by symptoms, or by X-ray appearance. Fifty-eight per cent of our patients have stone disease, much as the Western populations in the years 1961–79, when 39–78% had stones [7, 8]. Bone changes are fairly common, and the alkaline phosphatase is 580 ± 1178 units/L. In India, Gupta [13] noted stones and nephrocalcinosis in 82%, bone disease in 55%, hypertension in 27% and proximal myopathy in 18%.

Mechanism of stone formation in PHPT

Whilst excess calcium excretion has been held responsible for stone formation [1], stones can occur in the absence of overt hypercalciuria. Hyperuricosuria may contribute to stone formation. Ljunghall and Ackerstrom [23] have demonstrated correlations between serum calcium and 24 hour uric acid excretion. Others have noted a reduction in the stone inhibitory potential of urine.

Cost-effective detection and screening

PHPT is diagnosed by demonstrating concurrent elevated serum calcium and inappropriately raised PTH concentration. Serum phosphorus is low, but this is not diagnostic. In our patients, mean serum calcium was 12.23 ± 1.92 mg/dl, with a range from 9.6–18 mg/dl; and serum phosphorous was 2.3 ± 0.84 (1.2–5.3) mg/dl. The PTH level, normal in one patient, was elevated up to 2900 times the upper limit of normal values in the remainder. (The variation in the normal values of the various kits used over the nine-year period precludes the use of absolute units.)

As the removal of hyperfunctioning parathyroid tissue dramatically reduces recurrence, it is cost-effective to screen all stone patients for PHPT in spite of the low yield. The best screening test is a serum calcium (which costs Rs 60 – US\$ 2.00 in 1993 Rs value). Abnormal values of calcium lead to further investigations: serum PTH (US\$ 6) and simultaneous serum calcium and phosphorus (US\$ 2.00 each), to confirm PHPT.

Because of the low incidence in relation to the West, and elusive intermittent hypercalcaemia in PHPT, we felt that it was appropriate to repeat calcium investigations on subsequent yearly follow-up visits for check-up for recurrence. Seldom do we pick up PHPT from these numerous calcium investigations. It is necessary to calculate the corrected serum calcium, because low albumin levels are common in this part of the world, and ionized calcium estimations are not as yet practical.

Similarly, in the group of patients with low serum phosphorus levels, diligent follow-up has failed to detect PHPT if serum calcium levels have remained normal. Other causes such as decreased intake of phosphorus containing foods and phosphaturia should be sought as a cause. Idiopathic hypercalciuria with low serum phosphorus would be the main differential diagnosis in the West.

Should random screening of serum calcium be done in Pakistan to detect PHPT before it causes stone?

In the West and Japan, parathyroid disease is being detected more frequently by random biochemical screening. The beneficial effects of this include the reduction in the numbers of stone patients due to PHPT. Should we in Pakistan also adopt this approach of random screening of populations?

Biochemical screening of large populations seems attractive for the following reasons:

- Severe biochemical or pathological derangement can exist in the absence of symptoms.
- A third of asymptomatic patients may have decreased creatinine clearance, though the BUN and creatinine are normal.
- Hypercalcaemia increases the risk of premature death [3].
- As many as 4.6% of asymptomatic patients [18] to 5.7% of symptomatic ones [6] have carcinoma.

On this basis, one could argue for screening asymptomatic populations in the third world as in the West. However, the majority of cases will be detected in menopausal females. These patients will not have stone disease, and mass screening will not be cost-effective for stone prevention.

Additionally, the NIH consensus conference has suggested that most asymptomatic patients with mild hypercalcaemia and normal creatinine clearance, only require watching until they develop osteopaenia or alteration of creatinine clearance [24].

Mass screening of hospitalized patients is certainly not cost-effective for detecting PHPT. In this setting, the majority will have hypercalcaemia from malignancy or because of the administration of calcium carbonate as an antacid in chronic renal failure.

Shek *et al.* [25] found hypercalcaemia in 462 (1.6%) of 29 107 samples. Hypercalcaemia was confirmed in a second sample in 183 (60%) of 302 accessible patients of which 72% were due to malignancy, 6.0% due to tuberculosis and only 5.5% due to PHPT. Such examples demonstrate how as much as US$ 6500 may be spent to detect one parathyroid adenoma! In contrast, screening stone patients will cost 160 dollars for every detected patient, given an incidence of 1.25%.

In general, routine tests have a problem: they push costs of medical care significantly, without necessarily improving health care. Physicians may not see the results of routinely ordered tests. In one study, only 1 in 4 hypercalcaemics detected by routine biochemical test were noted and followed-up by physicians [26].

It is usually cost-ineffective to screen patients with tests ordered as a batch without reasoning out the need for the test, without knowing the accuracy of the test and its limitation, or without a definitive useful intervention when the result is abnormal.

Elucidating the cause of hypercalcaemia

In a stone patient, hypercalcaemia is probably due to PHPT, as the other causes such as vitamin D intoxication, malignancy and sarcoidosis, are infrequent [1]. Though often quoted as a cause, thiazide administration rarely causes hypercalcaemia except in patients with PHPT, and this can be confirmed as a cause from the history and by repeating a serum calcium after stopping the drug. Benign idiopathic familial hypocalciuric hypercalcaemia (IFHH) should be considered in differential diagnosis, especially in children, as PHPT is rare at this age. Raised serum calcium and normal urinary calcium will be found in other family members as well. IFHH is not associated with urinary tract stones.

A PTH level will establish the diagnosis of PHPT. Of the different assays available, intact PTH molecule (iPTH) is the best, particularly in the presence of renal impairment. We have only recently changed to measuring iPTH and our results reported here refer to mid-molecular assays. Assays for iPTH have a 97% sensitivity [27]. False negatives can be minimized by performing iPTH estimations after EDTA infusions [28], if clinical suspicion is strong and the iPTH results are normal.

The PTH estimation should be combined with a repeat serum calcium as this will detect the occasional patient with normal PTH levels and PHPT. The following case early in our experience with PHPT demonstrates this:

Mrs ZS. Recurrent stone former. Serum calcium 12.0, phosphorus 2.6 mg/dl max normal PTH 0.27 ng/ml. Whilst the PTH is in the normal range, one would expect the high calcium to suppress PTH levels, which it obviously has not done. This patient had an arteriogram which demonstrated a 3-cm adenoma. This was successfully removed. Today we operate on the basis of the biochemical evaluation and would not think of doing an arteriogram.

It is cost-ineffective to request a PTH estimation (cost US$ 6) in stone patients unless a (at times single) calcium estimation is abnormal.

Management

The patient with proven PHPT and stone disease should have a neck exploration and removal of the offending adenoma(s), or excision of 3.5 glands in hyperplasia (see below for alternative management). Any physician involved in the management of PHPT will need to address some of the issues that are discussed below.

Does treatment of PHPT reduce stone formation?

Parathyroidectomy in patients with PHPT is rewarding, as patients will remain stone free or show a decrease in the number of stones formed. Nephrocalcinosis and pre-existing stones may disappear. In McGeown's series, new stone formation reduced from 0.24 to 0.05/patient year [29] and in Deaconsons *et al.*'s from 0.36 to 0.02 per patient year [30]. Patients with adenoma have a greater tendency to remain stone free, but 45% of patients with hyperplasia may reform their stones [31]. In general 5.6% [30] to 11% [32] may reform a stone.

When does hypercalcaemia require urgent treatment?

Patients vary in their response to elevated serum calcium. Symptoms start at 11.5–12 mg (2.9–3 mmol). Serum calcium elevations above 15 mg should be promptly brought down, as at these levels there is risk of coma or cardiac arrest. Smaller elevations can be corrected by improving hydration by intravenous fluid therapy and furosemide which reduces calcium reabsorption in the ascending limb of the loop of Henle [1]. Salmon, and now human calcitonin can be used to bring down the calcium as a temporary measure before surgery. Bisphosphonates, such as plicamycin and pamidronate, can be used as additional measures.

Who should operate?

In the setting of renal stone disease, the urologist is primarily responsible for diagnosing PHPT. The exploration for PHPT should however be done by a person competent in surgery in the neck, particularly thyroid surgery, and familiar with neck anatomy. Where urology residencies train surgeons to do parathyroid explorations, or when urologists have had a full general surgical training before urology fellowships, it is appropriate that the urologist operates, but only if on a regular basis. The specialty of endocrine surgery is not developed in Pakistan. It is the urologist's responsibility to have the operation done by a competent person.

The disease is infrequently picked up, and most surgeons in Pakistan will be occasional operators (less than five operations per year). This is disadvantageous for the patient, and it is preferable to send all patients with PHPT to one tertiary hospital.

Preoperative localization

Examination of the neck may be revealing: the occasional adenoma is palpable, especially in Pakistan where the gland may be 3 cm long. More often there is a prominence of one or the other side of the neck in the region of the thyroid, best detected by using the thumb to palpate the neck, whilst sitting in front of the patient.

Localizing the gland preoperatively reduces operating time and allows the surgeon to exercise the option of unilateral neck exploration.

Preoperative localization is usually however reserved only for re-explorations [24]. No method of localizing parathyroid adenomas has a sensitivity of more than 70%. Sonography has a sensitivity of 43% [33] to 71.5% but the positive predictive value is 88% as compared to 38% for CT with drip infusion of contrast. CT in combination with sonography has a 78% sensitivity [18]. CT is more useful in identifying mediastinal adenomas where the initial exploration has failed because the gland was in the mediastinum. The use of Gd-DTPA increases the sensitivity of MRI by increasing the contrast of the parathyroid. In persisting hyperparathyroidism after failed surgery, ultrasound localization is helpful. Selective catheterization and estimation of PTH identifies the site in 63% [33].

Thallium–technetium (Th–Tc) scan has a 64% sensitivity [27], but only 45% of ectopic glands can be correctly recognized [34]. Th–Tc scan correctly predicted the side of the adenoma, but a third of those interpreted as lower parathyroids were in fact large drooping (ptosed) upper parathyroids [35]. Gallagher *et al.* [36] suggest the use of induced hypocalcaemia to increase the uptake of parathyroids in a Th–Tc scan. Dual radioactive toluidine blue – Tc-99 m thyroid scintigraphy has a sensitivity of 87%, a specificity of 94%, and an accuracy of 92% [37]. There is also a 98% success rate in localizing the small and ectopic glands.

We operate on few (3–7) parathyroids each year. We therefore requested Th–Tc scans to identify the site of the adenoma as suggested by Okerlund *et al.* [38]. We have found negative scans even with adenomas as large as 33 mm (long axis) and have not found the Th–Tc scan useful. It is cost-ineffective for the primary exploration. Initially available free, it now costs US$ 50 at government hospitals and US$ 260 at private institutions. It is generally agreed that preoperative localization be restricted to patients undergoing re-exploration.

As re-exploration of the neck is associated with a 41% incidence of hypoparathyroidism, 2% risk of death, and 6% risk of vocal cord paralysis [39], preoperative localization is justified before re-exploration. Re-exploration is poorly accepted by Pakistani patients. Compliance is low; additional costs have to be borne by individuals for the re-exploration. Therefore in Pakistan, it is necessary to reduce the negative primary exploration rate to as low a figure as possible by every possible means. In our series of 35 patients, we were unable to find the gland in two patients at initial exploration.

Peroperative localization of the glands

Peroperative localization of the glands by methylene blue is a useful adjunct for the occasional operator (less than ten operations per year). Methylene blue (6–8 mg/kg) given intravenously diluted in 200 ml of normal saline, half to one hour prior to operation, stains the glands grey–blue. The larger dose per kilogram is used for lean individuals with a higher muscle to fat ratio: muscle takes up more of the methylene blue than does fat. Infusion causes a dark blue pigmentation of the skin and interferes with the pulse oximeter readings during infusion. The dye is eliminated by renal excretion but is retained in the parathyroid glands. We have had one episode of bradycardia and hypotension, in a patient who was prone to vasovagal attacks and had similar attacks when taken for her previous eye surgeries (at which time, methylene blue had not been used).

We recommend using methylene blue for the occasional operator, because it reduces operating time from around five hours to less than two hours [12].

Intraoperative monitoring to test completeness of surgery

Serial monitoring of iPTH has been used in the West to detect the completeness of operation [40] as results are available in 15 min. Blood should be drawn 10 min after the removal of all abnormal tissue. However, it has been shown that patients may have normal levels of iPTH prior to surgery, and that levels fall after removal of the first adenoma; it is not therefore a substitute for bilateral exploration.

Urinary cyclic AMP is not feasible in the average clinical service laboratory. Intraoperative ultrasonography has been used by some.

Unilateral operation or bilateral exploration?

Tiblin *et al.* [41] noted long-term hypocalcaemia in 16% of patients who had bilateral exploration, compared to 4% in those who had unilateral exploration. Unilateral exploration requires less time for operation. For these reasons it is recommended by Yoshioda [18] who uses this approach for 86% of his patients.

In the third world, the operator cannot afford to miss a second adenoma (10% of all adenomas have a second adenoma), as the patient cannot afford to have a second operation for a condition that could have been so easily detected at the primary operation. As even intraoperative estimation of iPTH cannot rule out the presence of another gland, and there is no foolproof method of ensuring removal of all functioning tissue except by careful exploration and follow-up, we feel currently that a full exploration is advisable.

Histological proof of identification of parathyroid gland

Many (70% of surgeons questioned by Tiblin *et al.* [41]) consider intraoperative histological confirmation necessary, but biopsy of the remaining glands is practised regularly only in the US and Sweden. Much looks like parathyroid tissue and histological confirmation by biopsy is necessary to ensure that all glands are identified and fat lobules or thyroid nodules are not mistakenly identified as parathyroids. Visual identification is not enough.

A careful technique during biopsy of the remaining glands (see below) will not increase the incidence or severity or duration of hypocalcaemia. Tenting up one pole of the gland by a 5/0 prolene suture and snipping it off with an iris scissors can remove adequate tissue for biopsy confirmation (that the gland identified is a parathyroid gland) without lifting the entire parathyroid from its vascular bed.

Exploration for mediastinal parathyroid

Most mediastinal parathyroids are in the thymus and most can be removed through the neck, as the blood supply to the thymus is from the neck. A median sternotomy is not often required. However, if a Th–Tc scan detects a parathyroid in the chest, and a CT scan shows that this is a large, deeply seated mass, or the planes of the capsule are not clearly defined, the primary exploration must be through a median sternotomy.

In our series of 30 adenomas, two were intrathyroideal, four were mediastinal (three of these being intra-thymic), six right superior, three right inferior, four left superior, and 11 left inferior. The two carcinomas were right superior and right inferior. Of the mediastinal parathyroid adenomas, two were detected by radioisotope scan and confirmed by CT to require a thoracotomy. The others were removed through the cervical incision.

Alternatives to surgery

Ablation by deliberate injection of large dose of radiocontrast material into the artery that selectively perfuses the adenoma [42] is not cost-effective as an alternative to primary exploration. It requires a high level of skill, and whilst immediate success was obtained in 22 of 30 procedures in 27 patients, long-term control was obtained in 17 (63%) [42]. Percutaneous ethanol injection has been used in Japan and Italy. An approach with selective contrast ablation and surgical re-exploration only in failed cases appears attractive for recurrent disease in otherwise ill patients.

Simultaneous operation for PHPT with that for other diseases

Though parathyroid surgery may occasionally take a long time, it does not involve sudden shifts in intravascular volume. It is therefore safe to combine surgery for PHPT simultaneously or sequentially, with operations for other diseases. Serum calcium should be monitored intraoperatively during the second operation, as a patient with hungry bones and renal stones, requiring surgery for PHPT and say, renal stones, may drop serum calcium to alarmingly low levels (4 mg/dl in one of our patients). In such cases, where alkaline phosphatase and bone X-rays are suggestive of severe bone involvement, the surgeon may wish to do the additional procedure first, before the parathyroidectomy.

Farley *et al.* [43] have combined parathyroid exploration in 117 patients with other operations on the breast (25), biliary tract (21), female genitourinary tract (19), and intra-abdominal (18) and cardiothoracic (6) regions. The mean operating time was 155 min and hospital stay 7.6 days [43].

Prediction and management of severe postoperative hypocalcaemia

Facial tingling will alert the physician to the possibility of hypocalcaemia. In patients with extensive bone and stone disease, profound hypocalcaemia can occur and has required continuous drip infusion of calcium to maintain reasonable calcium levels.

Postoperative hypocalcaemia, which reaches its nadir around the morning of the first postoperative day in the West [1], or around the second to third day in our experience, results from a drop in the PTH levels as the remaining suppressed glands struggle to produce more hormone. The fat content of the gland has been taken to indicate the degree of suppression of the gland. On a histological section, up to 30% of the section of normal parathyroid tissue will consist of fat cells. Cusamano *et al.* [44] have noted that postoperative hypocalcaemia is more profound when the remaining glands show more extensive replacement of the gland by fat. In our study we were not able to confirm this and found no correlation between the amount of fat in the gland [45], and the degree of postoperative hypocalcaemia, which correlated with the extent of the bone disease as shown by alkaline phosphatase. Hypocalcaemia will be exaggerated by inadvertent interference with the blood supply of the remaining glands, or removal of an excess amount of glandular tissue in patients with hyperplasia. Profound postoperative hypocalcaemia is also seen in patients with extensive coexisting bone disease, and serum alkaline phosphatase is a good predictor of the amount of calcium required to maintain normocalcaemia. As calcium is deposited in bone, it carries magnesium with it. Magnesium is essential for the manufacture, release and peripheral action of PTH. Serum magnesium drops postoperatively in patients with bone disease, and low serum magnesium levels will predict more profound and prolonged hypocalcaemia. Magnesium sulphate orally or intramuscularly is effective in combating hypomagnesaemia. Bone remineralization takes a long time, and some noted no change in the dual photon absorptiometry in the bone density of lumbar spine at one year, though it increased in the femoral neck by 7.4%.

In the West, PHPT manifesting as renal stones is associated with minor changes in serum calcium, and small glands, and less marked changes in bone density.

Prevention of persistent postoperative hypocalcaemia

Persistent postoperative hypocalcaemia is likely to occur on a long-term basis without an end-point in patients with hyperplasia in whom too much tissue has been removed. It is therefore prudent to follow a procedure of removing all four parathyroids and then implant a portion of one-half of a gland in the forearm or sternomastoid. This will prevent hypocalcaemia, and if the remaining graft hyperfunctions, this can easily be detected by radioisotope scanning, and a part of the surviving transplant could be removed. It is preferable to transplant a portion of the parathyroid in the arm than to leave behind a half gland in the neck.

Cryopreservation of parathyroid grafts is another useful adjunct in treatment of hyperplasia patients. It allows replantation in those cases where serum calcium does not return to normal. Cryopreserved tissue can also be used in those 10% [46] of cases of hyperplasia where the initial autograft into the forearm fails or malfunctions [46]. Freezers used for storing bone marrow can be used. Tanaka *et al.* [47] have shown that the ratio of PTH levels in veins draining the implanted tissue and veins in the contralateral arm will be 1.5 after one week if the graft has taken.

Conclusion

PHPT is an uncommon cause of stones, but can be easily detected by screening stone patients, using serum calcium as an initial screening test, followed by iPTH assay in hypercalcaemic patients. Treatment for stone patients with PHPT is by operation, preferably in a tertiary centre. Stone formation decreases following successful parathyroidectomy.

References

1. Halabe A, Sutton RAL. Primary hyperparathyroidism as a cause of calcium nephrolithiasis. In: Coe FL, Favus M, editors. Disorders of bone and mineral metabolism. New York: Raven Press; 1992:671–84.
2. Heath HW III, Hodgson SF, Kennedy MA. Primary hyperparathyroidism; incidence morbidity and potential economic impact on the community. N Engl J Med 1980;302:189–93.
3. Ljunghall S, Hillman P, Rastad J *et al.* PHPT epidemiology diagnosis and clinical picture. World J Urol 1991;15:681–7.
4. Charig CR, Webb DR, Payne SR. Comparison of treatment of renal calculi by open surgery, PCNL and ESWL. Br Med J 1986;292:879–82.
5. Friedrichs R, Behrendt U, Graf K. PHPT studies of 4000 patients treated by ESWL. Helv Chir Acta 1991;58:327–30.
6. Talati J. Genitourinary surgery in Pakistan. In: Ahmed, Blanchard, Eckloff *et al.*, editors. Surgery for all. Lahore: Ferozesons, 1992:373.
7. Silverberg J. Nephrolithiasis and bone involvement in PHPT. Am J Med 1990;89:327–34.
8. Broadus AE, Horst RL *et al.* The importance of circulating 1,25 (OH) vitamin D in the pathogenesis of hypercalcemia and renal stone formation in PHPT. N Engl J Med 1991;302:421–6.
9. Derick FC. Renal calculi in association with hyperparathyroidism, a changing entity. J Urol 1982;127:226.
10. Su. Metabolic evaluation of active stone formers. Abstract 80, 2nd Asian Congress of Urology Abstracts; 1993.
11. Brasier AR, Nussbaum SR. Hungry bone syndrome: Clinical and biochemical predictors of its occurrence after parathyroid surgery. Am J Med 1988;84:654–60.
12. Hadfield J. The surgery of parathyroid glands: Personal series of 65 patients. Pak J Surg 1989;5:1–4.
13. Gupta MM. Primary hyperparathyroidism. J Assoc Phy India 1990;38:154–6.

14. Brown EM, Pollack M, Siedman CE *et al.* Calcium-ion-sensing cell-surface receptors. N Engl J Med 1995;234–9.
15. Fujiwara S. A review of 45 years of study of Hiroshima and Nagasaki atomic bomb survivors: Hyperparathyroidism. J Radiation Res Tokyo 1991;32:245–8.
16. Saxe AW, Gibson G. Lithium increases the tritiated thymidine uptake by abnormal parathyroid glands. Surgery 1991;110:1067–76.
17. Ackerstrom G, Rastad J, Ljunghall S *et al.* Cellular physiology and pathology of the parathyroid glands. World J Surg 1991;15:672–88.
18. Yoshioda. PHPT: Problems in surgical indications and treatment. Hinyokika Kiyo 1991;37:1185–90.
19. Obara T, Fujimoto Y. Diagnosis and treatment of patients with parathyroid carcinoma, an update and review World J Surg 1991;15:738–44.
20. van Heerden JA, Grant CS. Surgical treatment of PHPT an institutional perspective. World J Surg 1991;15:688–92.
21. Sandelin K, Thompson NW, Budeson L. Metastatic parathyroid carcinoma; dilemmas in management. Surgery 1991;110:978–86.
22. Middeki M, Klirglich M, Holzgrave H. Circadian blood pressure rhythm in primary and secondary hypertension. Chronobiol Int 1991;8:451–9.
23. Ljunghall S, Ackerstrom G. Urate metabolism in primary hyperparathyroidism. Urol Int 1982;37:73–8.
24. Consensus development conference panel. Diagnosis and management of asymptomatic primary hyperparathyroidism: Consensus development conference statement. Ann Int Med 1991;114:593–7.
25. Shek CC, Natkunam A, Tsang V *et al.* Incidence, cause and mechanism of hypercalcemia in a hospital population in Hong Kong. Quart J Med 1990;77:1277–85.
26. Frohlic A, MacNair P, Transbol I. Awareness of hypercalcemia in a hospital population. Scan J Clin Lab Invest 1991;51:37–41.
27. Livingstone JI, Tellez M, Burke M *et al.* A three year audit of the role of PTH assays and Th Tc isotope subtraction scan in preoperative investigation of PHPT. Postgrad Med J 1991;67:1055–8.
28. Bergenfelz, Valdermarrsson S, Ahren B. Measurement of intact parahormone in the diagnosis of hyperparathyroidism. Acta Endocrinol Copenhagen 1991;125:668–74.
29. McGeown MG. Effect of parathyroidectomy on the incidence of renal calculi. Lancet 1961;1:586–7.
30. Deaconson TF, Wilson SD, Lehman J Jr. The effect of parathyroidectomy on the recurrence of nephrolithiasis. Surgery 1987;102:910–13.
31. Siminowitch JMP, Caldwell BE Jr, Straffon RA. Renal lithiasis and hyperparathyroidism; diagnosis, management and prognosis. J Urol 1981;126:720–2.
32. Purnell DC, Smith LH, Scholz DA *et al.* PHPT, a prospective clinical study. Am J Med 1971;50:670–8.
33. Buhr HJ, Graf S, Herfarth C. Clinical aspects, diagnosis and surgical therapy of persisting PHPT. Chirurg 1992;63:103–8.
34. Summers GW. Parathyroid exploration. Arch Otolaryn Head Neck Surg 1991;117:1237–41.
35. Chan TY, Serpill JW, Chan O *et al.* Misinterpretation of upper parathyroid adenoma on thallium 201 Tc 99m subtraction scan. Br J Radiol 1991;64:1–4.
36. Gallagher SJ, Fraser WD, Logue FC, Boyle IT. Augmentation of parathyroid 201 Ti/99Tcm scanning by perfusion of trisodium edentate. Nucl Med Commun 1991;93:797.
37. Czerniak A, Zwaas ST, Shustik O *et al.* The use of radio iodinated toluidine blue for preoperative localization of parathyroids. Pathol Surg 1991;110:832–8.
38. Okerlund MD, Sheldon K, Corpuz E *et al.* A new method with high sensitivity and specified for localisation of abnormal parathyroid glands. Ann Surg 1984;200:381–8.
39. Lafferty FW, Hubay CA. Primary hyperparathyroidism: A review of the long term surgical and non surgical morbidities as a basis for a rational approach to treatment. Arch Intern Med 1989;149:780–96.

40. Robertson GS, Iqbal SJ, Bolia A *et al.* Intraoperative PTH estimation, a valuable adjunct to parathyroid surgery. Ann R Coll Surg Eng 1992;74:19–22.
41. Tiblin S, Bondesson AG, Uden P *et al.* Current trends in surgical treatment of solitary parathyroid adenoma, a questionnaire study from 53 surgical departments in 14 countries. Eur J Surg 1991;157:103–7.
42. Pas HI, Brennan MF, Norton JA *et al.* Results of a multidisciplinary strategy for management of mediastinal parathyroid adenoma in a case of persisting PHPT. Ann Surg 1992;215:101–6.
43. Farley DR, van Heerden JA, Grant CS. Are concomitant surgical procedures acceptable in patients undergoing cervical exploration for PHPT. Mayo Clin Proc 1991;66:681–5.
44. Cusamano RJ, Mahadevia P, Silver C. Intraoperative histological evaluation in exploration of parathyroid glands. Surg Gynaecol Obstet 1989;169:506–10.
45. Khan A, Shaikh H, Talati J. In primary hyperparathyroidism due to adenomas, post-operative hypocalcemia is not influenced by histology of remaining glands. In Ryall *et al.*, editors. Urolithiasis 2. New York: Plenum Publishers, 1994.
46. Wagner PK, Seesko HG, Rothmund M. Replantation of cryopreserved human parathyroid tissue. World J Surg 1991;15:751–5.
47. Tanaka Y, Tominaga Y, Hayashi S *et al.* Kinetics of PTH metabolism after parathyroidectomy and graft into forearm in patients with secondary hyperparathyroidism due to chronic renal failure. Nippon Geka Gakkai Zaashi 1991;92:57–63.

43. The role of diet in the prevention of urolithiasis

SALMA HALAI BADRUDDIN

Urolithiasis is associated with a group of urinary risk factors that potentially can promote the formation of urinary calculi. These include low urine volume, low pH, hyperoxaluria, hypercalciuria, hyperuricosuria and reduced urinary inhibitors of crystal formation. This chapter will review the potential role of diet in modifying the above mentioned factors.

Fluid

In a review of risk factors in calcium stone disease, Robertson *et al.* [1] state that the 24-hour urinary volume is more important as a biochemical risk factor than either oxalate or calcium excretion. Chronic dehydration has been identified as the major cause of stone disease in 13 to 19% of patients attending a stone clinic [2, 3]. The causes of chronic dehydration were hot climate 40%, hot occupation 29%, poor water intake 30%, sports 1%. The occurrence of chronic dehydration is very possible in a country like Pakistan which has a relatively hot climate and a large percentage of the population engaged in agricultural and other physically demanding occupations. In urban areas the unavailability of safe drinking water and the lack of public toilet facilities may both result in a voluntary restriction of fluid intake. Therefore proper prescription of fluid intake should form an integral part of the dietary management of urolithiasis. The objective should be to maintain a urine output of at least 2 l with a specific gravity of less than 1.015 through each 24-hour period. To accomplish this the patient must drink 3–4 l of liquid per day [4]. A higher intake will be required if there is excessive sweating or diarrhoea. Such a programme of high fluid intake has been reported to prevent new stone formation in approximately 60% of patients with idiopathic calcium urolithiasis [5].

Diet and urinary pH

Alkalization of urine is usually achieved by ingesting citrate salts, although the pH of urine may be changed by eating certain types of foods which will leave an alkaline residue in the body. Foods that produce an alkaline urine are: milk and cream; carbonated beverages; fruits except plums and prunes; all vegetables except corn;

J. Talati et al. (eds) The Management of Lithiasis, 289–295
© *1997 Kluwer Academic Publishers. Printed in Great Britain.*

lentils (dals) and beans; coconut and almonds; and baking soda and baking powder [4, 6].

Although there are no reports of specific foods (other than citrus fruit) that can increase the urinary citrate levels, several workers have reported that hypocitraturia can be induced by diets high in sodium and animal proteins [7–9].

Oxalate

Increased urinary oxalate excretion promotes the formation of stones. In normal urine the molar ratio of calcium to oxalate is usually 5:1. A ratio of 1:1 favours stone formation. Therefore increases in urinary excretion of oxalate have a greater effect on crystalline mass than increases in calcium [10].

About 10–20% of the urinary oxalate is derived from diet; the remainder comes from the metabolism of glycine and ascorbic acid [11]. Under normal circumstances the pathways for metabolism of ascorbic acid to oxalate are saturated, so that an increase in ascorbic acid intake does not result in increased urinary oxalate excretion. However in susceptible individuals large doses (1–2 g/day) of ascorbic acid result in an increase in oxalate excretion [12]. Excessive intake of ascorbic acid can also lead to a decreased urinary pH due to the high excretion of ascorbic acid, which may further facilitate stone formation. Deficiency of pyridoxine has also been reported to increase the formation and excretion of oxalate. Vitamin B_6 is a co-factor in the glyoxalate–glycine reaction. Decreased transamination of glyoxalate to glycine results in shunting it to oxalate [13].

Dietary restriction of oxalate is particularly indicated when there is increased intestinal absorption of oxalate. Hyperoxaluria frequently occurs as an adjunct to absorptive hypercalciuria, since the high intestinal absorption of calcium does not leave sufficient calcium to complex oxalate in the intestinal tract and prevent its absorption. Dietary restriction of calcium in the management of calcium oxalate urolithiasis further compounds the problem. Smith [10] reviewed several studies which suggest that urinary oxalate excretion is inversely related to dietary intake of calcium. Massey and Sutton [14] have recently shown that patients on a diet containing moderate amounts of calcium (650 mg/day) which was restricted in only eight high oxalate foods (rhubarb, beet, spinach, nuts, chocolate, berries, wheat bran and tea) excreted 392 μmol/day oxalate as compared to the urinary oxalate excretion of 432 μmol/day by patients who omitted all dairy products and consumed only 0.5 mmol/day (5.6 mg/day) oxalate. The patient should be helped to choose foods according to personal preference, such that intake does not exceed 50 mg/day [15].

A patient may have one 100-g serving of any one of the following foods which contain 5–50 mg oxalate per 100 g: liver, beans, corn, bell pepper (*Shimla Mirch*), red plums, coffee, ovaltine. The following, which contain more than 50 mg per 100 g, should be avoided as far as possible: tea (110–156 mg/200 ml cup), beetroot, okra (*Bindi*), spinach, squash (*Kaddu*), *phalsa* (Grewia asiatica), *jamun* (Syzygium cumini), nuts, sesame seeds, chocolate, cocoa powder. The stronger the tea the more the oxalate content [6, 15].

When advising patients regarding a low oxalate diet special mention should be made of the fact that tea is high in oxalates, and particularly harmful if taken without milk – the calcium in milk precipitates oxalate. Herbal and green teas have been reported to have less than half the oxalate content of regular tea and could be used as a substitute for black tea [16]. Since green leafy vegetables are high in oxalate, it should be borne in mind that chewing *pan* (betel leaf) may also add substantially to the oxalate intake.

Calcium

Dietary calcium restriction has been standard therapy for calcium stone formers; however the advisability of strict dietary calcium restriction is now being questioned. Low calcium intake leads to increased oxalate absorption, and is reported to be inversely related to the risk of calcium oxalate stones as well as negative calcium balance with bone resorption. In a cohort of 45 619 men the relative risk of kidney stones was 0.56 (P for trend < 0.001) in the highest quintile for calcium intake (more than 1050 mg/day), compared to the lowest quintile (less than 605 mg/day) [17]. Fuss *et al.* [18] determined the bone mineral content in 32 male renal stone formers, 18 presenting with idiopathic urolithiasis and 14 with primary hyperparathyroidism. The bone mineral content of the radius was reduced in patients with idiopathic urolithiases on a low calcium diet to a similar level as patients with primary hyperparathyroidism. A second study of patients with idiopathic urolithiasis showed that the bone mineral content of these radius was significantly lower in those on a diet that provided only 359 mg calcium/day [19]. These authors suggest that it may be safer to treat idiopathic hypercalciuria with thiazide diuretics which reduce the renal excretion of calcium rather than a low calcium diet.

The best approach may be selectively to restrict high oxalate foods and insure a moderate intake of calcium of 600–800 mg/day at least as the first step in the prevention of recurring stone disease. Milk and milk products are the major sources of calcium in the diet. An intake of two cups of milk or its equivalent will provide approximately 600 mg calcium. Most green leafy vegetables provide substantial amounts of calcium but are also rich in oxalate and should be avoided.

Protein

In addition to oxalate and calcium, patients with recurrent nephrolithiasis have been reported to be particularly sensitive to dietary intake of animal protein. Goldfarb [20] reviewed population and clinical studies to show that a clear correlation exists between the consumption of animal protein and prevalence of nephrolithiasis. A high protein intake of 2 g/kg/day has been reported to increase urinary calcium and uric acid levels and decrease urinary citrate levels [8], which results in a significant decrease in the ability of the urine to inhibit calcium oxalate monohydrate crystal agglomeration. Grover *et al.* [21] have also shown that addition of a sodium urate solution to urine samples resulted in the spontaneous precipitation of calcium oxalate dihydrate crystals. A high protein diet which increases urinary uric acid not only increases the risk of uric acid stones but may also increase the risk of calcium oxalate stone formation. The protein intake should be no more than 1 g/kg of ideal body weight. The intake of foods rich in purines which can be metabolized to uric acid, should also be restricted in patients with calcium oxalate urolithiasis. In general foods high in protein are high in purines; however some vegetables and grain products such as cauliflower, green beans, peas and oatmeal also contribute substantial amounts of purine to the diet [22].

Sodium

There is a close relationship between renal tubular calcium and sodium handling, and most factors that increase urinary sodium excretion also tend to increase urinary calcium excretion. Therefore dietary sodium may also be a risk factor for hypercalciuria and thus for calcium oxalate stone formation. It has been reported that diets high in sodium decreased the ability of urine to inhibit calcium oxalate monohydrate crystal agglomeration and this effect was more marked when subjects were on a high protein, high sodium diet [8]. In a study of 282 patients with calcium oxalate kidney stones, dietary sodium was found to be more important than dietary protein, purine, or oxalate, in contributing to calcium excretion on a free diet [23]. Restriction of dietary sodium in patients with hypercalciuria has been shown to have a beneficial effect on calcium excretion [24]; therefore patients should be advised to decrease their sodium intake by restricting their salt intake to not more than one teaspoon/day (approximately 2300 mg Na) and to avoid obviously salty foods such as chips and salted nuts.

Vitamin A and glycosaminoglycans

Glycosaminoglycans (GAG) have been reported to act as inhibitors of calcium oxalate crystal growth and aggregation [25] and significant differences in GAG excretion in urolithiasis patients and healthy subjects have been reported [26].

Epidemiological data show that lower urinary tract stones seen in various countries of south-east Asia are related to protein malnutrition [27]. High protein diets have been reported to increase excretion of GAG in normal subjects [26]. A reduction in GAG excretion of 60 to 80% has been observed in children with deficient protein and vitamin A intake as compared with a healthy control group; GAG excretion normalized with vitamin A supplements despite continued protein deficiency [28]. Since diets high in protein also tend to be high in vitamin A, it is possible that the association between low protein diets and urolithiasis may really be a reflection of the vitamin A content of these diets. Animal studies have provided further support for the hypothesis that vitamin A deficiency enhances risk of bladder stones by increasing crystal formation and reducing crystal growth inhibitors such as GAGs in the urine [29].

Table 43.1   Dietary plan

Food group	Foods that can be included in diet as indicated	Foods to be avoided
Cereal and grains	Rice, atta, maida, pasta – to meet caloric requirement	Sewje, oatmeal
Protein foods	Meat, fish, poultry Legumes 100 g/day (half a cup cooked/day)	Organ meat
Milk and milk products	Two cups milk/day or equivalent	
Vegetables	All except those in avoid column	Green leafy vegetables, okra, squash, sweet potato, cauliflower, beetroot
Fruits	All except those in avoid column	Phalsa, jamun, berries
Miscellaneous	Ovaltine not more than 1 cup/day or coffee not more than 2 cups/day; Carbonated beverages – as desired within limits	Tea, nuts, sesame seed, chocolate, cocoa

Diets that are restricted in animal protein, dairy products and green leafy vegetables in an attempt to prevent recurrent stone disease may not provide adequate intake of vitamin A unless a special effort is made to include fruits and vegetables which are high in vitamin A but not in oxalate, such as papaya, mango, carrot, etc.

Large trials to determine the impact of vitamin A supplementation on morbidity and child survival have been carried out in India and other developing countries. A study of the incidence or recurrence of urolithiasis in these children as compared to controls would provide more definitive data regarding the impact of vitamin A deficiency in urolithiasis.

In summary the patient with recurrent calcium oxalate urolithiasis needs the following dietary modifications:

- Energy: According to body size and activity. The major source of calories should come from the allowed cereal and grain products.
- Protein: 1 g/kg ideal body weight.
- Fat: May need restriction if steatorrhoea present.
- Sodium: Less than 100 mEq/day (approximately 1 teaspoon salt).
- Calcium: 600–800 mg/day.
- Oxalate: Not more than 50 mg/day.
- Purines: Less than 125 mg/day.
- Fluids (mainly water): Not less than 3 l in 24 hours.

These modifications can be achieved by following the plan given in Table 43.1.

References

1. Robertson WG, Peacock M, Heyburn PJ *et al.* Risk factors in calcium stone disease. In: Brockis JG, Finlayson B, editors. Urinary calculus. Littleton: PSG Publishing, 1981:265–73.

2. Rose GA. Other metabolic causes of stone. In: Clinical and laboratory aspects. Rose GA, editor. Urinary stones. Lancaster: MTP Press, 1982:235.

3. Embon O, Rose GA, Rosenbaum T. Chronic dehydration stone disease. Br J Urol 1990;66:357–62.

4. Hui YH. Diet in kidney disease. In: Human nutrition and diet therapy. California: Wadsworth Health Sciences Division, 1983:728–9.

5. Hosking DH, Erickson SB, Van Den Berg CJ *et al.* The stone clinic effect in patients with idiopathic calcium urolithiasis. J Urol 1983;130:1115–1118.

6. Gopalan C, Rama Sastri BV, Balasubramanian SL. Nutritive value of Indian foods. India: National Institute of Nutrition. Indian Council Med Res Hyderabad, 1985.

7. Breslau NA, Brinkley L, Hill KD *et al.* Relationship role of animal protein – rich diet to kidney stone formation and calcium metabolism. J Clin Endocrinol Metab 1988;66:140–146.

8. Kok DJ, Iestra JA, Doorenbos CJ, Papapoulos SE. The effects of dietary excesses in animal protein and in sodium on the composition and the crystallization kinetics of calcium oxalate monohydrate in urines of healthy men. J Clin Endocrinol Metab 1990;71:861–7.

9. Pak CYC. Citrate and renal calculi. New insights and future directions. Am J Kidney Dis 1991;17:420–5.

10. Smith LH. Diet and hyperoxaluria in the syndrome of idiopathic calcium oxalate urolithiasis. Am J Kidney Dis 1991;17:370–5.

11. Wyngaarden JB, Elder TD. Primary hyperoxaluria and oxalosis. In: Stanbury JB, Wyngaarden JB, Fredrickson DS, editors. The metabolic bases of inherited disease. New York: McGraw-Hill, 1966:189.

12. Tiselius HG, Alugard LE. The diurnal excretion of oxalate and effect of pyridoxine and ascorbate on the oxalate excretion. Eur Urol 1977;3:41.

13. Harrison AR, Kasidas GP, Rose GA. Hyperoxaluria and recurrent stone formation apparently cured by short courses of pyridoxine. Br Med J 1981;282:2097–8.

14. Massey LK, Sutton RAL. Low oxalate, moderate calcium diet lowers urinary oxalate in calcium kidney stone-formers (abstract). J Am Diet Assoc 1992;92:A–9.

15. Ney DM, Hofmann AF, Fischer C, Stubblefield N. The low oxalate diet book. San Diego: University of California, 1981.

16. McKay DW, Seviour JP, Comerford A *et al.* Herbal tea: An alternative to regular tea for those who form calcium oxalate stones. J Am Dietetic Assoc 1995;95:360–1.

17. Curhan GC, Willett WC, Rimm EB, Stampfer MJ. A prospective study of dietary calcium and other nutrients and the risk of symptomatic kidney stones. N Engl J Med 1993;328:833–8.

18. Fuss M, Pepersack T, Bergman P *et al.* Low calcium diet in idiopathic urolithiasis: A risk factor for osteopenia as great as primary hyperparathyroidism. Br J Urol 1990;65:560–3.

19. Fuss M, Pepersack T, Van-Geel J *et al.* Involvement of low-calcium diet in the reduced bone mineral content of idiopathic renal stone formers. Calcif Tissue Int 1990;46:9–13.

20. Goldfarb S. The role of diet in the pathogenesis and therapy of nephrolithiasis. Endocrinol Metab Clin N Am 1990;19:805–20.

21. Grover PK, Ryall RL, Marshall VR. Effect of urate on calcium oxalate crystallization in human urine: Evidence for a promotory role of hyperuricosuria in urolithiasis. Clin Sci 1990;79:9–15.

22. Pennington JAT, Church HN. Food values of portions commonly used. Philadelphia: JB Lippincott, 1985.

23. Burtis WJ, Gay L, Insogna KL *et al.* Dietary hypercalciuria in patients with calcium oxalate kidney stones. Am J Clin Nutr 1994;60:424–9.

24. Silver J, Friedlander MM, Rubinger D *et al.* Sodium-dependent idiopathic hypercalciuria in renal stone formers. Lancet 1983;2:484.

25. Bowyer RC, Brockis JG, McCulloch RK. Glucosaminoglycans as inhibitors of calcium oxalate crystal growth and aggregation. Clin Chem Acta 1979;95:23–8.

26. Caudarella R, Rizzoli E, Malavnotta M. Clinical and metabolic aspects of urinary glycosaminoglycans excretion in calcium stone formers. In: Inhibitors of crystallization in renal lithiasis and their clinical application. Acta Med Roma 1988:187–92.

27. Anderson DA. Environmental factors in the etiology of urolithiasis. In: Civuentes-Delatte A, Rapado A, Hodgkinson A *et al.*, editors. Urinary calculi. Basel: Karger, 1973.
28. Danes BS, Bearn AG. The effect of retinol (vitamin A alcohol) on urinary excretion of mucopolysaccharides in Hurler syndrome. Lancet 1967;1:1027–31.
29. Kancha RK, Anasuya A. The effect of vitamin A deficiency on urinary calculus formation in rats. J Clin Biochem Nutr 1990;8:51–60.

44. Systematic follow-up of patients with recurrent nephrolithiasis: A guide for the practising urologist

NOSHIR F. DABHOIWALA

Recurrence is common in stone disease. In the past, urologists attempted to prevent recurrence by correcting anatomic defects, restoring good urinary drainage and treating concomitant infections. An improved understanding of the basic underlying pathophysiology of nephrolithiasis allows the urologist to incorporate a basic screening and therapy programme for the recurrent stone-former in his post-therapy management of the patient. The practising urologist struggling against time in a busy outpatient service or office practice can always liaise with a local laboratory and a nephrologist with similar interests. In the majority of cases he can then provide his patients with suitable guidelines for therapy and monitoring their progress under therapy.

In every patient with recurrent renal stone disease a three-pronged approach is advocated: Stone, dietary and laboratory analysis.

Stone analysis

Some form of stone analysis is essential to enable the clinician to understand and treat effectively the underlying metabolic pathophysiological process. It is important to impress on a patient the necessity of salvaging any stone fragments he may pass spontaneously. Spectroscopic analysis or X-ray diffraction studies of even small stone fragments is possible and available. But such studies are generally expensive and also not universally available. An infrared spectroscopy equipment can easily cost DM50 000. Under less sophisticated health care conditions, a simple analysis is preferable to none, as from a study of stone composition, appropriate preventive strategies can be derived.

In a struvite or large, predominantly phosphate-containing stone, the primary underlying pathology is usually infection and not metabolic. For such patients:

- Associated anatomical abnormalities of the urinary tract causing poor urinary drainage should be corrected.
- Vesico-ureteral reflux should be corrected if present.
- Specific urine-culture-guided antibiotic therapy may be required on a long-term basis.
- A good urinary volume of more than 1500 ml per day should be ensured.

J. Talati et al. (eds) The Management of Lithiasis, 297–300
© *1997 Kluwer Academic Publishers. Printed in Great Britain.*

– Acidifying agents (such as enteric coated ammonium chloride tablets) should be used judiciously to limit bacteriuria, and should be avoided in renal failure.
– Every effort should be made to eliminate residuals.

These measures stabilize and improve overall kidney function in addition to preventing recurrence.

Renal stones such as cystine and xanthine stones caused by rare metabolic diseases are diagnosed through stone analysis. In these latter cases it is best to seek advice and help for these patients at a specialist centre at an early stage.

Dietary analysis

Every patient should receive advice from a dietician who is aware of the habits, traditions and customs of the local population. The dietician must be instructed to obtain from the patients a detailed analysis of the diet with special emphasis on the intake of calcium, purines, oxalates and fluids. The type of fluid ingested and the timing of fluid intake are important. It is amazing to note from the analysis that most patients, in spite of repeated stone problems, frequently have an insufficient fluid intake. The vast majority (more than 80%) of patients have to be frequently cajoled and persuaded to increase consistently their urine production to more than 1500 ml per day. The second major problem encountered frequently in the Western world is that people are not often used to drinking plain water. This forms a major hurdle which needs to be overcome.

The effects of modern day lifestyles and advertising can sometimes lead to unfortunate repercussions. Milk is considered to be good for health, and one encounters regularly misguided patients who, in addition to a good diet which includes cheese, chocolate in one form or another, as well as other calcium containing food products, also further overload the system by ingesting a litre or more of milk per day. To make matters worse, such an individual often concomitantly reduces his daily fluid intake proportionally as milk is considered to be a fluid. Other examples of excess can be found in patients who are compulsive nibblers or have a sweet tooth. Some of these recurrent stone-formers regularly have a large daily intake of chocolate. With a pre-existent underlying defect of calcium metabolism being present in a patient it is easy to see that stone recurrence would be facilitated in such cases. Some health care faddists take large doses of multi-vitamins without any advice or supervision from a local doctor. Others use various diets for dubious reasons, herbal medicines, and powders or potions of questionable therapeutic value on the advice of 'health care shops' and practitioners of 'alternative forms of medicine', which is allowed by law in The Netherlands. Some of these therapies contain large amounts of calcium and often sodium as well. All these diverse but important inputs into the daily life of a patient need to be evaluated meticulously in conjunction with the dietician. A good dietician can also help with the further monitoring of a patient during follow-up as well as providing encouragement to the patient and the necessary feedback to the urologist.

Metabolic work-up

All recurrent stone-formers should, in addition to a stone analysis, have a good laboratory work-up which can and should be undertaken easily on an outpatient basis. Recurrent stone-formers, for the purposes of the current discussion, are patients who have been known to be symptom-free and radiologically and/or ultrasonographically disease-free for at least six months before a stone is again demonstrated. In our opinion, patients with a significant family history of urolithiasis in the immediate family, need also to be investigated as extensively as recurrent stone-formers, even after the first episode of stone disease. Under ideal circumstances it is perhaps advisable to have the patient symptom-free before undertaking a metabolic work-up, but in practice this is often difficult and not cost-effective.

In our experience, there is a preponderance of male patients with recurrent stone disease. This seems to be the observation generally, not only in the Western world, but also in developing countries. Whether an underlying genetic factor plays any role in a sexual bias is unknown.

From experience, it seems sufficient to have a single serum analysis of the diverse components unless repetition is specifically indicated on clinical grounds i.e. suspicion of hyperparathyroidism. On the other hand, analysis of 24-hour urine collections must be done at least twice or preferably three times. The patient should be properly instructed to collect all urine passed during a 24-hour period into a specially provided container for the consecutive collection days. On this basis an accurate analysis of not only the total volume passed, but also of the chemical composition of the urine can be made with a reasonable degree of accuracy. The containers provided to the patient must be clean and sufficiently large (approx. 3 litres) to accommodate all the urine produced during a 24-hour period. The container should also have a good screw-top lid so that no urine is lost in transport and the patient is not inconvenienced by either leakage or unpleasant smells during transportation to the laboratory. The patient should be instructed to store the containers in a cool place or preferably in the refrigerator, especially in warmer climates, and when delivery to the laboratory on a daily basis may not be possible.

Diagnosis, therapy and follow-up

On the basis of the above investigations provisional conclusions can be drawn and further investigation initiated where applicable. From the information obtained from the dietician it is easy to see whether dietary factors need to be redressed and above all whether the patient has a sufficient fluid intake. Twenty-four-hour urine volume study also confirms the dietician's finding and may be helpful in convincing a reluctant patient of the importance of improving fluid intake. Care must be taken in explaining to patients the importance of not only increasing their fluid intake but also not overdoing it. Special attention needs to be drawn to the fact that the fluid intake should as far as possible be well spread out during the waking hours and emphasis must be placed on the large intake of water in one form or another, as well as cautioning against ingestion of milk or drinks made from milk in calcium stone-formers. However some calcium intake is necessary in stone-formers. Adjustments of diet and regular check-ups are best left in the capable hands of the dietician with whom the patient can liaise on a regular basis. The dietician must keep in touch with the physician.

Incomplete forms of renal tubular acidosis can often pre-exist with urolithiasis. Detection may be difficult but suspicion should be aroused in patients who have low citrate levels. These patients need to be investigated further by an internist before receiving therapy with sodium bicarbonate or a similar agent.

When hyperuricosaemia or hyperuricosuria is a problem the first priority must be to also check the urinary pH repeatedly. Levels below 6.0 are typical in stone-formers. A small proportion of calcium stone-formers may have hyperuricosuria. The vast majority will however have hypercalciuria, often idiopathic.

All patients with recurrent nephrolithiasis require long-term treatment and follow-up. As a simple rule of the thumb, follow-up in straightforward cases can be undertaken at three monthly intervals in the first year, then at six-monthly intervals during the following two years, provided a stable disease situation exists. Thereafter yearly check-ups are advised. At every follow-up visit serum and 24-hour urinary biochemistry should be repeated as an ongoing evaluation of therapy and patient compliance. Depending on available facilities, X-ray and ultrasonographic studies should also be carried out at these check-ups. The importance of long-term therapy and follow-up cannot be emphasized strongly enough. Patient compliance with the instituted regimes does tend to wane with time. The moral support, encouragement and supervision provided by regular follow-up visits to the urologists are important aspects in this ongoing battle to achieve a long recurrence-free interval. The two main objectives of therapy for all recurrent stone-formers are a good diuresis pattern (more than 1500 ml per day), and correction of dietary imbalance. In addition, pharmacotherapy also plays an important role, especially in the case of uric acid and calcium stone disease. The standard therapy for the former is allopurinol if alkaline therapy and dietary restrictions fail, and thiazide diuretics for the latter. During long-term therapy, care should be taken to detect side-effects related to both drugs. Potassium depletion is uncommon after thiazide therapy in recommended doses (e.g. 25 mg chlorthalidone per day), but can be treated effectively and simply by oral supplements of potassium. If under thiazide medication, a persistent and significant rise of serum calcium above normal levels is observed, it is essential that primary hyperparathyroidism be excluded.

Systematic management and long-term care of the patient with recurrent stone disease can be very effective in reducing recurrent stone disease.

45. Follow-up of urolithiasis patients: A guide for urologists in developing countries

JAMSHEER TALATI

Recurrence is the bane of stone disease. The physician in Pakistan has to determine how best to prevent recurrence in a patient who earns perhaps less than US$ 40 a month and feeds four. Treatment costs will have consumed much of his/her resources and financial assistance from patient welfare funds. Investigations which enquire into causes of stone formation in the patient must be carefully chosen by the urologist, who will have to assume the role of adviser, friend, nephrologist and dietician, in addition to the traditional 'surgical' role.

Stone analysis, serum calcium and 24-hour urinary excretion rates are important when designing a prophylactic regime. This should target the patient's lifestyle – fluid and eating habits. Collecting three 24-hour urines is difficult and costly. To give the best fit data, urine should be collected whilst the individual is eating the average weekday meal, especially if the weekend meals are different. Two or three urine collections and analyses are difficult; even one specimen is produced only after repeat reminders (see Table 45.1). Under such circumstances, analysis of spot urines and calculation of creatinine ratios may be considered.

Twenty per cent of our patients do not or cannot comply with our request for a 24-hour sample of urine. Can we do without further investigation of the aetiology of the stone? It costs nothing to tell patients to drink enough water to produce in excess of 1.5 L urine and to space out fluid intake over the 24 hours. This will prevent further stone formation in 60% of patients [1]. It costs little to ensure that that advice is followed. The office worker will have to take boiled water with him/her as the sewage contaminated tap water available in the office may lead to diarrhoea.

Dietary advice

It costs little to obtain a diet history. It is cost-ineffective to advise fancy diets to villagers. It is foolish to expect compliance with advice on diets that a villager or

Table 45.1 Difficulties in obtaining compliance in collecting 24-hour urines

Month total	Patients on recall	Missing data incomplete	Completed	Remain
February	25	12	9	3
March	34	12	3	9
April	37	21	14	7

J. Talati et al. (eds) The Management of Lithiasis, 301–303
© *1997 Kluwer Academic Publishers. Printed in Great Britain.*

poor man cannot access or afford. The physician must know what his patient can buy – he must advise whole wheat chapatti, not brown bread or esphagul husk or isogel. The physician must understand his local population's eating habits, traditions, and customs in order to be effective.

It is cost-effective to restrict excess milk intake in hypercalciurics, and in the southern towns in Punjab where people drink a litre or more a day. It is inappropriate and counter-productive to restrict milk in populations that drink little milk, have low normal calcium excretions and yet produce oxalate stones. Restricting proteins in a patient with uric acid stone is inappropriate if the patient's consumption is less than 1 g protein per kilogram body weight, but it is more cost-effective to lower uric acid excretion by reducing meat intake than by advising allopurinol. A change of lifestyle is better than a prescription for medicines which achieves poor compliance.

It is however inappropriate to give dietary advice unless there are obvious serious dietary indiscretions detected on diet history, or the 24-hour urine indicates abnormal excretion rates.

Diet therapy is cheaper than drugs, but drugs will be needed in some patients. Especially in Pakistan, we are becoming aware of the extent of hypocitraturia, which will require alkali in any form. But how sure are we that the effects of various drug therapies are really the effects of drug and not of concerned continuous supervision of adequate fluid intake? This is an important question, because though metabolic survey can cost up to Pak Rs 1000 (more than US\$ 33), treatment of a new stone can cost Pak Rs 15 000 (US\$ 500). (In the US, the cost of metabolic survey is US\$ 1000, the cost of medical prophylaxis less than US\$ 300, and the cost of therapy US\$ 5000–10 000.) In this context, potassium citrate has been clearly shown in a prospective study to reduce recurrences in hypocitraturic patients better than a placebo.

It costs nothing to advise patients and their siblings to marry outside their families, and break tight inbreeding. But at this time there is insufficient evidence to prove genetic predisposition, and the best policy may be simply to present information on familial incidence to the patients and allow them to make their own decisions. Such advice is probably justified when a large number of family members are involved, and in groups where marriages are arranged within the tribe.

Problems of follow-up

It is unclear whether yearly follow-up with a KUB X-ray (or ultrasound if the stone is a urate one) and urinalysis are cost-effective. It is more important to ensure that the patient has access to a doctor as soon as he gets a colic. The logistics of follow-up in a unit treating 700 patients a year become formidable (to the extent of impossibility) within ten years. Family practitioners working closely with the urology unit can lessen this burden. Continuing medical education encourages them to undertake good prophylactic management and follow-up at their practice and reduces the workload on the tertiary facility.

Conclusion

The physician should ensure that all stone particles are eliminated. Effective treatment by extracorporeal shock wave lithotripsy, surgery or endoscopy may leave the patient with little cash to pay for the metabolic work-up, but money must be found, because specific treatment directed to correct aetiological factors – metabolic, infective or other – provides a good insurance against stone recurrence, especially in infected stones. The need for a high fluid intake and altered dietary habits should be explained to the patient. This may all reduce or eliminate the need for drugs. Centralized sophisticated laboratories should be set up to analyse stones.

Reference

1.   Hosking DH, Erickson SB, Van Den Berg CJ *et al.* The Stone Clinic effect in patients with idiopathic calcium urolithiasis. J Urol 1983;130:1115–18.

Section VI
Paediatric Urolithiasis

46. Urolithiasis in children

ZAFAR NAZIR and FARHAT MOAZAM

Urolithiasis is relatively uncommon in children in the industrialized world, but it remains a major source of morbidity in the stone belt countries that stretch from Turkey and Egypt in the West to Indonesia in the East. Approximately 100 new cases of urolithiasis in children are reported in the entire United Kingdom each year [1]. In the United States, urolithiasis is responsible for one in 7600 paediatric hospital admissions [2]. In contrast, in a single government hospital in Pakistan, over a one-year period, 1 out of 73 admissions was related to urolithiasis, the majority being bladder stones [3]. In Afghanistan, suprapubic cystolithotomies account for approximately 20% of all surgical procedures performed on children [4].

Aetiology

The aetiology and location of urinary tract calculi in children varies in different parts of the world. In the West, stones tend to be located in the upper urinary tract and are largely calcium oxalate or struvite in composition [5, 6]. These are often related to urinary tract infections, inherited metabolic defects and underlying congenital anatomical anomalies or vesicoureteral reflux [2, 7–9]. In non-industrialized countries, urinary tract calculi in children are often located in the lower tract and the composition is predominantly ammonium acid urate and/or calcium oxalate [6]. The feeding pattern in infants, including a diet high in oxalate precursors and depleted in phosphate, have been implicated in the aetiology of bladder stones [5, 10]. In studies from Thailand, supplementation of the diet with phosphate buffers appears to decrease crystalluria, and, it is postulated, may decrease stone formation [11]. Other predisposing factors in some countries include recurrent infections, schistosomiasis and dehydration secondary to the high ambient temperature, and recurrent gastroenteritis. Recent studies from South Africa and Iran appear to indicate a change in these trends with renal stones becoming more frequent as these countries become more affluent [12, 13].

Management

The management of a child with urolithiasis requires identification and control of the acute presenting symptoms including infection, as well as identification of any

J. Talati et al. (eds) The Management of Lithiasis, 307–313
© *1997 Kluwer Academic Publishers. Printed in Great Britain.*

predisposing metabolic and anatomical abnormalities. The subsequent management must include a plan to eliminate the calculi, provide appropriate dietary and pharmacologic manipulation if needed, as well as correct any underlying urinary tract anomalies to prevent stasis and recurrent stone formation. In children with calcification on a plain abdominal film, compatible with urinary calculi, a complete blood count, urinalysis, urine culture and a biochemical profile are indicated. When blood urea nitrogen (BUN) and creatinine levels are normal, the entire anatomy of the urinary tract must be visualized. In the absence of allergy to intravenous contrast, an intravenous urogram (IVU) should be obtained to determine the location of the stone, the degree of obstruction, the relative level of renal function and whether there is an underlying anatomical abnormality. A renal ultrasound can be used as the primary imaging procedure in a child with renal insufficiency and for follow-up of children after clearance of the stone. An analysis of a 24-hour urine collection for calcium, oxalate, uric acid, citrate and creatinine is best undertaken when the patient is asymptomatic and on a normal fluid intake and diet. A nitroprusside test on a urine aliquot will test for cystine. If the patient has a history of recurrent urinary tract infections, a voiding cystourethrogram (VCUG) is indicated to rule out reflux. Urodynamic studies, if available, may be useful in patients suspected of lower urinary tract dysfunction. It is important that investigations take into account the cost–benefit ratio. Laboratory evaluations should be appropriate to the nature of the stone in the patient presenting for management. This is of particular importance in developing countries with limited resources and few third party payers.

The indications for stone removal in children are similar to those in adults. Stones producing obstruction, infections and renal damage need intervention. Currently, options available for stone elimination include open surgical lithotomy, transurethral stone destruction, percutaneous nephrolithotomy and extracorporeal shock wave lithotripsy (ESWL). Each of these approaches has its own indications and contraindications; however these therapeutic modalities are not mutually exclusive and should be regarded as adjunctive modes of therapy, to be used in concert. With the advent of endoscopic techniques and ESWL in the 1980s, open surgery has been relegated to a secondary role in the treatment of urinary tract stones in children. Open surgical procedures for stone disease have become the exception rather than the rule in industrialized countries, with only 2–4% of patients with urolithiasis undergoing traditional surgery [5]. The ideal management of paediatric urolithiasis should include techniques which combine efficient and complete removal of the stone, in addition to ensuring minimal morbidity and renal damage. In children, the choice of therapy is dependent on the patient size, the anatomy of the urinary tract, the stone burden, and the composition and location of the stone. In the third world, non-availability of appropriate technology and expertise in the use of modern treatment modalities in children may be limiting factors, and surgical interventions will continue to play a greater role than in the West.

The major advance in the treatment of paediatric urolithiasis, which is now available worldwide, is the use of ESWL. This has been projected as the treatment of choice for the majority of upper urinary calculi in children. Third generation lithotriptors which employ small focal points and ultrasound for localization and monitoring of stone fragmentation, are particularly attractive for use in children. By eliminating radiation hazards and reducing the pain associated with the procedure, ESWL has become popular for elimination of a majority of upper urinary tract stones in infants as young as four months of age [14]. Children and adolescents appear to pass stone fragments quite easily with minimal morbidity. Complications of ESWL, including skin bruising at the entrance and exit sites, fever, distal ureteral obstruction caused by columns of stone fragments (*steinstrassen*) and perirenal haematoma, are rare. Although a young, unco-operative patient may require general anaesthesia, intravenous sedation is usually sufficient. A stone clearance rate in the range of 75 to 97% has been reported with ESWL [14–17]. Less suitable for ESWL are large calcium oxalate and cystine calculi which are quite hard, and large branched struvite (staghorn) calculi. For such stones, percutaneous debulking or open nephrolithotomy may be more appropriate as the initial or definitive treatment.

Although the efficacy of ESWL for stone clearance is well established, a number of concerns have surfaced regarding the use of this form of treatment in immature kidneys. An 8–10% incidence of hypertension, transient proteinuria and nephrotic syndrome secondary to glomerular membrane damage, reduction in renal function immediately after treatment as well as renal fibrosis as a sequela of intraparenchymal haemorrhage, have been reported in experimental and clinical studies [18–22], although no long-term ill effects on renal function have been demonstrated to date. A causal relationship between the number of shocks administered, as well as the kilovoltage employed during lithotripsy, have been postulated as the cause of renal damage [21, 23–25]. There is general agreement that long-term follow-up of patients undergoing ESWL is essential. Due to uncertainties regarding long-term effects in children, use of ESWL should be restricted to small stones that do not require an excessive number of high energy shock waves. Overzealous and prolonged treatment should be avoided and it may be safer to stage the treatment rather than deliver high energy shock waves to the kidney in one treatment session. If not properly shielded, gonads in the male patient may be at risk of shock wave damage in the case of ureteric and bladder stones. ESWL is currently not recommended for females with child-bearing potential if the stone is located in the true pelvis [26].

The current trend in medicine is rapid export of technology from the West to the third world. With the potential of ESWL for delayed side-effects necessitating long-term follow-up, this may produce difficulties in densely populated, less affluent countries with poorly developed health systems [27]. Ironically many such countries provide the most fertile market for this new technology, raising the ethical dilemma of the use of technology in countries where assessment of long-term risks is difficult.

The techniques of percutaneous nephrolithotomy and ureteroscopic retrieval of ureteric calculi have achieved a high success rate in adults. With the recent availability of small size endoscopes and the ultrasonic, electro-hydraulic and laser (EHL) probes, these options are also becoming attractive for the management of urolithiasis in children [6, 10, 28, 29]. Major advantages over the open surgical techniques include shorter hospital stay and convalescent period. With increase in expertise, simultaneous correction of coexisting anatomic abnormalities such as endoscopic incision of calyceal neck and endopyeloplasty for pelviureteric junction obstruction is also possible. Reported complications include haemorrhage, need for multiple procedures to render the patient stone-free, sepsis, extravasation of urine, vesicoureteric reflux and ureteric strictures due to over-dilation of the ureter. Due to the relatively smaller size of paediatric patients, mobility of the kidney within the Gerota's fascia, and a smaller collecting system, the possibility for error in children is much greater than in adults. Considerable experience in the use of these techniques must be considered a prerequisite for attempting these procedures in children.

Although advances in instrumentation and technology have swung the pendulum away from open surgery, the latter remains an acceptable approach to large staghorn calculi and in patients where orthopaedic deformities prevent proper positioning for ESWL or percutaneous access to the kidney. In addition, in less affluent societies, open surgery may be the most cost-effective modality, permitting simultaneous correction of associated anatomical abnormalities (see Figures 46.1 and 46.2). It can be performed safely with excellent stone clearance and minimal postoperative morbidity and mortality [27]. Although in the last decade reports of experience with surgical management of urolithiasis have become infrequent, stone

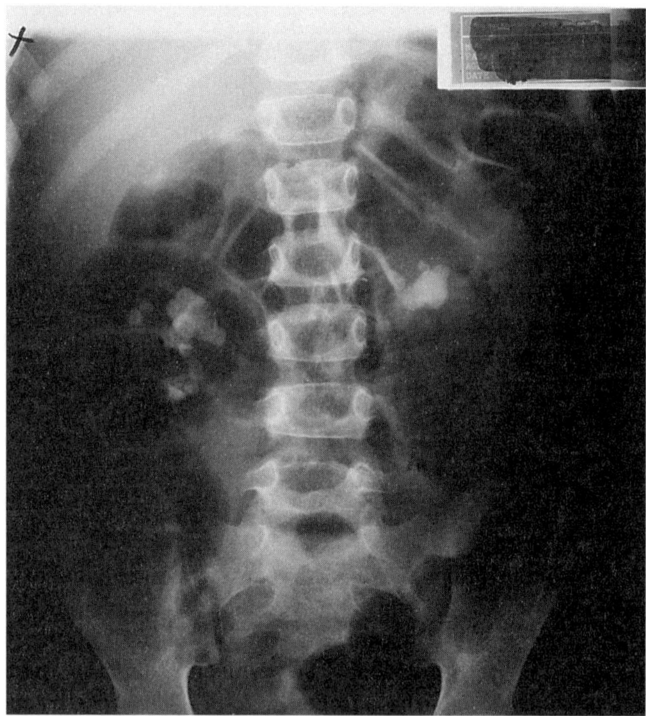

Figure 46.1 Plain X-ray of abdomen of a five-year-old child, showing multiple and bilateral renal calculi

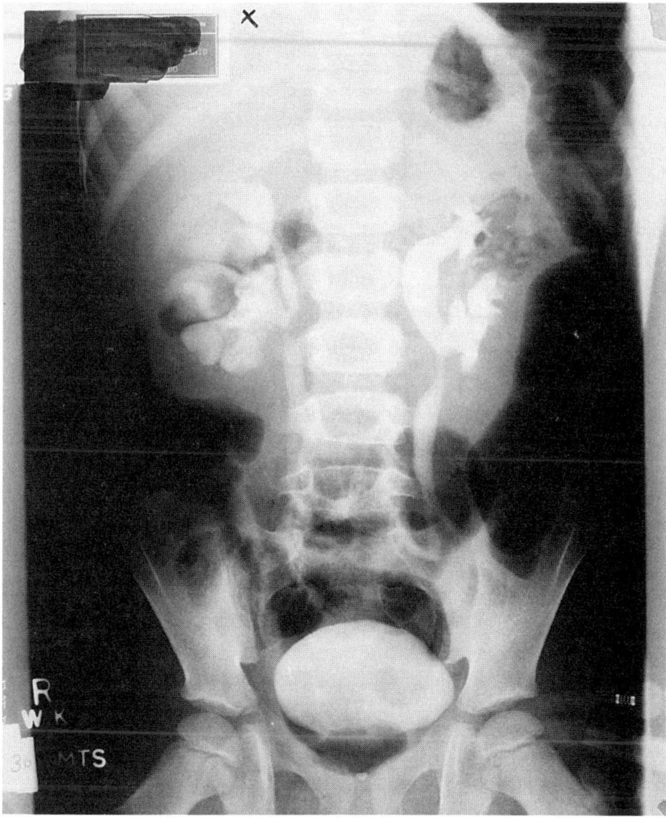

Figure 46.2 IVP of the same patient as shown in Figure 46.1, showing bilateral pelviureteric junction obstruction, confirmed at surgery

clearance rates remain comparable to those achieved with ESWL and endoscopic procedures [8, 27, 30]. In a third world setting with limited resources, open surgery remains an effective mode of treatment of urinary calculi, particularly in children. Teaching hospitals which provide manpower for rural settings must continue to train residents in these techniques. Use of lithotriptors should be ideally selected for children with small stones and those who have undergone prior renal surgery.

Whatever the mode selected for stone clearance, long-term follow-up (a minimum of five years) is advisable in view of an 8–44% recurrence rate reported in the paediatric patient [6, 23, 31, 32]. The highest recurrence rate is reported among patients with metabolic disorders and underlying anatomical abnormalities [7, 9, 32]. Other factors contributing to recurrence include urinary tract infections, functional abnormalities, multiple stones, incomplete stone clearance, malnutrition and dehydration. These lithogenic factors must be actively investigated and eradicated as an essential part of the management of urolithiasis in children.

References

1. Thornhill JA, Moran K, Mooney EE *et al.* Extracorporeal shock wave lithotripsy monotherapy for pediatric urinary tract calculi. Br J Urol 1990;65:638.
2. Gearhart JP, Herzberg GZ, Jeff RD. Childhood urolithiasis: Experience and advances. Pediatrics 1991;87:445.
3. Khan MN, Islam S, Afzal S *et al.* Urolithiasis in children – a comparison of Western and Pakistani data. Pak J Surg 1991;7:57.
4. Srivastava RN, Hussainy MAA, Goel RG *et al.* Bladder stone disease in children in Afghanistan. Br J Urol 1986;58:374.
5. Smith LH, Segura JW. Urolithiasis. In: Kelalis PP, King LR, Belman AB, editors. Clinical pediatric urology. 3rd ed., Philadelphia: WB Saunders, 1992:1327–52.
6. Woodhouse CRJ. Renal anomalies and diseases. In: Woodhouse CRJ, editor. Longterm pediatric urology. London: Blackwell Scientific Publications, 1991:37–47.
7. Diamond DA. Clinical pattern of pediatric urolithiasis. Br J Urol 1991;68:159.
8. Choi H, Snyder HM, Duckett JW. Urolithiasis in childhood: Current management. J Pediatr Surg 1987;22:158.
9. Diamond DA, Rickwood AMK, Lee PH *et al.* Infection stones in children: A twenty year review. Urology 1994;43:525.
10. Levin RK, Hensle TW. Pediatric urolithiasis. In: Asheraft KW, editor. Pediatric urology, Philadelphia: WB Saunders, 1990:461–88.
11. Valyasevi A, Van Reen R. Pediatric bladder stone disease: Current status of research. J Pediatr 1968;72:546.
12. Cifuentes JM, Pourmand G. Mineral composition of 103 stones from Iran. Br J Urol 1983;55:465.
13. Buckes GJ, de Bruiyn H, Vermaak WJH. Effect of change in epidemiological factors on the composition and racial distribution of renal calculi. Br J Urol 1989;60:387.
14. Marberger M, Turk C, Steinkogler I. Piezoelectric extracorporeal shock wave lithotripsy in children. J Urol 1989;142:349.
15. Newman DM, Coury T, Lingeman JE *et al.* Extracorporeal shockwave lithotripsy experience in children. J Urol 1986;136:238.
16. Kroovand RL, Harrison LH, McCullogh DL. Extracorporeal shockwave lithotripsy in childhood. J Urol 1987;138:1106.
17. Wilbert DM, Schofer O, Riedmiller H. Treatment of pediatric urolithiasis by extracorporeal shock wave lithotripsy. Eur J Pediatr 1988;147:579.
18. Lingeman JE, Wood JR, Toth PD. Blood pressure changes following extracorporeal shock wave lithotripsy and other forms of treatment for nephrolithiasis. J Am Med Assoc 1990;263:1789.
19. Araque A, Alamo C, Fraile B *et al.* Nephrotic syndrome after extracorporeal shock wave lithotripsy. Nephron 1994;68:393.
20. Newman R, Hackett R, Senior B *et al.* Pathologic effects of ESWL on canine renal tissue. Urology 1987;29:194.
21. Kaude JV, Williams CM, Millner MR *et al.* Renal morphology and functions immediately after extracorporeal shock wave lithotripsy. Am J Roentgenol 1985;145:305.
22. Corbally MT, Ryan J, Fitzpatrick J *et al.* Renal functions following extracorporeal lithotripsy in children. J Pediatr Surg 1991;26:539.
23. Nijman NJM, Ackaert K, Scholtmeijer RJ *et al.* Longterm results of extracorporeal shock wave lithotripsy in children. J Urol 1989;142:609.
24. Kaji DM, Xie HW, Hardy BE *et al.* The effects of extracorporeal shock wave lithotripsy on renal growth, function and arterial blood pressure in an animal model. J Urol 1991;146:544.
25. Thomas R, Frentz JM, Harmon EP *et al.* Effects of extracorporeal shock wave lithotripsy on renal function and body height in pediatric patients. J Urol 1992;148:1064.
26. Harmon EP, Neal DE, Thomas R. Pediatric urolithiasis: Review of research and current management. Pediatr Nephrol 1994;8:508.
27. Moazam F, Nazir Z, Jafarey AM. Pediatric urolithiasis: To cut or not to cut. J Pediatr Surg 1994;29:761.

28. Hill ED, Segura JW, Patterson DE *et al.* Ureteroscopy in children. J Urol 1990;144:481.
29. Callaway TA, Lingardh G, Basata S *et al.* Percutaneous nephrolithotomy in children. J Urol 1992;148:1067.
30. Androulakakis PA, Micheal V, Polychronopoulou S *et al.* Pediatric urolithiasis in Greece. Br J Urol 1991;67:206.
31. Androulakakis PA, Barratt TM, Ransley PG *et al.* Urinary calculi in children: A 5 to 15 year follow up with particular reference to recurrent and residual stones. Br J Urol 1982;54:176.
32. Diamond DA, Menon M, Lee PH *et al.* Etiological factors in pediatric stone recurrence. J Urol 1989;142:606.

Section VII
Biliary Tract Stones

47. ESWL in gallstone therapy: History, current status and expectations

LUCAS GREINER

Acoustic energy can be a strong destructive force, as is for example demonstrated by the breakdown of the walls of ancient Jericho by the mere sound of trumpets. Acoustic energy can be especially effective under two special conditions: first, when the sound waves are focused; and second, when they hit an interface between two substances with highly different capabilities of propagating sound waves (as the interface between liquid and stone material). With the exception of Jericho, no further military applications of destructive sound energy are reported. In medical technology, however, the therapeutic use of extracorporeally produced shock waves for lithotripsy (ESWL) is extremely successful in urology [1] – and shock waves are high energy sound waves. Even before the first human application of ESWL in kidney stones in 1980, our early *in vitro* series had demonstrated the capability of shock waves to disintegrate gallstones as well (though only at higher energy levels) [2]; the first clinical reports however [3, 4], pointed out that biliary ESWL would not become as much an overwhelming success as had lithotripsy in urology.

This chapter intends to highlight both the past and the present, as well as the future expectations in biliary ESWL.

History

As early as in 1979, our first systematic *in vitro* trials of shock wave application to gallstones were carried out at the Dornier laboratories. Subsequently, animal experiments with implanted gallstones were conducted in dogs by Brendel and Enders [2]. During this period of careful preclinical evaluation – lasting for six years – one of the crucial questions was how to aim at the gallstones. Initially, X-ray control of targeting the stone and monitoring its disintegration was favoured, since fluoroscopy had been chosen for ESWL of urinary tract stones. Subsequently, however, ultrasonography was accepted – even by older physicians who had trained in the pre-ultrasound era and who were involved in the project of biliary ESWL – to be the method of choice to defect gallstones in the gall-bladder, to direct focused shock wave energy at these stones, and to monitor their process of disintegration.

This period of preclinical studies turned out to be a very interesting and fruitful phase of co-operation between physicians and their 'tool-makers' in medical tech-

J. Talati et al. (eds) The Management of Lithiasis, 317–327
© *1997 Kluwer Academic Publishers. Printed in Great Britain.*

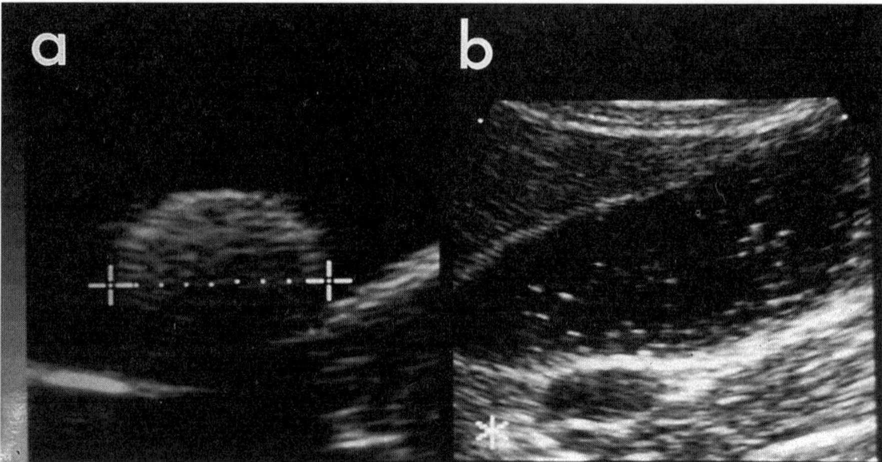

Figure 47.1 (a) Solitary stone before ESWL; (b) residual minor fragments 18 hr later. The patient was stone-free after one month with additional lythic therapy

nology, which led to the first clinical applications of ESWL in a patient with a solitary gall-bladder stone in 1985 by Paumgartner *et al.*; and by our working group treating the first bile-duct and gall-bladder stones in 1985 and 1986, respectively (4, 5) (see Figure 47.1). These early clinical experiences were gained with the prototype GM1-lithotriptor, an underwater spark-gap type of machine. It was a rather simple modification of the famous HM3-bathtub lithotriptor, the first machine used for kidney stones. The GM1-prototype lithotriptor had two modifications. First, the steering component was no longer X-ray fluoroscopy, but a small, effective, real-time ultrasound device with a 3.5 MHz sector probe mounted coaxially to the central axis of the shock wave field. Second, the patient's position was changed from the supine (as usual in kidney stone ESWL) to the prone, allowing propagation of the shock wave energy to the gall-bladder stone by the shortest pathway possible. The other main features of the HM3 apparatus remained unchanged (water immersion of the patient's body with an optimum of shock wave transmission, the position of the shock wave generator at the bottom of the tub, etc.). The first treatments demonstrated clearly that it was possible to destroy gall-bladder stones *in vivo* by ESWL even without general anaesthesia. The incidence of side-effects due to fragment migration was much lower than feared, before starting the clinical evaluation of our new therapy of gallstones. This was the good news. The bad news, however, was a limited disintegration capability of the shock waves, leaving the gall-bladder with fragments not able to leave the gall-bladder spontaneously, even after repeated exposures in repeated ESWL-sessions (see Figure 47.2). Therefore, adjuvant lytic therapy was necessary from the start of gall-bladder stone ESWL. This restricted its application to stones with a chemical composition allowing non-invasive peroral lytic therapy with bile acids (ursodeoxycholic and chenodeoxycholic acid). These agents are effective in cholesterol stones only. In bile-duct stones, on the other hand,

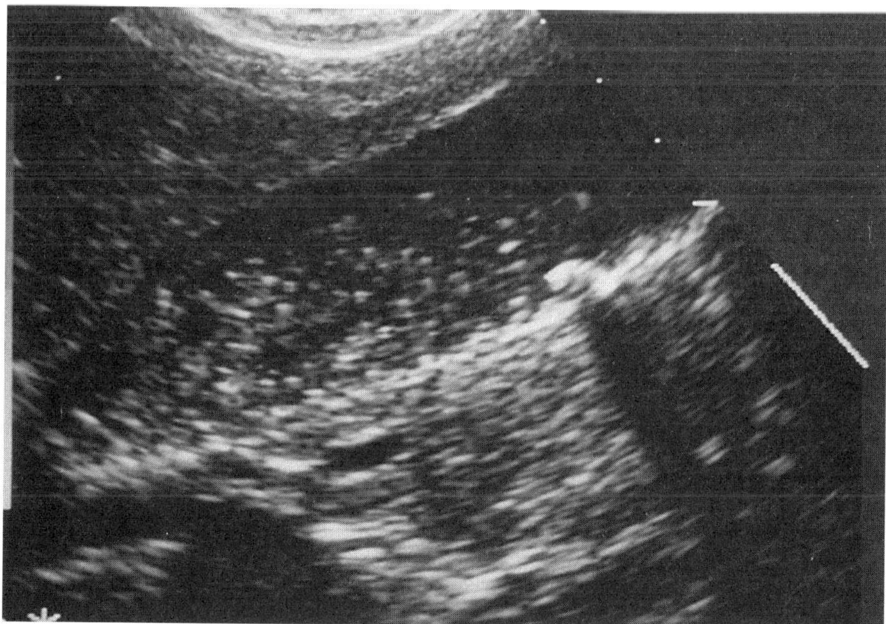

Figure 47.2 Two days after ESWL of two stones of 15-mm size: minor fragments and one 6-mm residual (disappeared after re-ESWL)

the chemical composition of the calculi is of no major importance because the fragments are accessible to endoscopic extraction procedures.

It was clear from the start that this new therapeutic approach to gallstone disease would raise both an enormous interest and criticism [6–8]. The levels of hope and expectation in this new medical technology were rather high [3, 8, 9], and in numerous local and international congresses, the pros and cons were debated vividly and controversially. At the beginning of the period 1985–88, clinical data were only available from the two initiating centres in Germany [3, 4, 6, 8], but then a rapid accumulation of further clinical experience was published. These data demonstrate clearly that biliary ESWL is a good non-operative treatment option only for highly selected cases of gall-bladder and bile-duct stones. The selection criteria for these two groups of calculi are quite different: in gall-bladder stones, stone volume and composition as well as gall-bladder contractility are the main criteria; whereas in bile-duct stones, only those stones which are not treatable by operative endoscopy should be submitted to ESWL.

Gall-bladder stone ESWL

The ideal stone candidate for gallbladder ESWL may be characterized by the four S-words: the symptomatic, solitary, sonolucent stone (see Figure 47.3) in a sufficiently contracting gall-bladder. Whether a stone is symptomatic or not can be

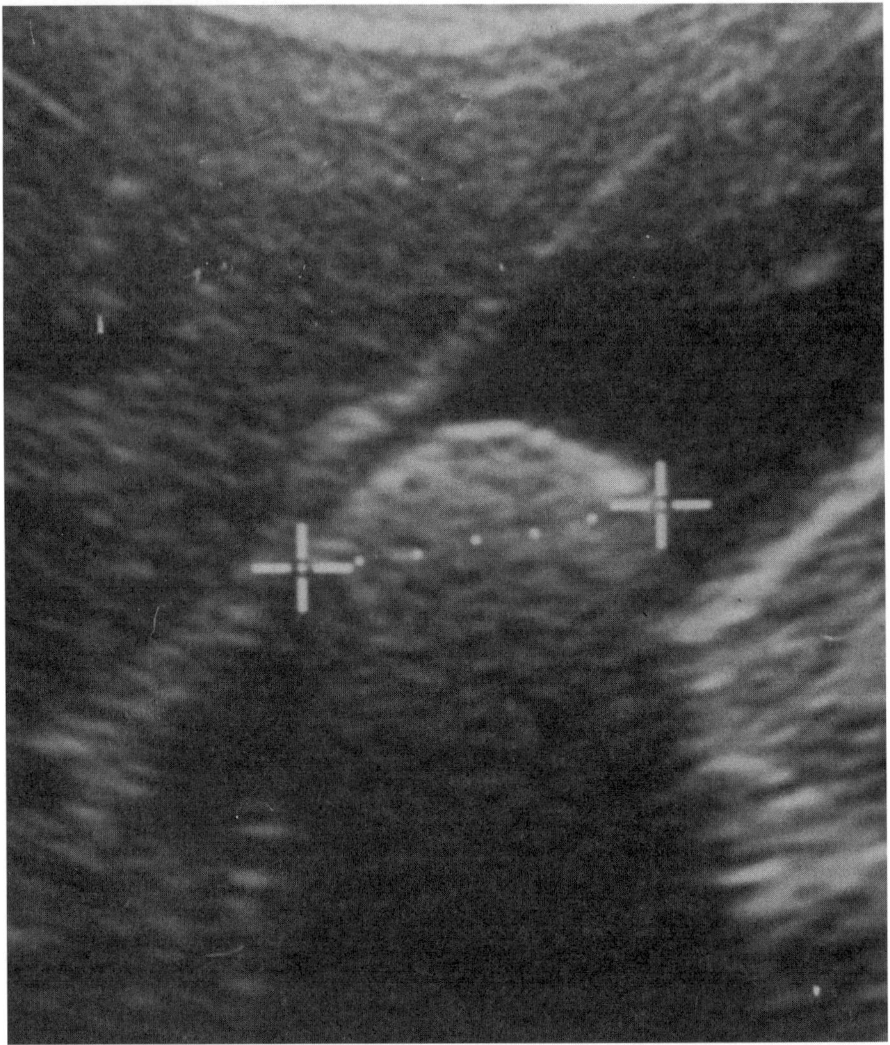

Figure 47.3 Ideal ESWL candidate – solitary, symptomatic, sonolucent stone, medium sized (19 mm)

determined easily in most patients; sometimes, however, it might be difficult or even impossible to distinguish between symptoms attributable to an irritable gut syndrome or concomitantly existing stones [7]. The stone number can be evaluated easily by carefully conducted ultrasonography; ultrasound examination is also the method of choice for evaluating the stone volume and gall-bladder characteristics such as contractility and wall thickness (excluding patients with chronic inflammatory gall-bladder changes) (see Figure 47.4). The highly sonolucent stone (Figure 47.3) with a homogeneous echo pattern and a low amplitude entrance echo corresponds very well to a non-calcified so-called pure cholesterol stone [10]; evaluation

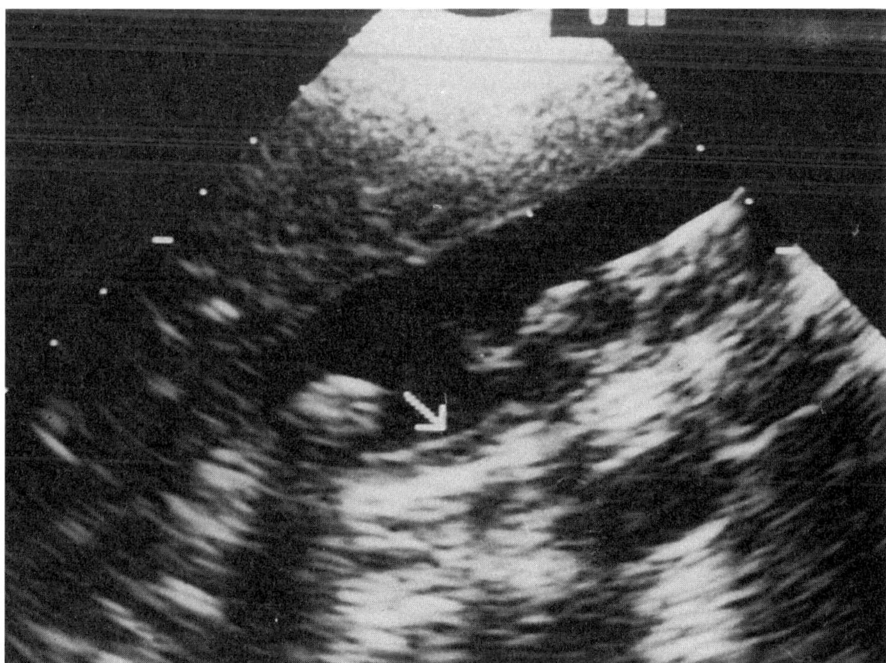

Figure 47.4 Another ideal ESWL candidate – however, the gallbladder shows wall thickening due to chronic inflammation (arrow); no non-operative treatment possible

of these criteria of echogenicity, however, demands a very high degree of ultrasound experience, usually not substituting the conventional X-ray study for excluding stone calcification.

Results

In six years we have treated over 1400 gall-bladder stones patients with ESWL and subsequent lytic therapy with ursodeoxycholic and chenodeoxycholic acid in combination; 76% of the patients treated were female, and average age was 46 years (range 17–73 years). The results evaluated to date are shown in Table 47.1.

Table 47.1   Results of gall-bladder ESWL – initial six years' experience

	Percentage freedom from stones			
	Months after ESWL[a]			
	1	6	12	18
Solitary ≤20 mm	12	41	60	66
Solitary ≥21 mm	?	12	31	42
Several (2–5)	5	15	34	45
Multiple (6–15)		9	20	37

n = 1400, of which 812 were solitary.
[a] After ESWL, patients received continuous lytic therapy.

The poor initial results in gallbladder ESWL in the USA [10] can be possibly explained by the fact that the study was multicentre, the use of shock wave energies which were too low [8], and an inadequate experience in clinical ultrasound.

The term 'freedom from stones' is the most important criterion whenever the treatment results of different working groups are compared. The demonstration of genuine freedom from calculi is, however, problematic, demanding optimized sonographic conditions such as an experienced investigator, 5-MHz transducers, and variable patient positioning. The more meticulous the follow-up ultrasound examinations, the lower the true rate of success in terms of real freedom from stones will be; stubborn small and very small residual (probably pigment) stones can only be detected after determined repositioning of the patient, e.g. examination in the left lateral or upright position. These minimal remainders are frequently overlooked. It is conceivable (and in our view even probable) that high rates of renewed stone formation after termination of oral dissolution treatment can be explained as renewed growth of such residual mini-fragments in gall-bladders erroneously considered to be stone-free. In such cases – which are naturally hard to define – the term 'pseudo stone recurrence' would be more appropriate. In carefully conducted studies, the true recurrence rate observed ranged from 5–10% during the first year after termination of lytic therapy, with an additional rate of renewed stone formation of 3–5% during each year of further follow-up.

Complications and serious side-effects of ESWL are rare (see Table 47.2). There have been no fatalities. The most serious complications observed have been liver haematoma/haematobiloma in three cases, necessitating surgical intervention in one patient. Severe biliary colic as a result of fragment migration occurs in 5–10% of all patients treated and just under 1% require endoscopic sphincterotomy. Figure 47.5 demonstrates that even 8 mm fragments may pass into the gut, though as a rule fragment size in faeces varies from 1 to 3 mm. A further 15–20% of patients report 'biliary' complaints and pain. True colic, pain and 'biliary' discomfort are almost always rare or singular events; about 75% of all patients treated convincingly report a (marked) improvement of their biliary problems as compared to the status before ESWL – even when fragment remainders are still present. The attitude of the patients to the post-ESWL complications and complaints is determined decisively by the information they receive before undergoing the procedure. However, an adequate understanding of the anatomical and (patho-)physiological background of gall-bladder ESWL is only achievable in a minority of patients, despite intensive efforts to provide appropriate information and counselling.

During follow-up, there may be compliance problems with respect to taking the oral dissolution medication and attending follow-up appointments. These problems

Table 47.2   Complications of gall-bladder ESWL

Genuine biliary colic	5–10%
Biliary complaints	15–20%
Cystic duct obstruction	3%
Biliary pancreatitis	2%
Need for endoscopic sphincterotomy	1%

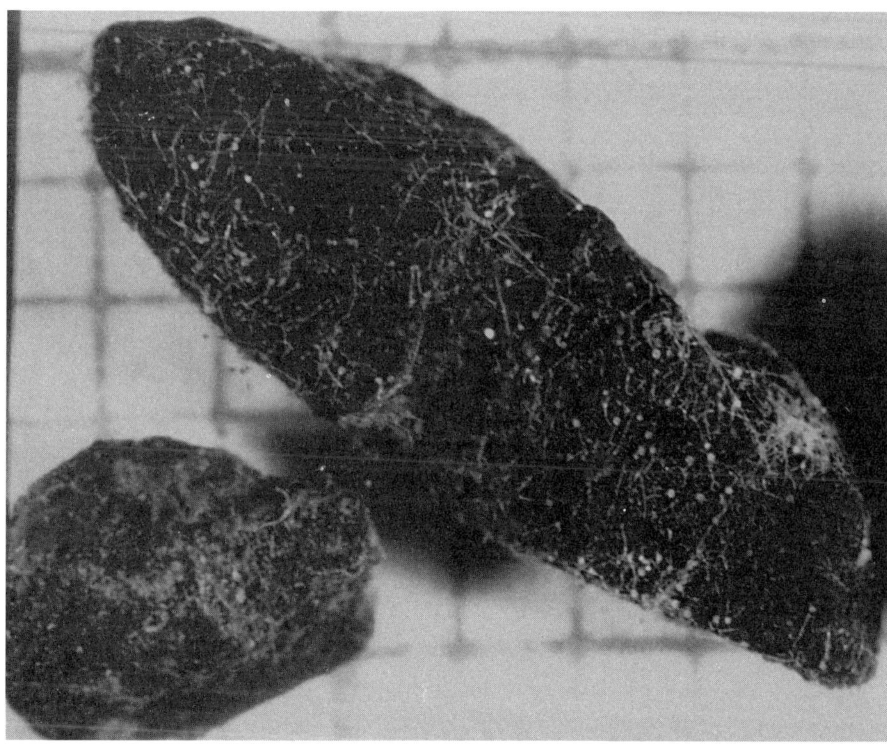

Figure 47.5 Fragments (8-mm) found one day after ESWL in the stool. These unusually big pieces passed asymptomatically [6]; as a rule, fragment size in the faeces varies between 1 and 3 mm

may increase with time since ESWL; in individual groups up to 25% are lost to follow-up each year.

The drawbacks, disappointments and – in some cases – problematic experiences presented here should not be allowed to detract from the success of our new non-operative procedure in diminishing the number of cholecystectomies by a simple and gentle procedure requiring no anaesthesia, leaving a stone-free gall-bladder in a high percentage of (carefully selected) cases with a low number of genuine relapses.

Extrahepatic and intrahepatic bile-duct stones

ESWL of extrahepatic and intrahepatic bile-duct stones is indicated when the usual endoscopic–operative procedures fail or are not possible (see Figures 47.6–47.8, Table 47.3) [3, 6].

Extrahepatic bile-duct stone ESWL requires lithotriptors which allow both ultrasonic and radiographic stone localization as only about half of the common bile-duct stones can be detected and localized by expert ultrasonography; moreover, the

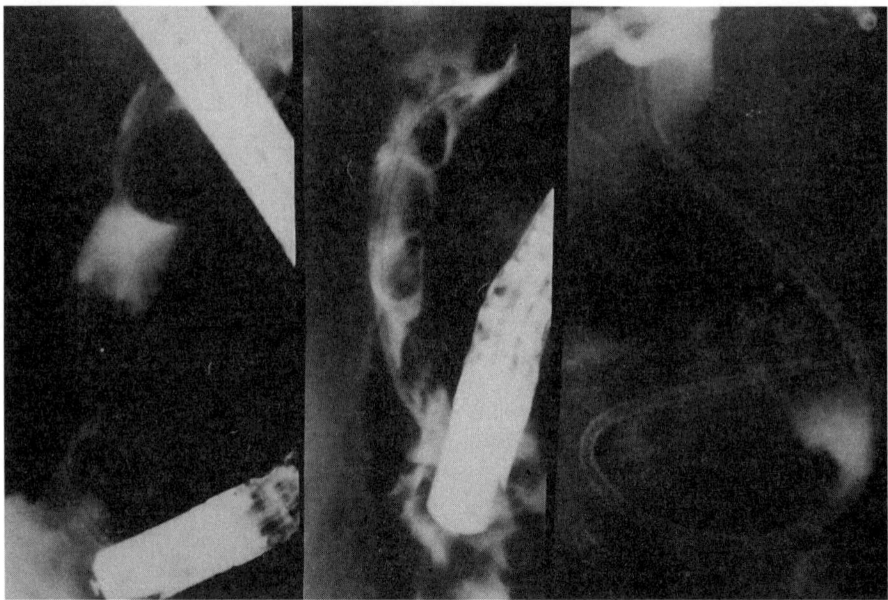

Figure 47.6 Bile duct stone not treatable by endoscopy: (a) before; and (b) after ESWL; (c) stone-free bile-duct system after endoscopic fragment extraction

Table 47.3   ESWL in problematic (endoscopy-resisting) extrahepatic and intrahepatic bile-duct stones

Endoscopic stone removal impossible because:
  Stones are too large
  Stones resist mechanical fragmentation
  Large sphincterotomy carries too great a risk

Endoscopic sphincterotomy impossible or not helpful because:
  Bile-ducts not accessible (partial/total gastrectomy,
  Roux-en-Y-anastomosis)
  Stones not accessible (bile-duct strictures,
  intra-hepatic stones)

air filling of bile-ducts subsequent to endoscopic sphincterotomy can render ultrasonographic (but not X-ray) stone visualization impossible. For intra-hepatic stones (hepatolithiasis), ultrasonographic localization alone is far superior to radiographic localization (Figure 47.8). Repeat sessions may be necessary in both extrahepatic and intrahepatic stones.

Complete freedom from stones can be achieved in almost all cases of problematic extrahepatic bile-duct stones [5]. As a rule, fragments are extracted endoscopically after successful stone disintegration. In the case of intra-hepatic stones [11], particularly in dilated intrahepatic bile-ducts, it is not uncommon for small stones or fragments to remain after ESWL; these residuals are neither washed out nor cleared spontaneously. Bile-duct obstruction, however, is in almost all cases

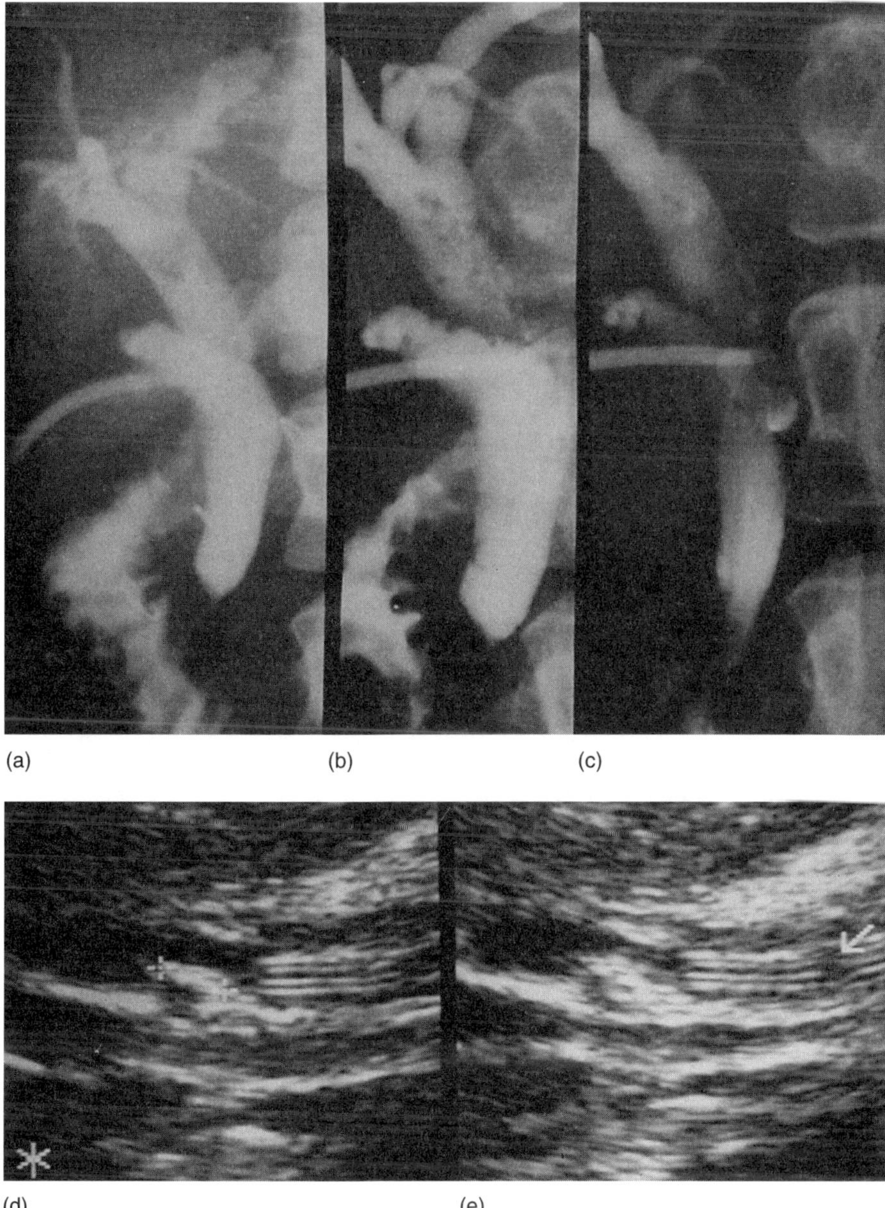

(a)   (b)   (c)

(d)   (e)

Figure 47.7 'Residual' (forgotten) stone after laparoscopic cholecystectomy before (a), immediately after (b), and two hours after ESWL (c) without endoscopic sphincterotomy; (d) ultrasonographical imaging of the stone (cross-marks) (d) and the T-tube (arrow) (e) before ESWL.

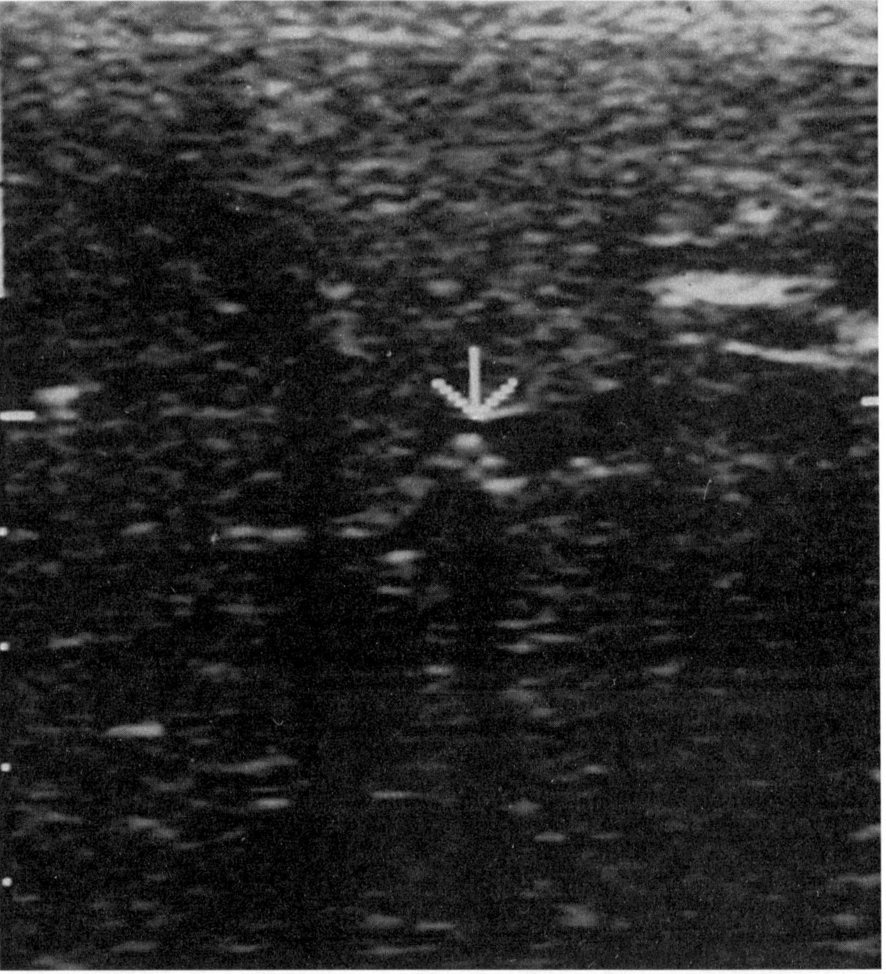

Figure 47.8 Fragments of hepatolithiasis (arrow) after ESWL in a slightly distended intrahepatic bile-duct

resolved by ESWL. Residual fragments may be submitted to additional lytic therapy with ursodeoxycholic acid.

Conclusions and expectations

Today ESWL is still a treatment option for the solitary symptomatic sonolucent [12] gall-bladder stone up to 20 mm in a sufficiently contractile gallbladder [3, 4]. The number of gall-bladder stone patients suitable for ESWL can be expected to increase in the future with the more widespread use of qualified ultrasonography, revealing younger stones (in younger patients) before chronic damage to the gall-bladder has occurred. Improvements in the shock-wave therapy itself can be

expected from an improved pre-ESWL analysis of the stones (for example by optimized ultrasound procedures) [11] (Figure 47.3), improved shock-wave qualities
and a considerably more generous use of repeat ESWL sessions with higher shockwave energies.

In extrahepatic bile-duct stones not treatable by endoscopy, ESWL has become
as successful as in urinary stone treatment [5]. In intrahepatic bile-duct stones,
ESWL is the method of choice to resolve biliary obstruction. Bile-duct stone
surgery has become a rarity due to operative endoscopy and ESWL.

ESWL has made surgeons think about something new [13] in biliary surgery,
provoking the development of laparoscopic [14] cholecystectomy; biliary ESWL is
an important non-operative therapeutic option in selected cases of both gall-bladder
and bile-duct calculi.

References

1. Forssmann B, Hepp W, Chaussey C *et al.* Eine methode zur berueh-rungsfreien zertruemmerung
   von nierensteinen mit stosswellen. Biomed Tech (Berlin) 1977;22:164.
2. Brendel W, Enders G. Shock waves for gallstones: Animal studies. Lancet 1983;i:1045.
3. Sauerbruch T, Delius M, Paumgartner G *et al.* Fragmentation of gallstones by extracorporeal shock
   waves. N Engl J Med 1986;314:818.
4. Greiner L, Wenzel H, Jakobeit C. Biliary shock wave lithotripsy – fragmentation and lysis: A new
   method. Dtsch Med Wschr 1987;112:1893.
5. Wenzel H, Greiner L, Jakobeit C. Extracorporeal shock wave lithotripsy in problematic bile duct
   stones. Dtsch Med Wschr 1989,114:738.
6. Greiner L, Muenks C, Heil W *et al.* Gallbladder stone fragments in feces after biliary extracorporeal
   shock wave lithotripsy (ESWL). Gastroenterology 1990;98:1620.
7. Fromm H, Greiner L. Combination of extracorporeal shock wave fragmentation and bile acid dissolution treatment of gallstones: Further data and experience. Gastroenterology 1988;94:1512.
8. Sackmann M, Delius M, Sauerbruch T *et al.* Shock wave lithotripsy of gallstones: The first 175 patients. N Engl J Med 1988;318:393.
9. Ponchon T, Barkun AN, Pujol B *et al.* Gallstone disappearance after extracorporeal lithotripsy and
   oral bile acid dissolution. Gastroenterology 1989;89:457.
10. Schoenfield LJ, Berci RL, Carnovale W *et al.* The effect of ursodiol on the efficacy and safety of
    extracorporeal shock wave lithotripsy of gallstones. New Engl J Med 1990;323:1239.
11. Nakayama F, Soloway R, Nakama T *et al.* Hepatolithiasis in East Asia. Retrospective study. Dig
    Dis Sci 1986;31:21.
12. Tsuchiya Y. Ultrasonographic properties of gallstones. Differentiation between cholesterol stones
    and pigment stones. Bil Tract Pancr 1986;7:1438.
13. Langenbuch C. Ein fall von exstirpation der gallenblase wegen chronischer cholelithiasis. Heilung.
    Berliner Klin Wschr 1882;19:123.
14. Holohan TV. Laparoscopic cholecystectomy. Lancet 1991;338:795.

48. Current management of gallstone disease: Perspective from a developing country

MUSHTAQ AHMED and TURAB PISHORI

At the Aga Khan University Medical Center (AKUMC) in Karachi, which is a non-governmental, private, fee-for-service institution, cholecystectomies constituted 20% (222/1133) of the general surgical procedures in 1995 and ranked first in frequency. By comparison, in one general surgical unit of a government hospital, the Civil Hospital, Karachi, which caters for an indigent population, the frequency of cholecystectomies was 9% (67/753) during that year [1]. It appears that gallstone disease is common to all socioeconomic groups in Karachi. Cholecystectomy however, did not feature as a common procedure in a survey of district hospitals in rural Pakistan [2].

The mean age of our patients at AKUMC was 46 years ($n = 536$), compared with 50 years observed in a series from Germany [3] and 52 years in a series from the UK [4].

A female preponderance of 3:1 was similar to that seen in the West [3, 4]. Mixed stones were the commonest. Analysis has revealed calcium and mucoprotein in the core of 76% of the stones in Karachi suggesting an infective aetiology [5]. In addition to conventional surgery the available techniques for the management of gallstones include medical dissolution therapy, extracorporeal shock wave lithotripsy, transcutaneous removal of gallstones, endoscopic sphincterotomy for common bile-duct stones, and laparoscopic cholecystectomy. In a developing country like Pakistan, conventional surgery remains the mainstay of management of gallstone disease in government hospitals with constrained resources. However, in some private hospitals, minimally invasive procedures such as laparoscopic cholecystectomy (LC) and endoscopic sphincterotomy (ES) are available. While one may argue in favour of an equitable distribution of advanced technology, the fact is that open surgery is safe and cost-effective in low surgical risk patients with uncomplicated disease. Therefore, to optimize the use of resources, it is recommended that only patients who are at high surgical risk and/or have serious complications should be referred to specialized centres. This policy would also ensure the availability of training sites for open surgery. It seems sensible therefore, to discuss separately the management of:

1. Symptomatic, low surgical risk patients, including those with uncomplicated common bile-duct (CBD) stones.

J. Talati et al. (eds) The Management of Lithiasis, 329–335
© 1997 Kluwer Academic Publishers. Printed in Great Britain.

2. Symptomatic, high surgical risk patients including those with serious complications of CBD stones.
3. Asymptomatic patients.

Symptomatic low surgical risk patients

In developed countries LC has virtually replaced open cholecystectomy (OC) as the gold standard. LC is better tolerated, reduces hospital stay and permits early rehabilitation. There is some evidence of a diminished metabolic response following LC [6] as compared with OC. In view of the patients' demand for LC it is not possible to run a large enough randomized controlled trial to demonstrate its safety in comparison with OC. However, data from large multicentre trials in the US, UK and Europe show acceptable rates of complications with LC [7–9]. Significantly, however, major complications as a result of errors in technique, e.g. haemorrhage, bowel and bile-duct injury are more frequent in LC than in OC. Bile-duct injury is a major stigma for LC, its frequency being 1.5–2.5 times greater than in OC [10]. Bile-duct injuries sustained during LC tend to be more severe [11], more than half requiring anastomotic repair [12]. There is also a suggestion that recognition of bile-duct injury at the time of operation is less frequent in LC than in OC [13]. There is good evidence that the incidence of bile-duct injury from errors in technique in LC is related to the learning curve period [13]. It should be possible to obviate this problem by proper training and credentialling of surgeons for LC. However, both these functions may be deficient in developing countries.

Even though LC may be intended for all symptomatic patients with gallstones, a selection bias is unavoidable. Patients with acute cholecystitis and those who are extremely obese, have had upper abdominal surgery or are pregnant, constitute relative contraindications. There is also a small though persistent rate of conversion from LC to OC engendered by difficulty in dissection. In Kum *et al.*'s series [14] of 66 patients with histologically proven acute cholecystitis, 30% needed conversion from LC to OC. The main reason was difficulty in identifying the cystic duct. LC does not lend itself to additional abdominal procedures; CBD exploration is rarely undertaken as an adjunctive procedure. The limited application of LC as compared with OC explains the lower overall morbidity and mortality associated with LC [7].

CBD stones in low risk patients

The advent of LC has forced a re-evaluation of the policy on detection and removal of CBD stones. An overzealous approach in the past has given way to circumspection in the light of knowledge about the natural history of bile-duct stones and the difficulties and hazards involved in CBD exploration by ES, LC or open technique [15]. The points to consider are:

1. The majority of CBD stones are migratory from the gall-bladder. Their incidence rises with age [16].

2. There is good evidence that stones pass spontaneously into the duodenum and that expectant treatment is successful [17]. A relatively small proportion of CBD stones (15–25%) become symptomatic over the years.
3. Narrow ducts, not more than 6 mm in diameter, are more liable to damage by ES or open CBD exploration [18]. The bile-duct diameter increases with age.

The popularity of LC has caused younger patients with narrower bile-ducts to come forward for treatment. A strong argument can be made for expectant management of patients with silent bile-duct stones whose bile ducts are not more than 6 mm in diameter. In these patients, even routine intraoperative cholangiography may be questioned, especially if the value of this investigation in outlining biliary anatomy for prevention of bile-duct injury is discounted [19].

Only patients who are symptomatic (history of obstructive jaundice or acute pancreatitis) or are suspected to have CBD stones should be considered for ES or open CBD exploration. Additionally, a CBD diameter of more than 6 mm strengthens the case for exploration. Bile-duct stones may be predicted fairly accurately by non-invasive methods [20]. When indicated ES may precede LC if facilities are available. ES may also follow LC when stones have been confirmed on intraoperative cholangiography. Intraoperative ES together with LC is another possible option [21]. A highly skilled endoscopist, whose success rate is 90%, should be available [22].

However, in the low surgical risk patient the outcome in terms of morbidity, residual stones and mortality is no different following open CBD exploration as compared with ES [23]. Indeed open surgery is a more acceptable option in low resource conditions. In order to reduce the incidence of residual stones, intraoperative choledochoscopy and cholangiography are necessary.

The advantages of conventional surgery are that it caters for a wider range of pathological possibilities including acute cholecystitis and CBD stones. No special training is required and the instruments are readily available.

The high risk patient

Technology for managing medically compromised patients with gall-bladder stones is deficient. Percutaneous techniques are not widely practised due to lack of facilities and expertise. However, in special centres in the West, a recurrence rate of 31% and a symptomatic recurrence rate of 14% have been reported with transcutaneous techniques of gall-bladder stone extraction in medically compromised patients [24].

The cirrhotic with gallstones

The mortality associated with acute cholecystitis in cirrhotics is up to 50% [25]. On the other hand up to 80% of cirrhotics with gallstones remain asymptomatic [25]. The recommendation, therefore, is to perform elective surgery in cirrhotics as soon as symptoms supervene. Either LC or OC may be offered. Open subtotal cholecystectomy has also been recommended. The cirrhotic with choledocholithiasis also constitutes a high risk for surgery in whom ES has proved to be valuable [26].

Surgery in the unsuspected cirrhotic poses yet another problem in countries like Pakistan. The prevalence of HBV and HCV related cirrhosis is high [27, 28]. We have shown that in unsuspected cirrhotics whose liver function is well preserved, mortality is not increased following cholecystectomy even though operative blood loss is higher [29].

The diabetic with gallstones

A higher mortality from acute cholecystitis in diabetics demands that surgery is undertaken as soon as the patient becomes symptomatic.

CBD stones in high risk patients

Independent risk factors associated with poor outcome in patients with CBD stones have been identified. They are: a raised serum total bilirubin, co-morbidity, and a dual approach at stone removal including ES and surgery [30]. It seems that in medically compromised patients ES alone should be advised. If ES is unlikely to be successful it should not be attempted and in this event surgery should be the only definitive treatment. Eighty per cent of patients who have stones in an *in-situ* gallbladder following extraction of CBD stones by ES, remain asymptomatic for 5–10 years [31]. Therefore, cholecystectomy need not necessarily follow ES stone extraction in medically compromised patients.

The indication *par excellence* for ES is the patient with residual CBD stones following previous open CBD exploration. In comparison with surgical re-exploration, the morbidity and mortality of ES are significantly lower [31]. In contrast with residual stones, primary CBD stones are a different problem and necessitate sphincteroplasty or biliary-enteric anastomosis.

ES and nasobiliary drainage have dramatically improved outcome in patients with acute suppurative cholangitis and septicaemia. In the Hong Kong randomized controlled trial, mortality was threefold lower with ES and nasobiliary drainage ($n = 4/41$) compared with immediate operative intervention ($n = 13/41$) [32]. Similarly, urgent ES within 24 hours of onset of illness, has improved outcome in severe acute gallstone pancreatitis [33]. ES with stone extraction ($n = 195$) was able to reduce morbidity and mortality 2.5-fold and 9-fold respectively, compared with conventional management ($n = 121$), probably by averting pancreatic necrosis [34]. By contrast early open CBDE resulted in a significantly increased morbidity and mortality in severe acute gallstone pancreatitis [35].

Intrahepatic bile-duct stones are uncommon in Pakistan. In south-east Asia a combination of open surgical and endoscopic techniques has been used for their management [36].

There is no doubt that ES has considerably improved the management of CBD stones in high risk patients, and in those with serious complications. There is therefore good reason to refer such patients to tertiary centres where multidisciplinary care is available.

Asymptomatic patients

The study of the natural history of gallstone disease has shown that only 15% of asymptomatic patients become symptomatic over 10–20 years [37]. It used to be generally accepted that patients should be offered surgery only when they became symptomatic. Biliary pain is the harbinger of future complications such as acute cholecystitis and migration of stones into the CBD. However, the ready acceptance of LC by patients seems to have caused a reversal of this strategy and cholecystectomy rates have gone up considerably since the advent of LC [7]. It may be argued that LC early in the course of gall-bladder disease may prove cost-effective if it reduces the incidence of complications such as those resulting from stone migration to the CBD. Controlled prospective studies should justify this approach. A high incidence of gall-bladder cancer related to stones [38] and *Salmonella* infection in endemic areas [39] may further strengthen the argument in favour of LC for asymptomatic stones.

On the other hand, unbridled enthusiasm for LC in the young, asymptomatic patient with a functioning gall-bladder may result in disturbance of upper GI physiology, e.g. impaired antroduodenal motility and reflux bile gastritis [40]. Reduction in bile salt pool may cause post-cholecystectomy diarrhoea from subclinical fat malabsorption [41]. A higher risk of right sided colon cancer has been demonstrated both experimentally and clinically [42, 43], although this is controversial. Relief of atypical symptoms such as flatulent dyspepsia is less satisfactory than the relief of typical biliary pain following cholecystectomy [44, 45]. For all these reasons the indiscriminate use of LC may be unwise. The economic burden of operating on asymptomatic patients should also be carefully considered in developing countries.

Conclusion

In view of the comparable safety of conventional surgery and minimal access surgery (ES and LC) in the low risk patient, it would seem sensible to encourage the former in low resource government hospitals. Conventional surgery is more comprehensive and effectively takes care of acute cholecystitis and uncomplicated CBD stones. It is technically less demanding; no special training is required. The technology is readily available and unlikely to change. An added advantage is that peripheral hospitals will be preserved as training sites for conventional surgery. This policy may appear to be unjust if one insists that modern technology should be available to everyone irrespective of social class. This is impractical. Where resources are constrained it is essential to establish a referral system such that modern technology is not denied those who need it most.

By contrast, high risk surgical patients and patients with serious complications of CBD stones should be referred to specialized centres where a multidisciplinary approach including surgery, gastroenterology and radiology is available. Morbidity and mortality are significantly reduced in these patients with the use of minimally invasive techniques. It is important that the surgeon performing LC and perhaps ES should also be adept at conventional surgery in order to deal with the complications and treatment failures associated with newer techniques. Postgraduate programmes should build in rotations for the trainees in government hospitals where open surgery of a high quality is practised.

References

1. Sultan N. 1996, Personal communication.
2. Blanchard RJW, Blanchard MEE, Toussignant P, Ahmad M, Smythe C. The epidemiology and spectrum of surgical care in district hospitals in Pakistan. Am J Pub H 1987;77:1439–45.
3. Ure BM, Troidl H, Spangenburger W *et al.* Long term results after laparoscopic cholecystectomy. Br J Surg 1995;82:267–70.
4. Martin IG, Holdsworth PJ, Asker J *et al.* Laparoscopic cholecystectomy as a routine procedure for gallstones: Results of an 'all comers' policy. Br J Surg 1992;79:807–10.
5. Sadruddin A, Zuberi SJ. Histochemical staining of gall stones. Indian J Gastroenterol 1987;6:159–60.
6. Jakeways MSR, Mitchell V, Hasim IA, Chadwick SJD, Shenkin A, Green CJ. Metabolic and inflammatory responses after open or laparoscopic cholecystectomy. Br J Surg 1994;81:127–31.
7. Deziel DJ, Millikan KW, Economou SG, Doolas A, Ko S-T, Airan MC. Complications of laparoscopic cholecystectomy: A national survey of 4292 hospitals and an analysis of 77,604 cases. Am J Surg 1993;165:9–14.
8. Dunn D, Nair R, Fowlez S, McCloy R. Laparoscopic cholecystectomy in England and Wales: Results of an audit by The Royal College of Surgeons of England. Ann R Coll Surg Engl 1994;76:269–75.
9. Cuschieri A, Dubois F, Mouiee J *et al.* European experience with laparoscopic cholecystectomy. Am J Surg 1991;161:385–8.
10. McMahon AJ, Fullarton G, Baxter JN, O'Dwyer PJ. Bile duct injury and bile leakage in laparoscopic cholecystectomy (review). Br J Surg 1995;82:307–13.
11. Roy AF, Pass RB, Lapointe RW, McAlista VC, Dagenais MH, Wall WJ. Bile duct injury during laparoscopic cholecystectomy. Can J Surg 1993;36:509–16.
12. Gouma DJ, GO PM. Bile-duct injury during laparoscopic cholecystectomy and conventional cholecystectomy. J Am Coll Surg 1994;253:229–33.
13. The Southern Surgeon's Club, Moore MJ, Bennett CL. The learning curve for laparoscopic cholecystectomy. Am J Surg 1995;170:55–9.
14. Kum K, Goh MY, Isaac JR, Tekant Y, Ngoi SS. Laparoscopic cholecystectomy for acute cholecystitis. Br J Surg 1994;81:1651–4.
15. Perissat J, Huibregste K, Keane FBV, Russell RCG, Neoptolemos JP. Management of bile duct stones in the era of laparoscopic cholecystectomy (review). Br J Surg 1994;81:799–810.
16. Hermann RE. The spectrum of biliary stone disease. Am J Surg 1989;158:171–3.
17. Murison MSC, Garteu PC, McGinn FP. Does selective peroperative cholangiogram result in missed common bile duct stones (Abstract). Br J Surg 1989;76:1343.
18. Shermans, Ruffolo TA, Hawes RH, Lehman GA. Complications of endoscopic sphincterotomy. Gastroenterology 1991;101:1068–75.
19. Lorimer JW, Fairful Smith R. Intra operative cholangiography is not necessary to avoid duct injuries during laparoscopic cholecystectomy. Am J Surg 1995;169:344–7

20. Barkun AN, Barkun JS, Fried GM, *et al.* Gallstone Treatment Group. Useful predictors of bile duct stones in patients undergoing laparoscopic cholecystectomy. Ann Surg 1994;220:32–9.

21. Siddiqui MN, Hamid S. Per-operative endoscopic sphincterotomy during laparoscopic cholecystectomy (letter). Br J Surg 1995;82:1435.

22. Cotton PB. Endoscopic retrograde cholangiopancreatography and laparoscopic cholecystectomy. Am J Surg 1993;165:474–8.

23. Pitt IIA. Role of open choledochotomy in the treatment of choledocholetithiasis. Am J Surg 1993;165:483–6.

24. Donald JJ, Cheslyn-Curtis S, Gillams AR, Russell RGC, Lees WR. Percutaneous cholecystolithotomy: Is gallstone recurrence inevitable? Gut 1994;35:629–5.

25. Orozco H, Takahashi T, Mercado A, Prado E, Borunda D. Asymptomatic cholelithiasis in the cirrhotic. Am J Surg 1994;168:232–4.

26. Sugiyama M, Atomi Y, Kuroda A, Muto T. Treatment of choledocholelithiasis in cirrhosis: Surgery or endoscopic sphincterotomy. Surgery 1993;218:68–73.

27. Malik A, Luqman M, Ahmad A *et al.* Sporadic non-A, non-B hepatitis: A seroepidemiological study in an urban population. J Pak Med Assoc 1987;37:190–2.

28. Qureshi H, Zuberi SJ, Lodhi TZ, Alam E. Clinical features, course, viral markers and followup of young non-alcoholic cirrhotics – a retrospective study. Digestion 1989;42:110.

29. Hamid S, Siddiqui M, Jafri W, Shah H, Khan H, Ahmed M. Outcome of biliary tract surgery in unknown cirrhotics. Ann R Coll Surg Eng 1993;75:434–6.

30. Neoptolemos JP, Shaw DE, Carr-Locke DL. Multivariate analysis of preoperative risk factors in common bile duct stones. Am J Surg 1989;209:157–61.

31. Leese T, Neoptolemos JP, Carr-Locke DL. Successes, failures, early complications and their management following endoscopic sphincterotomy: Results in 394 conservative patients from a single centre. Br J Surg 1985;72:215–19.

32. Lai ECS, Mok FPT, Tan ESY, Fan S, You K, Wong J. Endoscopic biliary drainage for severe acute cholangitis. N Engl J Med 1992;326:1582–6.

33. Fan Sheung-Tat, Lai ECS, MokFPT, Lo CM, Zheng SS, Wong J. Early treatment of acute biliary pancreatitis by endoscopic pepillotomy. N Engl J Med 1993;328:228–32.

34. Carr-Locke DL, London NJ, Bailey IA, James D, Fossard DP. Controlled trial of urgent endoscopic retrograde cholangiopancreatography and endoscopic sphincterotomy versus conservative treatment for pancreatitis due to gallstones. Lancet 1988;ii:979–83.

35. Kelly TR, Wagner DS. Gallstone pancreatitis: A prospective randomized trial of timing of surgery. Surgery 1988;104:600–5.

36. Chijiiwa K, Yamashita H, Kuroki S, Tanaka M. Current management and long term prognosis of hepatolithiasis. Arch Surg 1995;30:194–7.

37. McSherry CK, Ferstenberg H, Calhoun WF *et al.* The natural history of diagnosed gall stone disease in symptomatic and asymptomatic patients. Ann Surg 1985;202:59.

38. Godrey PJ, Bates T, Harrison M, Kingh B, Padley NR. Gallstones and mortality: A study of all gall stone related deaths in a single health district. Gut 1984;25:1029–33.

39. Freitag JL. Treatment of chronic typhoid carries by cholecystectomy. Publ Health Repo 1964;79:567–70.

40. Johnson AG. Pyloric function and gall stone dyspepsia. Br J Surg 1972;59:449–54.

41. Thaysen EH, Pederson L. Idiopathic bile acid catharsis. Gut 1976;17:965–70.

42. Werner B, Detter K, Mitschke H. Cholecystectomy and carcinoma of colon. Z Krebsforsch Klin Oncol 1977;88:223–30.

43. Turunen MJ, KiviLaakso EO. Increased risk of colorectal cancer after cholecystectomy. Ann Surg 1981;194:639–41.

44. Fenster F, Longborg R, Thirlby RC, Traverso LW. What symptoms does cholecystectomy cure? Am J Surg 1995;169:553–8.

45. Bates T, Ebb SR, Harrison M, A'Horn RP. Influence of cholecystectomy on symptoms. Br J Surg 1991;78:964–7.

Epilogue

JOHN H. DIRKS

In this review dealing with epidemiology, risk factors and stone formation, the varying choices of management and related issues of effectiveness and cost are well described. Not forgotten is the key issue of prevention of calculi which, in a technical era in which the stone is zapped as soon as it is discovered, can all too easily be ignored. The issue of prevention remains highly relevant to all patients with previous stone formations, and particularly in developing countries where the technology may not be readily available to treat the next occurrence.

In looking to the future, it is most important that we develop significant clinical academic groups, composed not only of skilled clinical investigative urologists and specialists in metabolism and nephrology, but also of epidemiologists and basic scientists. There is a continuing need to establish sounder information on epidemiology of urolithiasis in a more rigorous and deliberate fashion in countries like Pakistan and its cities and provinces, and in other developing nations. This has to be based on investigation and sound laboratory and radiological work. There is a need to apply more prospectively measures for the prevention of urolithiasis, which is often difficult because communities are isolated and the Third World problems of poverty, illiteracy, malnutrition, limited dietary fare, poor income and poor housing, among other issues, still prevail. Nevertheless, the challenge must not be ignored and it will be necessary to develop a cadre of interdisciplinary groups in the regions of the world that are not well networked, at least within their own country. The level of hydration and calcium, oxalate and citric acid excretion, among others, remain important issues.

ESWL has made a tremendous difference to the treatment of stones, reducing morbidity and enhancing the effectiveness of treatment of urolithiasis considerably. However, the technology remains unavailable, inadequate, or poorly manned for so many cities and towns. Therefore, there must be a continuing drive to develop even simpler technologies that are non-interventional and allow maintenance of the effectiveness of therapy while minimising the cost. Government and international development agency support for such programs are often necessary. Not to be lost in this is the training of high quality manpower in different regions of the world, at a high standard, in training centers all linked internationally yet certainly independent and self-sufficient.

In addition to technology for crushing stones, improvements in stone therapy by medical and pharmaceutical means need to be made. The use of agents such as

I. Talati et al (eds) The Management of Lithiasis, 337–338
© 1997 Kluwer Academic Publishers. Printed in Great Britain.

diazides and citrate has been of great benefit in prophylaxis. However, there is room for further medical therapeutic strategies to enhance therapy results from, say, ESWL.

The fundamental challenge that remains is not diagnosing, treating and preventing urolithiasis, but the issue of more globalized facilities in the various regions that can deal with education, training and research. The goal of every nation should be to improve its educational and health care status in such a way that various medical conditions such as urolithiasis can be effectively dealt with in their own domain. I believe that Dr. Talati's and his colleagues' endeavours will serve to make that progress in the field of urolithiasis.

John H. Dirks, MD
July 1996
Former Dean and Rector,
The Aga Khan University, Karachi, Pakistan
Former Dean and Professor of Medicine,
Toronto University, Toronto, Ontario, Canada

Appendix   Non-visual laser lithotripsy

T.K. SHAH, Z.X. JIANG and G.W. WATSON

Non-visual or blind laser lithotripsy (NVLL) is laser fragmentation of the calculi without direct or endoscopic vision. Strictly speaking the process is not completely blind since it is controlled by a spectroscopic feedback. Laser lithotripsy for ureteric stones under direct ureteroscopic vision is widely practised. It is generally safe and well established; however there is some morbidity and the procedure has some limitations.

The main cause of morbidity due to the procedure is documented to be the trauma to the ureter produced during the passage of the ureteroscopes rather than the application of the laser itself [1–4]. The large-sized ureteroscopes which are still being used quite extensively produce significant mucosal tears, particularly when their introduction has to be preceded by dilatation of the ureteric orifice. This problem to some extent has been rectified by the introduction of the newer generation of ureteroscopes with much smaller diameters [5]. Most of these can now be passed into the ureter without the need for prior dilatation. The use of the ureteroscope is however still restricted in certain situations. There are a number of cases where even the very fine ureteroscope (diameter 6.8–7.5) can fail to gain access, for example strictures or stenoses at the uretero-vesical junction or of ureter distal to a calculus, upper third of some ureters and in particular ureters in children. These are some of the situations in which the use of non-visual laser lithotripsy may be useful.

Similar ideas in laser lithotripsy have been explored previously with the different objectives of preventing damage to tissues during laser lithotripsy and identifying the composition of the stone or for laser fragmentation of the stone precluding the need for ureteroscopes. The systems employed so far have relied upon either the analysis of laser-induced fluorescence, acoustic signals, spectral analysis of the plasma emission or on photo-thermal radiometry. We advanced the concept of NVLL by analyses of the plasma emission spectrum with the objectives of *in-vivo* identification of the stone from a non-stone target and fragmentation of the stone without direct visual aid [6]. Laser, when applied to the stone, causes absorption of the energy which produces vaporization and subsequent release of ions and electrons from the stone surface. The plume of these charged particles, called the plasma, absorbs a large portion of the laser pulse energy resulting in its rapid expansion and subsequent production of a strong shock wave on the stone surface, leading to the fragmentation of the stone [7, 8].

J. Talati et al. (eds) The Management of Lithiasis, 339–343
© *1997 Kluwer Academic Publishers. Printed in Great Britain.*

All urinary stones exhibit a characteristic spectrum, including the uric acid calculi which have calcium in their shells but not in their cores. The exceptions are the cystine stones which only rarely produce a calcium spectrum. Other targets which can be encountered in the ureter either produce no plasma and therefore no spectrum, such as the damaged and normal ureter and blood clots, or in other instances although a plasma and a spectrum is produced, it does not contain the distinct calcium emission or absorption lines. This is observed in case of ureteric stents, catheters and guide wires. The whole process is monitored as a continuous display during fragmentation. A negative spectrum means that the stone is not being targeted and the fibre needs re-positioning.

When applying this technique in the patients, the laser fibre sheathed in the delivery catheter is advanced into the ureter through a cystoscope.

Radiological control by an image intensifier helps in getting the fibre close to the target. Laser pulses at low frequency are delivered while the fibre is manipulated in the ureter. The target is identified by the appearance of the typical spectrum when the fibre comes in contact with the stone. Laser pulses are then delivered at a frequency varying between 1–10 Hz and the fragmentation process is monitored by continuous displays of the spectra. The results of our first 12 patients done by this technique are shown in Table 1. In 9 of the 12 patients the target was positively identified as stone on the appearance of the spectrum. Among the three failures, one was a cystine stone (patient 3) which produced no spectrum, the second one was a stone trapped in a peri-vesical ureteric diverticulum (patient 5) to which the fibre could not be directed, and in the third patient (patient 10) the sharp fibre end perfo-

Table 1   Result of Non-visual Laser Lithotripsy in 12 patients

Patient No.	Stone site	Biochemical composition *in vivo*	Non-visual identification spectral display	Fragmentation monitored visually	Procedure completed
1.	Lower ureter	Ca, oxalate	Yes	Yes	Yes
2.	Upper ureter	Ca, oxalate	Yes	No. Stone flushed back in the kidney	No
3.	Lower ureter	Cystine	No	No	Yes
4.	Mid ureter	Ca, Mg, NH_4	Yes	Yes	Yes
5.	Lower ureter	Ca, oxalate	No. Stone in ureteric diverticulum	Yes, after Ureteroscopic visualization	Yes
6.	Mid ureter	Ca, oxalate	Yes	Yes	Yes
7.	Upper ureter	Ca, Mg, NH_4	Yes	Yes	Yes
8.	Mid ureter	Ca, oxalate	Yes	Yes	Yes
9.	Lower ureter	Ca, oxalate	Yes	Yes	Yes
10.	Lower ureter	Mg, NH_4, PO_4 CO_3	No, blind fibre advancement perforated the ureter	Yes, after ureteroscopic localization	Yes
11.	Lower ureter	Not known	Yes	Yes	Yes
12.	Mid ureter	Not known	Yes	Yes	Yes

rated the ureteric wall which was confirmed on ureteroscopy. All of these stones were eventually located on ureteroscopy.

In all the patients the fragmentation process was monitored by continuous display of the spectra except in one of the upper ureteric stones (patient 2) which was flushed into the kidney and in the cystine stone (patient 3) which required fragmentation under vision with electrohydraulic lithotripsy. In the last two patients we were trying new designs of the laser delivery catheter. These did not prove very effective and the procedure was completed under ureteroscopic vision.

However, the main difficulty encountered during these procedures is the significant time lost in re-positioning the fibre onto the target which considerably slows down the process. To expedite, all the procedures were finally completed under ureteroscopic visual control.

In 1987 Teng *et al.* [9] looked at the possibility of stone detection by analyzing the laser-induced plasma spectrum on an optical multichannel analyzer (OMA). Jiany *et al.* [10] and Bhatta *et al.* [11] carried out independent experiments making use of the acoustic and optical plasma emission signals recorded on a digital storage oscilloscope to identify the stones and other targets. The main drawback with their work was that simultaneous recording of both the plasma emission and the acoustic signals for a positive and confident identification of the various targets makes it a relatively difficult proposition for clinical application. Rosen [12] successfully recorded the plasma optical emissions *in vivo* on a digital storage oscilloscope and used it to monitor the fragmentation process; however since this was not spectrally resolved the distinction between certain objects, e.g. guide wire, catheters etc., was not possible. Identification of the composition of a calculus using laser-induced fluorescence of the re-emitted light and plasma spectrum analysis has been carried out with quite encouraging results by several other workers [13–16].

Shah and Jiang [6, 17] have developed a system of inducing the plasma on the target using pulsed dye laser (coumarin 504). The same laser delivery fibre (300 μm core diameter) is used to retrogradely transmit the light emission of the plasma through a series of coupling lenses and beam splitter to collimate and re-focus onto a collecting fibre 91 μm core diameter plastic fibre. The collecting fibre feeds this plasma emission via a filter to the OMA. The filter allows the wavelength range of 350–450 nm to enter the OMA where the spectrum is analysed and displayed on a monitor.

The real-time spectral analysis of this plasma emission is used to identify the target and to monitor the process of fragmentation. Since the aim is not the identification of the composition of the target, we restrict the spectrum to the selected wavebands of 350–450 nm only. This waveband reviews distinctively the calcium ions' and atoms' absorption and emission line spectra. The positive identification is therefore dependent upon the presence of calcium in the target.

The basis of applying this technique is established from the *in-vitro* and *ex-vivo* experimental studies done earlier [6, 17]. The findings of these studies are presented in Table 2. It helped in establishing that the most apparent calcium absorption lines are at 393 nm, 397 nm and 423 nm. The most apparent calcium emission line, although not very specific, is seen around 428–430 nm. These absorption and emission lines

Table 2   Results of *in-vitro* and *ex-vivo* experiments at 40–60 mJ and 1–4 Hz frequency

Target	Composition	OMA recording absorption spectra	Oscilloscope signal	Recording signal
Urinary stone	Ca, oxalate	+++++	++	++
Urinary stone	Ca, oxalate	++	++	++
Urinary stone	Ca, Mg, NH$_4$, PO$_4$	+	+	+
Urinary stone	Cystine	+	+	+
Urinary stone	Cystine	–	–	–
Urinary stone	Urate	+	+	+
Urinary stone	Urate	+	+	+
Gallstone	Bile salt, bilirubin Cholesterol	+++	+++	+++
Gallstone	Metal	–	+	++
Ureteric catheter	PTEE	–	+	+
Blood clot	Blood	–	–	+
Bruised ureter	Mucosa	–	–	+/–
Normal ureter	Mucosa	–	–	–
Fibrous plaque	Fibrous tissue	–	Not done	Not done
Calcified plaque	Calcium-containing	+	Not done	Not done

are consistent and appear in all the traces in which calcium containing stones are present. Objects not containing calcium do not demonstrate this calcium-specific spectrum. These lines can therefore be used confidently for the detection of the target. In brief, plasma emission from a calcium-containing stone displays a spectrum which is very distinct and the main problem encountered during NVLL is to keep the fibre on the target during laser delivery. After every few shots the spectrum disappears and the fibre requires re-positioning. This is time-consuming and delays the whole procedure. Also, when the stone is incompletely fragmented the smaller fragments are not easy to relocate blindly. This problem is not unique to NVLL, as even under visual control only about 60% of the pulses would be a direct hit on the stone. This is both our experience and others' [6], and the process has to be interrupted every so often for re-positioning which is more difficult at this stage of development. It is expected that with improved catheter designs, perhaps incorporating trapping mechanisms, this problem can be satisfactorily resolved. The fragments which are small enough not to require further fragmentation should drop off from in front of the main stone bulk to allow the fibre to pass on to the larger fragments, quite similar to how the procedure is carried out under visual control.

The concept of non-visual or blind laser lithotripsy is theoretically very attractive. By obviating the use of endoscopes the effective diameter of instruments to deliver laser and fragment the stone can be reduced to under 5 Fr. The benefits that can arise from such a small diameter are obvious. We do not propose the NVLL to be a replacement of the ureteroscopic laser lithotripsy but rather an addition to the armamentarium of the surgeon to be employed in situations where ureteroscopic lithotripsy has failed or is unsuitable.

Our current work involves modifying and re-designing the delivery catheters for a more successful application of this technique. Another improvement that would make the technique more applicable is in modifying the OMA. With a specially designed OMA constructed for NVLL the response time can be reduced to synchronize with every plasma emission even if the laser pulse repetition rate is 10 Hz or more. With such a specifically designed OMA even the cost of the equipment could be brought down considerably.

References

1. Watson GM, Murray, Dretler SP, Parish. The pulsed dye laser for fragmenting urinary calculi. J Urol 1987;138:195.
2. Dretler SP. Laser lithotripsy: A review of 20 years of research and clinical applications. Lasers Surg Med 1988;8:341.
3. Coptcoat MJ, Ison KT, Watson GM, Wickham JEA. Lasertripsy for ureteral stones: 100 cases. J Endurol 1987;1:119.
4. Watson GM, Wickham JEA, Mils TN, Bown SG, Swain P, Salmon PR. Laser fragmentation of renal calculi. Br J Urol 1983;55:613.
5. Watson GM, Wickham JEA. The development of a laser and miniaturised ureteroscope system for ureteric stone management. World J Urol 1989;7:147.
6. Shah TK, Watson GM, Jiang ZX, King TA. Non-visual Laser Lithotripsy aided by plasma spectral analysis: Viability study and clinical application. J Urol 1993;149:1431–6.
7. Jiang ZX, Whiterhurst C, King TA. Basic mechanisms in laser lithotripsy. Vol. 1, Opto-acoustic Mechanical Analysis. Lasers Med Sci. 1991;6:443.
8. Nishioka NS, Teng P, Deutsch TF, Anderson RR. Mechanisms of laser induced fragmentation of urinary and biliary calculi. Lasers Life Sci 1987;1:231.
9. Teng P, Nishioka NS, Anderson RR. Optical studies of pulsed dye laser fragmentation of biliary calculi. Appl Phys B 1987;42:73.
10. Jiang ZX, Whitehurst C, King TA. Fragmentation methods in laser lithotripsy. Journal of Lasers in Urology, Laparoscopy and General Surgery 1991;1421:88.
11. Bhatta KM, Rosen D, Watson GM, Dretler SP. Acoustic and plasma guided lasertripsy (APGL) of urinary calculi. J Urol 1989;142:433.
12. Rosen D. (Personal communication, Aug. 1992)
13. Helfman J, Berline HP, Brozinsky T, Dorschel K, Scholz, Miller G. Identification of body concrements by fast time resolved spectroscopy of laser induced plasma. In: Stiener R, editor. Laser lithotripsy. Berlin, Heidelberg: Springer Verlag; 1988:31–40.
14. Engelhardt R, Meyer W, Hering P. Spectroscopy during laser induced shock wave lithotripsy, SPIE. Opt Fibres Med III 1988;906:200.
15. Holden D, Whiteburst C, Rao PN, King TA, Blacklock NJ. Identification of urinary stone composition by pulsed dye laser. Br J Urol 1990;65:441.
16. Muschter R, Knipper A, Maghraby H, Thomas S. Laser lithotripsy experience with different laser systems in the treatment of urinary calculi, SPIE. Laser Surgery: Advanced Characterization, Therapeutics and Systems. 1990; Vol. 1200:118.
17. Jiang ZX, King TA, Shah TK, Watson GM. Spectroscopic feedback in laser lithotripsy and laser angioplasty, SPIE. Opt Fibres Med VII 1992;1649:106.

Index

Developments in Nephrology

1. J.S. Cheigh, K.H. Stenzel and A.L. Rubin (eds.): *Manual of Clinical Nephrology of the Rogosin Kidney Center.* 1981   ISBN 90-247-2397-3
2. K.D. Nolph (ed.): *Peritoneal Dialysis.* 1981 ed.: out of print, 3rd revised and enlarged ed. 1988 (not in this series)   ISBN 0-89838-406-0
3. A.B. Gruskin and M.E. Norman (eds.): *Pediatric Nephrology.* 1981   ISBN 90-247-2514-3
4. O. Schück: *Examination of the Kidney Function.* 1981   ISBN 0-89838-565-2
5. J. Strauss (ed.): *Hypertension, Fluid-electrolytes and Tubulopathies in Pediatric Nephrology.* 1982   ISBN 90-247-2633-6
6. J. Strauss (ed.): *Neonatal Kidney and Fluid-electrolytes.* 1983   ISBN 0-89838-575-X
7. J. Strauss (ed.): *Acute Renal Disorders and Renal Emergencies.* 1984   ISBN 0-89838-663-2
8. L.J.A. Didio and P.M. Motta (eds.): *Basic, Clinical, and Surgical Nephrology.* 1985   ISBN 0-89838-698-5
9. E.A. Friedman and C.M. Peterson (eds.): *Diabetic Nephropathy.* Strategy for Therapy. 1985   ISBN 0-89838-735-3
10. R. Dzúrik, B. Lichardus and W. Guder: *Kidney Metabolism and Function.* 1985   ISBN 0-89838-749-3
11. J. Strauss (ed.): *Homeostasis, Nephrotoxicy, and Renal Anomalies in the Newborn.* 1986   ISBN 0-89838-766-3
12. D.G. Oreopoulos (ed.): *Geriatric Nephrology.* 1986   ISBN 0-89838-781-7
13. E.P. Paganini (ed.): *Acute Continuous Renal Replacement Therapy.* 1986   ISBN 0-89838-793-0
14. J.S. Cheigh, K.H. Stenzel and A.L. Rubin (eds.): *Hypertension in Kidney Disease.* 1986   ISBN 0-89838-797-3
15. N. Deane, R.J. Wineman and G.A. Benis (eds.): *Guide to Reprocessing of Hemodialyzers.* 1986   ISBN 0-89838-798-1
16. C. Ponticelli, L. Minetti and G. D'Amico (eds.): *Antiglobulins, Cryoglobulins and Glomerulonephritis.* 1986   ISBN 0-89838-810-4
17. J. Strauss (ed.) with the assistence of L. Strauss: *Persistent Renalgenitourinary Disorders.* 1987   ISBN 0-89838-845-7
18. V.E. Andreucci and A. Dal Canton (eds.): *Diuretics.* Basic, Pharmacological, and Clinical Aspects. 1987   ISBN 0-89838-885-6
19. P.H. Bach and E.H. Lock (eds.): *Nephrotoxicity in the Experimental and Clinical Situation,* Part 1. 1987   ISBN 0-89838-997-1
20. P.H. Bach and E.H. Lock (eds.): *Nephrotoxicity in the Experimental and Clinical Situation,* Part 2. 1987   ISBN 0-89838-980-2
21. S.M. Gore and B.A. Bradley (eds.): *Renal Transplantation.* Sense and Sensitization. 1988   ISBN 0-89838-370-6
22. L. Minetti, G. D'Amico and C. Ponticelli: *The Kidney in Plasma Cell Dyscrasias.* 1988   ISBN 0-89838-385-4
23. A.S. Lindblad, J.W. Novak and K.D. Nolph (eds.): *Continuous Ambulatory Peritoneal Dialysis in the USA.* Final Report of the National CAPD Registry 1981–1988. 1989   ISBN 0-7923-0179-X

Developments in Nephrology

Kluwer Academic Publishers – Dordrecht / Boston / London